Osteoarthritis Research and Treatment

Osteoarthritis Research and Treatment

Edited by Shawn McLean

hayle
medical

New York

Hayle Medical,
750 Third Avenue, 9th Floor,
New York, NY 10017, USA

Visit us on the World Wide Web at:
www.haylemedical.com

ISBN: 978-1-63241-714-5

Cataloging-in-Publication Data

Osteoarthritis research and treatment / edited by Shawn McLean.
    p. cm.
Includes bibliographical references and index.
ISBN 978-1-63241-714-5
1. Osteoarthritis. 2. Osteoarthritis--Research. 3. Osteoarthritis--Treatment.
I. McLean, Shawn.
RC931.O67 O77 2019
616.722 3--dc23

Table of Contents

Preface

This book has been an outcome of determined endeavour from a group of educationists in the field. The primary objective was to involve a broad spectrum of professionals from diverse cultural background involved in the field for developing new researches. The book not only targets students but also scholars pursuing higher research for further enhancement of the theoretical and practical applications of the subject.

Osteoarthritis is a common form of arthritis. It usually occurs with age. It is a joint disorder which results from the breakdown of joint cartilage and underlying bone. Its symptoms include joint pain, swelling, stiffness, weakness in the joints and reduced motion. Joints near the ends of the fingers, knees, hips and lower back are some of the most commonly affected joints. A genetic involvement is usually found in most of the cases. However, excess body weight, joint injury and abnormal limb development are the most common causes of osteoarthritis. Osteotomy, hemiarthroplasty, joint replacement surgery, arthroscopic surgery and total shoulder arthroplasty are some effective treatment methods for the treatment of osteoarthritis. This book presents the complex subject of osteoarthritis in the most comprehensible and easy to understand language. It presents researches and studies performed by experts across the globe. The extensive content of this book provides the readers with a thorough understanding of the subject.

It was an honour to edit such a profound book and also a challenging task to compile and examine all the relevant data for accuracy and originality. I wish to acknowledge the efforts of the contributors for submitting such brilliant and diverse chapters in the field and for endlessly working for the completion of the book. Last, but not the least; I thank my family for being a constant source of support in all my research endeavours.

Editor

1

Local Therapies for Osteoarthritis

Sarah Karrar and Charles Mackworth-Young

1. Introduction

Osteoarthritis (OA) is the most common chronic joint condition affecting an estimated 8 million people in the UK alone. It manifests as localised joint pain, stiffness and occasionally swelling. Osteoarthritis can be secondary to pre-existing joint damage - commonly inflammatory arthropathy or previous injury - or primary with no known pre-existing damage. Risk factors for primary OA include old age, female sex and family history and obesity.

The disease can be restricted to a particular joint or generalised, affecting multiple joints. In severe cases, it can be progressive eventually leading to loss of function and deformity.

Treatment has mainly focused on symptomatic relief from pain, physical approaches such as rehabilitation and physiotherapy, disease modifying treatment (such as hydroxychloroquine) and surgery. Pain relief with systemic drugs has drawbacks. In particular the use of non-steroidal anti-inflammatories (NSAIDs) has been associated with significant adverse events including gastritis and increased risk of cardiovascular disease. In view of this, there has been increased interest in localised treatments for OA.- i.e. therapies that are administered to the joint itself, or in the region of the joint. These can be divided into topical treatment, such as anti-inflammatory gels and creams and thermotherapy, and more invasive local treatment including joint aspiration, and intra-articular joint injection with corticosteroid and hyaluronans.

2. Topical treatments

2.1. Thermotherapy

Thermotherapy refers to the application of either heat or cold (cryotherapy) to affected joints in an attempt to improve pain, stiffness and swelling.

Ice massage and ice packs application have both been studied in knee osteoarthritis [5-10]. In one review [7], cryotherapy was found to reduce pain, stiffness and oedema. Regular ice massage, given 5 times a week, was found to have a clinically significant effect on all three symptoms as well as function (11% improvement relative difference), strength (29% improvement) and range of movement (8% relative difference) over a short period of time [8]. However, these improvements were not replicated with less frequent applications (3 times per week) [9] and there are no data to indicate a more long term effect of cold therapy on osteoarthritis as these studies looked at short term results. It is likely that most of the effects of cryotherapy are related to the induction of local vasoconstriction and the reduction of local blood flow resulting in reduced swelling.

Common methods of superficial heat administration are electrical heating pads, application of hot packs, towels or wax, or immersion in warm water or wax baths. In some early trials, heat application was not found to improve function or symptoms [8,9]. In recent years, however, there has been an explosion of studies looking at different modalities of local heat therapy[10-13]. These include the application of heat packs [12], ultrasound [13 11] and diathermy. The application of local heat packs has been found to provide short-lived benefit in terms of pain relief [12, 14]; and in particular, wet heat has been found to be better than dry heat [15] for symptomatic improvement. In one study [12] 18 patients were treated with either steam generating heat sheets for 6 hours daily or with quadriceps strengthening exercises only for a total of 12 weeks. At the end of the study, patients in the heat treated group reported statistically significant improvements in symptoms as well as the Timed Up and Go time (a measure of function). The mechanism of heat therapy in osteoarthritis is unclear, although *ex vivo* studies of cartilage [15, 16] have indicated raising chondrocyte temperature might increase their metabolism and production of proteoglycans. This in part, maybe secondary to increased blood flow to the chondrocytes.

On the whole, the data suggest that thermotherapy maybe useful as an adjunct in the treatment of osteoarthritis although long-term benefits have not been established.

2.2. Local ultrasound therapy

The role of ultrasound (US) in diagnosis of musculoskeletal problems has been well established. Its popularity in large part due to the low cost and non-invasive nature of the modality. In recent years, there has been growing interest in its application for therapeutic purposes [13,18-20]. In theory direct treatment with US leads to local heating of the tissue at depths not achieved by applying heat packs. There are two methods for doing this: continuous US which leads to a rise in temperature of the treated tissues; and pulsed wave treatment which harnesses other properties of US. *In vitro* and animal studies [18, 19] have suggested that pulsed wave US can increase collagen production and reduce expression of membrane metallo-proteinase, suggesting a protective role. This has failed to translate to clinical benefit as recent randomised controlled studies [13, 20] comparing continuous, pulsed and sham US on knee osteoarthritis symptoms and joint function, have shown no difference in pain scores nor 15m-walk time. In general, the safety of US has been established but evidence is scarce for any therapeutic advantage [13,20].

2.3. Laser therapy

Laser beam therapy directs intense light to treated tissue. Two types of laser therapy have been trialled in osteoarthritis: low-level and high intensity. Low- level laser therapy uses red and infra-red light whilst high intensity laser therapy uses higher wavelengths of radiation for deeper tissue penetration. Low level laser therapy has been found to reduce pain, possibly by modulating the local inflammatory process In a rat model of osteoarthritis, laser therapy caused a reduction in neutrophil migration, oxidative stress, altered levels of cyclo-oxygenase-2 and other pro-inflammatory mediators) [21]. Other than providing symptomatic relief, there is also some evidence that laser promotes fibroblast proliferation, collagen synthesis and bone regeneration [22-26]. In a rabbit model of osteoarthritis, six weeks of treatment with laser therapy not only resulted in improved pain but also histological evidence of reduced inflammation as well as a reduction in cartilage damage [27]. This suggests that laser therapy could have disease-modifying as well as symptomatic benefits.

So far, the results of early clinical trials have been mixed [28]. More recent studies have tended to be more positive with those treated with laser therapy and exercise doing better than those treated with exercise alone on pain measurements as well as function [29, 30]. These studies suggest that laser in combination with standard physiotherapy could have advantages over standard therapy. We have little evidence regarding long term effect and whether the cellular effects noted results in halting disease progression. The use of low-level laser therapy has now been approved by the US Food and Drug Agency (FDA) and so we are likely to see an expansion in its use in the coming years.

2.4. Topical non-steroidal anti-inflammatory drugs

Non-steroidal anti-inflammatory drugs (NSAIDS) work by blocking the action of cyclo-oxygenases responsible for prostaglandin synthesis, the latter being known mediators of inflammation [31]. Locally this reduces pain, swelling and heat. NSAIDs also have central analgesic actions, possibly by reducing brain prostaglandin synthesis although alternative mechanisms include the induction of endogenous opioid peptides and blockade of serotonin release. From this, it can be seen why systemic NSAIDs have long been used for osteoarthritis. However, significant side effects including gastritis, renal impairment and increased risk of cardiovascular disease has meant that their long-term use has been limited. It is on this background that topical NSAID use has been promoted, theoretically providing analgesic and anti-inflammatory benefits without systemic adverse effects.

There are many types of topical NSAID. There are preparations containing diclofenac, ibuprofen, piroxicam, ketoprofen or felbinac as the active ingredient. Some include a penetration enhancer such as menthol or dimethylsulfoxide (DMSO). Gels and sprays tend to be more penetrative than cream preparations. Once applied, a topical NSAID must be absorbed by the underlying tissue or enter the local blood stream. Studies have shown that the absorption of NSAIDs into the underlying tissue gives rise to therapeutic local concentrations of the drug without significant systemic absorption [32,33]. An estimated 3-7% of the applied dose is thought to be absorbed systemically [33] with plasma concentrations being approximately 5% of those achieved with oral administration [33].

The skin seems to act as a reservoir from which the drug disseminates to the deeper tissue. Peak concentrations in the skin are achieved 2 hours after application with a further spike at about 19 hours later, likely secondary to systemic absorption. Further proof of their local action is the absence of analgesic effect at joints distant to the point of application [34].

There have been many studies looking into the effectiveness of topical NSAIDs in treating osteoarthritis [35-41]. These on the whole have found that topical NSAIDs were superior to placebo in the treatment of chronic pain. Most of the initial studies found no benefit beyond two weeks of treatment [35-41] but larger randomised controlled trials found long term benefit for up to 3 months when compared to placebo [42-43].

When compared to oral NSAID use, the results have been variable. A meta-analysis in 2004 [41] found that topical NSAIDs were less effective than systemic NSAIDs. Since then, however, there have been several studies showing comparable effectiveness. Two studies comparing oral diclofenac with a topical preparation of the drug [44,45] found that there was no difference in pain scores or physical function. They also found that those in the topical treatment arm had a much lower incidence of severe gastrointestinal side effects, deranged liver function tests and abnormal creatinine clearance [44,45]. These results were replicated in another study comparing oral and topical treatment with ibuprofen for knee osteoarthritis, which also found no difference in pain and function scores between the two arms [43].

On the whole, topical NSAID use is associated with fewer systemic adverse events [35, 39, 44, 45] as compared to oral preparations. The main adverse event associated with topical NSAID use is local skin irritation, which has been reported in up to 39.3% of patients [46]. However, these skin reactions occur with placebo gel application with equal frequency indicating that it may not be related to the drug itself [39]. Other studies also suggest that skin reactions may be more common with solutions containing DMSO than DSG [37]. There is some contradictory evidence regarding their safety in older patients as some studies have found the rate of GI side effects in the over 50s to be as high as 15% [46].

Overall the data suggest that topical NSAIDs may be considered as first line therapy for osteoarthritis as they appear to be efficacious and associated with fewer adverse events. There should be caution about their long term use in the elderly as these patients may be more prone to adverse events.

2.5. Other topical treatments

Topical capsaicin cream has been used to treat a multitude of different painful conditions including osteoarthritis, inflammatory arthritis and neuropathic pain. Derived from chilli peppers, capsaicin is a lipophilic alkaloid that acts as a local irritant. It activates local pain receptors (c-nociceptors) leading to the release of substance P [47]. This in turn causes local irritation in the initial phase of treatment. With repeated use, however, levels of substance P are depleted, leading to desensitisation of the pain fibres and hypoalgesia [48]. In clinical practice, capsaicin is better than placebo for the treatment of chronic pain but compares less favourably with other treatments. In a meta-analysis comparing capsaicin with plaster, capsaicin was found to be only marginally effective [49]. Other drawbacks include the need to apply the cream four times a day for maximum benefit, as well as local irritation and intense burning sensation (occurring in uto 40% of patients) [50]. These problems lead 10% of patients to discontinue treatment [49]. In view of this, topical capsaicin should be used in conjunction with more traditional treatments.

Other topical treatments include the use of salicylate or nicotine esters, which acts as a local counter-irritant or rubefacient. These cause localised vasodilatation and reddening of the skin. This results in a local sensation of warmth, which often palliates pain. Theories of mechanisms of action include irritation of the sensory nerve endings in underlying muscle and tissue [51] as well as activation of the transient receptor ion channels involved in relaying thermal and pain sensation [52,53]. Clinical studies have shown modest benefits with regular use [54,55]. Compared to placebo, 16% achieved ≥50% improvement in pain scores at 2 weeks [54]. However, when compared to topical NSAIDs, counter-irritants performed poorly [55]. On the whole, counter-irritants are well tolerated and may be useful as adjuvants to standard therapy or patients in whom standard analgesics are contra-indicated [55]. There are no data to support their long term use and they are not recommended as continuing therapy.

3. Local injections

3.1. Intra-articular corticosteroids

Intra-articular (IA) corticosteroid injections are frequently used to treat osteoarthritis. In common practice, they are diluted in local anaesthetic to provide immediate relief, ensure accurate drug delivery and allow even dispersal of the drug within the joint due to the larger volume [57]. Commonly used corticosteroids in IA injections include hydrocortisone acetate (HCA), methylprednisolone acetate (MPA) and triamcinolone acetonide (TCA). These vary in solubility with the former being more soluble than the latter. Less soluble preparations are longer acting and theoretically provide more long term relief. In one randomised control trial comparing MPA (more soluble and shorter acting) and TCA in knee osteoarthritis, greater improvement in pain scores was found in the TCA group at 3 weeks compared to MPA [56]. Interestingly, there was no difference between the 2 groups at 8 weeks despite TCA being longer acting. There was also no significant difference in functional scores [56].

Several studies have looked into whether intra-articular steroid injections have symptomatic or functional benefit in knee osteoarthritis [58-61]. These have shown short term (lasting between 1-4 weeks) improvement in pain but not function in these patients following injections when compared to placebo. Follow up beyond 4 weeks did not show longer lasting benefits as compared to placebo. These results were further corroborated in a Cochrane systematic review [62]. This suggests that IA steroid injections should be used as a short term bridging treatment to resolve acute painful flares pending further intervention such as surgery or physiotherapy. Trials looking IA injections in the hip echo the results of the studies done in the knee: patients gained rapid and short lived pain relief following injection but that these benefits were not maintained beyond 1 month [63,64].

Other studies, looking at 1st carpo-metacarpal joint (CMC) injections found more mixed results in terms of long term relief. In one study of 40 patients, no benefit was observed between steroid injection when compared to placebo [65]. Patients less likely to have sustained long term benefits were those with worse radiographic appearances (increased number of osteophytes and more advanced joint space narrowing) [66]. In patients with less advanced disease, IA 1st CMC joint injection could provide symptomatic relief up to 18 months following injection and splinting [66].

IA steroid injections work locally via anti-inflammatory effects, inhibiting the inflammatory cascade at multiple points. Local injection avoids the systemic problems associated with steroid use and allows delivery of high doses to the affected tissue. Response to IA injection, however, does not appear to be dependent on inflammation in the affected joint itself [61]. Further studies looking at whether inflammation detected on ultrasound predicted clinical response found that those without inflammatory change fared better in response to IA injection than those with evidence of inflammation. The presence of synovial thickening, synovial fluid volume and white cell count did not predict better response to IA injection [60, 61]. In knee OA, joint aspiration prior to IA injection appears to provide greater symptomatic benefit [60]. This is partly due to confirmation of correct position by prior aspiration and more concentrated drug delivery due to a lower volume [67].

Although IA injections avoid the toxic side effects of systemic steroids, they are not without risks themselves. All patients undergoing IA injection should be consented for the risk of infection, although this is a rare event (incidence reported between 1 in 3,000 to 1 in 50,000) [68] and may be clinically difficult to differentiate from an injection-induced crystal arthritis which can occur in 2-6% of patients [58, 60]. In general, septic arthritis following IA injection occurs 3 to 4 days post procedure. There is a risk of lipoatrophy at the site of injection (estimated 0.6% of patients) [69]. The risk of this is reduced by using shorter-acting preparations and doing imaging-guided injections where possible. Other serious local adverse events include tendon rupture, muscle wasting and local depigmentation. The risk of these can also be minimised by using guided injections where possible.

Systemic adverse events are rare with local corticosteroid injections. The most common is flushing (up to 40%) [69]. There have been reported incidents of unstable diabetic glycaemic control post injection but this tends to be minor and usually settles [70]. There is evidence for systemic absorption of intra-articular steroids [71]. Studies looking at the endocrine axis in patients who had received intra-articular steroid injections found that serum cortisol dipped 24-48 hours after IA injection and took up to 4 weeks to return to baseline [71]. Major complications, such as steroid induced osteoporosis, have not been observed however [72].

Studies in animals have suggested that intra-articular steroids can induce chondrocyte degeneration [73] but prospective clinical trials where patients were receiving regular IA injections have failed to demonstrate increased rate of cartilage loss [74]. There are also limited data to support significant increased risk of osteonecrosis in injected joints. Repeated IA injections offer no long-term benefit [67] and should generally be avoided but short-term use may provide rapid pain relief and can be used as a bridging treatment pending further intervention.

3.2. Intra-articular hyaluronic acid/hyaluronan

Hyaluronic acid is a large glycosamino-glycan molecule found in synovial and cartilage extra cellular matrix (ECM). It is produced by synoviovytes, chondrocytes and fibroblasts and functions as both lubricant as well as a means to maintain hydration within the joint [75]. Studies have shown that osteoarthritic joints have decreased hyaluronan content in the synovial fluid [76] and therefore IA injection with a synthetic analogue was developed to restore the function in degenerative joints.

Synthetic preparations of hyaluronic acid closely mimic endogenous molecules. Later preparations contain cross linked hyaluronin in order to achieve greater elasticity and viscosity. In theory this confers greater intra-articular durability of the solution. Preparations with a higher molecular weight also seem to be more beneficial than those with a lower weight [78]. This may be related to the difference in volume required for injection as well as the number of injections required and the intra-articular durability of the solution.

Multiple studies have been conducted into the effectiveness of IA injections of hyaluronans in osteoarthritis, mostly of the knee. These have found mixed evidence to recommend their use. In general, hyaluronans appear to be better than placebo in improving pain scores, function and patient global assessment when used in knee osteoarthritis [77]. The greatest clinical benefit is achieved at week 5-13 after a course of treatment of several injections. Part of the problem with interpreting the data is wide variability in trial design, frequency of injections and molecular weight of the synthetic product being used. In hip OA, hyaluronan injections were not superior to placebo nor corticosteroid injections in reducing pain or improving function [79]. These results were echoed in studies looking at its use in hand OA [80].

These injections are relatively safe and tend to provide longer term relief than corticosteroid injections. Its use, however, is restricted by the relatively high cost of the treatment [75]. IA hyaluronan injection is generally reserved for knee osteoarthritis and is offered either as a holding measure until more definitive treatment can be undertaken (e.g. surgery), or in patients for whom such treatment is inappropriate.

3.3. Subcutaneous and soft tissue injections

Trigger points are localised areas of tenderness and thickening in the soft tissues. They are typically found proximal to an inflamed or painful joint such as the rectus femoris in patients with knee OA and paraspinal regions in the cervical and lumbar spine [81]. They have also been described as interstitial fibrositis, myofasciitis and myofascial trigger points [82-84]. The aetiology and pathogenesis of these trigger points is unknown.

Trigger point injection has been used as a way of alleviating pain and discomfort associated with these areas of thickening. This can be direct injection of a substance (e.g. local anaesthetic or corticosteroid) into the point or indirect needling of the soft tissue in that area. The trigger point is identified as the maximal area of tenderness in the muscle and the point is then isolated by the thumb and forefinger to prevent movement in the underlying muscle. A small sterile needle is then introduced into the area and the substance injected directly into it (or alternatively it can be dry needled). If the injection is performed correctly, there is usually an acute worsening of pain associated with muscle spasm [85].

A systematic review of trigger point injection in the management of chronic musculoskeletal pain found an improvement in symptoms when used exclusively [86]. This was irrespective of the injectant used [86]. The addition of a local anaesthetic, however, has been found to reduce the pain and irritation of the caused by the procedure [84].

There are limited data on the efficacy of trigger point injection in the treatment of osteoarthritis. One study found that trigger point injection in conjunction with IA corticosteroid was more effective than IA injection alone in both pain and functional scores [87]. Other studies have looked at trigger point injections as sole treatment and this does not reflect clinical practice. Overall, trigger point injections are safe and can be used as additional therapy in OA.

Drugs used for trigger point injections have included local anaesthetic, corticosteroids, anti-inflammatories such as acetylsalicylate and ketorolac as well as saline and water [84, 88-92]. There have also been several studies looking at the use of subcutaneous salicylate therapy for OA. In one trial 40 patients with OA of the 1st CMC joint [93] were randomised into either sham injection or subcutaneous injection with salicylate into trigger points. Patients were assessed blind at 3, 7 and 13 weeks. Pain scores and tenderness were significantly lower in those treated with salicylate compared to sham injections [93].

The mechanism of action of subcutaneous salicylate injections is unclear, particularly as the site of injection is distant from the affected joint. One theory is that salicylate may alter central sensitisation and this is supported by the immediate relief patients report following injection. An alternative model would be that the local effect of salicylate modifies the neurogenic control of inflammation, which may be abnormal in diseases that affect musculoskeletal structures [94, 95]. Changes in the expression and transport of neurogenic peptides might be induced by the local irritant effect of salicylate [96]. Systemic anti-inflammatory effects are unlikely, since the benefits are not observed in distant sites [93].

There is, however, a degree of overlap with acupuncture in that the injection sites are standard acupuncture locations. Acupuncture involves the insertion of fine filiform needles at or near the painful site, or sometimes at distant acupuncture "points". In a variation of this, the needles are sometimes stimulated electronically or with heat. Patients typically receive six or more sessions for a complete course of treatment. A systematic review of 393 patients with osteoarthritis found that acupuncture significantly improved pain but not function when compared to sham acupuncture [97-104]. In addition, it was not better than standard treatment with physiotherapy or being on a waiting list to receive acupuncture [97,100]. There was also no additional benefit of including acupuncture to standard therapy with exercise and advice [103]. Moreover, there is little evidence for long term benefit following treatment with improvements in symptoms lasting up to 12 weeks only [97,100]. Acupuncture is relatively safe, however, with minimal risks of serious side effects [101-104].

4. Splinting/support

Osteoarthritic joints may be helped by various forms of external support. Benefit can be obtained by adjusting alignment, modifying stress or load, providing shock absorption, or simply resting the joint. Orthoses (including braces, splints and elasticated sleeves) are frequently used in OA of the hand and knee and hand.. For hand OA they include thumb and wrist splints; for the knee they include rest orthoses, knee sleeves and unloading braces. Medial patellar strapping may be specifically helpful for patellar maltracking [105]. Shoe insoles may be particularly helpful for OA affecting the ankle and knee, and can sometimes alleviate symptoms from OA of the hip: they include cushioned or neutral insoles, which act as a shock absorbers; and wedged insoles, which also modulate mechanical stress.

For OA of the knee and ankle the main purpose of orthoses and insoles is to support joint that is unstable, and to help correct alignment [106]. They can modify load bearing and contribute to pain reduction, and they often improve physical function. There is also evidence that they can improve proprioception [107] and that they may slow disease progression [108]. They are especially useful for mild or moderate uni-compartmental knee OA [109-110, 42] where there may be varying degrees of instability and mal-alignment. Unloading knee braces are designed to reduce the load transmitted to the diseased compartment by applying an external valgus or varus force. Symptomatic relief is achieved by stabilizing the joint, increased joint opening and reduced local muscle contraction [108]. One study [111] demonstrated that patients treated with unloading knee braces had better functional and symptomatic outcomes at 6 months with medial compartment knee OA. These results were not replicated in other studies [112] although there is evidence that they can improve quadriceps strength and gait symmetry [113]. The main disadvantage of these braces is poor tolerability due to the weight and heat of the device. In one study, 41% of patients complained of skin irritation [114] and up to 20% of patients discontinue use within 6 months [115].

Splinting of the thumb carpometacarpal (CMC) joint has also been found to be helpful in improving function and pain [116]. CMC joint OA contributes more to pain and disability than inter-phalangeal joint OA [117] and thus splinting of the CMC joint makes sense. In a systematic review in 2010, CMC splinting was found to improve function and grip strength [116]. Further RCT data has corroborated this finding and showed sustained benefit at 12 months [118]. However, these splints are inevitably somewhat cumbersome to wear, and inhibit many day-today functions of the hand.

In general, splinting might be useful for symptomatic relief and may even improve function with prolonged use in appropriately selected patients.

5. Conclusion

There are a number of different local treatments for osteoarthritis which focus on symptomatic relief. Choice of treatment should, therefore, be guided by patient response and personal preference. Most local therapies are safe, avoiding any major systemic side effects. In general, these therapies should be used as adjuncts to physiotherapy and systemic analgesia. Although some of these treatments are well established and have been used in clinical practice for many years (e.g. intra-articular injections and orthoses), newer approaches are being developed such as local laser therapy and subcutaneous sodium salicylate injections. There is limited data to show any benefit for long term outcome for any of these local therapies and further studies are required to establish this.

Author details

Sarah Karrar and Charles Mackworth-Young*

*Address all correspondence to: c.mackworth-young@imperial.ac.uk

Department of Rheumatology, Charing Cross Hospital, Fulham Palace Road, London, UK

References

[1] Felson DT, Zhang Y. An update on the epidemiology of knee and hip osteoarthritis with a view to prevention. Arthritis Rheum. 1998; 41(8): 1343-55.

[2] Zhang Y, Niu J, Kelly-Hayes M, Chaisson CE, Aliabadi P, Felson DT. Prevalence of symptomatic hand osteoarthritis and its impact on functional status among the elderly: The Framingham Study. Am. J. Epidemiol. 2002; 156(11): 1021-7.

[3] Arden N, Nevitt M. Oeseoarthritis: Epidemiology. Best Pract. Res. Clin. Rheumatol. 2006; 20(1): 3-25.

[4] Haq I, Murphy E, Dacre J. Osteoarthritis. Postgrad Med. J. 2003; 79(933): 377-83.

[5] Cameron MH. Physical agents in rehabilitation. From research to practice. Philadelphia: WB Saunders Company, 1999.

[6] Arthritis Foundation. Conditions and treatments. Disease Centre. http://www.arthriitis.org/conditions/DiseaseCenter/Oa.asp., 2003

[7] Brosseau L, Yonge KA, Robinson V, Marchand S, Judd M, Wells G, Tugwell P. Thermotherapy for treatment of osteoarthritis. Cochrane Database Syst. Rev. 2003; (4): CD004522.

[8] Yurtkuran M, Kocagil T. TENS, Electroacupuncture and Ice Massage: Comparison of Treatment for Osteoarthritis of the Knee. Am. J. Acupunct. 1999; 27(3-4): 133–40.

[9] Clarke GR, Willis LA, Stenner L, Nichols PJR. Evaluation of Physiotherapy in the Treatment of Osteoarthrosis of the Knee. Rheumatol. Rehabil. 1974; 13(4): 190–7.

[10] Hecht PJ, Backmann S, Booth RE, Rothman RH. Effects of Thermal Therapy on Rehabilitation after Total Knee Arthroplasty : A Prospective Randomized Study. Clinical Orthopedics and Related Research 1983; 178: 198–201

[11] Boyaci A, Tutoglu A, Boyaci N, Aridici R, Koca I. Comparison of the efficacy of ketoprofen phonophoresis, ultrasound and short-wave diathermy in knee osteoarthritis. Rheumatol. Int. 2013 Nov;33(11): 2811-8

[12] Ochiai S, Watanabe A, Oda H, Ikeda H. Effectiveness of thermotherapy using a heat and steam generating sheet for cartilage in knee osteoarthritis. J. Phys. Ther. Sci. 2014, 26 :281-284

[13] Cakir S, Hepguler S, Ozturk C, Korkmaz M, Iseleten B, Atamaz FC. Efficacy of therapeutic ultrasound for the management of knee osteoarthritis : a randomised controlled and double-blind study. Am. J. Phys. Med. Rehabil. 2014 May ;93(5) :405-12

[14] Michlovitz S, Hun L, Erasala GN. Continuous low-level heat wrap therapy is effective for treating wrist pain. Arch. Phys. Med. Rehabil. 2004, 85 :1409-1416

[15] Petrofsky JS, Bains G, Raju C. The effect of moisture content of a local heat source on the blood flow response of the skin. Arch. Dermatol. Res. 2009, 301 :581-585

[16] Brand HS, De Koning MH, Van Kampen GP. Effect of temperature on the metabolism of proteoglycans in explants of bovine articular cartilage. Connect. Tissue Res. 1991, 26 :87-100

[17] Kocaoglu B, Martin J, Wolf B et al. The effect of irrigation solution at different temperatures on articular cartilage etabolism. Arthroscopy 2011,27 :525-531

[18] Li X, Li J, Cheng K, Lin Q, Wang D, Zhang H, An H, Gao M and Chen A. Effect of low-intensity pulsed ultrasound on MMP-13 and MAPKs signaling pathway in rabbit knee osteoarthritis. Cell Biochem. Biophys. 2011 Nov;61(2):427-34

[19] Naito K1, Watari T, Muta T, Furuhata A, Iwase H, Igarashi M, Kurosawa H, Nagaoka I, Kaneko K. Low-intensity pulsed ultrasound (LIPUS) increases the articular cartilage type II collagen in a rat osteoarthritis model. J. Orthop. Res. 2010 Mar;28(3):361-9

[20] Ulus Y1, Tander B, Akyol Y, Durmus D, Buyukakıncak O, Gul U, Canturk F, Bilgici A, Kuru O. Therapeutic ultrasound versus sham ultrasound for the management of patients with knee osteoarthritis: a randomized double-blind controlled clinical study. Int. J. Rheum. Dis. 2012 Apr;15(2):197-206.

[21] Pallotta RC1, Bjordal JM, Frigo L, Leal Junior EC, Teixeira S, Marcos RL, Ramos L, Messias Fde M, Lopes-Martins RA. Infrared (810-nm) low-level laser therapy on rat experimental knee inflammation. Lasers Med. Sci. 2012 Jan;27(1):71-8.

[22] Barushka O1, Yaakobi T, Oron U. Effect of low-energy laser (He-Ne) irradiation on the process of bone repair in the rat tibia. Bone. 1995 Jan;16(1):47-55.

[23] Grassi FR1, Ciccolella F, D'Apolito G, Papa F, Iuso A, Salzo AE, Trentadue R, Nardi GM, Scivetti M, De Matteo M, Silvestris F, Ballini A, Inchingolo F, Dipalma G, Scacco

S, Tetè S. Effect of low-level laser irradiation on osteoblast proliferation and bone formation. J. Biol. Regul. Homeost. Agents. 2011 Oct-Dec;25(4):603-14.

[24] Saito S[1], Shimizu N. Stimulatory effects of low-power laser irradiation on bone regeneration in midpalatal suture during expansion in the rat. Am. J. Orthod. Dentofacial Orthop. 1997 May;111(5):525-32.

[25] Almeida-Lopes L[1], Rigau J, Zângaro RA, Guidugli-Neto J, Jaeger MM. Comparison of the low level laser therapy effects on cultured human gingival fibroblasts proliferation using different irradiance and same fluence. Lasers Surg. Med. 2001;29(2):179-84

[26] Kreisler M[1], Christoffers AB, Al-Haj H, Willershausen B, d'Hoedt B. Low level 809-nm diode laser-induced in vitro stimulation of the proliferation of human gingival fibroblasts. Lasers Surg. Med. 2002;30(5):365-9

[27] Wang P, Liu C, Yang X, Zhou Y, Wei X, Ji Q, Yang L, He C. Effects of low level laser therapy on joint pain, synovitis, anabolic and catabolic factors in a progressive osteoarthritis rabbit model. Laser Med. Sci. 2014 June 3

[28] Brosseau L, Welch V, Wells G, deBie R, Gam A, Harman K, Morin M, Shea B, Tugwell P. Low level laser thearpy (class I, II and III) for the treatment of osteoarthritis. Cochrane Database Syst Rev. 200;(2):CD002046.

[29] Al-Rashoud AS, Abboud RJ, Wang W, Wigderowitz C. Efficacy of low-level laser therapy at acupuncture points in knee osteoarthritis :a randomised double blind comparative trial. Physiotherapy. 2014 Sep;100(3) :242-8

[30] Soleimnapour H, Gahramani K, Taheri R, Golzari SE, Safari S, Esfanjani RM, Iranpour A. The effect of low-level laser therapy on knee osteoarthritis :prospective, descriptive study. Laser Med Sci. 2014 Sep; 29(5):1695-700

[31] Cashman JN. The mechanisms of action of NSAIDs in analgesia. Drugs 1996; 52 Suppl. 5: 13-23

[32] Haroutiunian S, Drennan DA, Lipman AG. Topical NSAID therapy for musculoskeletal pain. Pain Med. 2010 Apr;11(4): 535-49.

[33] Anon. Topical analgesics: A review of reviews and a bit of perspective. www.jr2.ox.ac.uk/Bandolier/Extraforbando/Topextra3.pdf 2005.

[34] Sioufi A, Pommier F, Boschet F, Godbillon J, Lavoignat D, Salliere D. Percutaneous absorption of diclofenac in healthy volunteers after single and repeated topical application of diclofenac Emulgel. Biopharm Drug Dispos. 1994; 15(6): 441–9.

[35] Massey T, Derry S, Moore RA, McQuay HJ. Topical NSAIDs for acute pain in adults. Cochrane Database Syst Rev. 2010 Jun 16;(6): CD007402

[36] Brunner M, Dehghanyar P, Seigfried B, Martin W, Menke G, Müller M. Favourable dermal penetration of diclofenac after administration to the skin using a novel spray gel formulation. Br. J. Clin. Pharmacol. 2005; 60(5): 573–7

[37] Barthel HR, Haselwood D, Longley S 3rd, Gold MS, Altman RD. Randomized controlled trial of diclofenac sodium gel in knee osteoarthritis. Semin. Arthritis Rheum. 2009; 39(3): 203-12.

[38] Moore RA, Tramer MR, Carroll D, Wiffen PJ, McQuay HJ. Quantitative systematic review of topical applied non-steroidal anti-inflammatory drugs. Brit. Med. J. 1998; 316(7168): 333-8

[39] Mason L, Moore RA, Edwards JE, Derry S, McQuay HJ. Topical NSAIDs for chronic musculoskeletal pain: systematic review and metaanalysis. BMC Musculoskeletal Disord. 2004; Aug 19;5: 28

[40] Lin J, Zhang W, Jones A, Doherty M. Efficacy of topical non-steroidal anti-inflammatory drugs in the treatment of osteoarthritis: meta-analysis of randomised controlled trials. Brit. Med. J. 2004; 329(7461): 324

[41] Biswal S, Medhi B, Pandhi P. Longterm efficacy of topical nonsteroidal antiinflammatory drugs in knee osteoarthritis: Metaanalysis of randomized placebo controlled clinical trials. J. Rheumatol. 2006; 33(9): 1841–4

[42] Roth SH, Shainhouse JZ. Efficacy and safety of a topical diclofenac solution (Pennsaid) in the treatment of primary osteoarthritis of the knee: a randomized, double-blind, vehicle-controlled clinical trial. Arch Intern Med. 2004; 164(18): 2017-23

[43] Underwood M, Ashby D, Cross P, Hennessy E, Letley L, Martin J, Mt-Isa S, Parsons S, Vickers M, Whyte K. Advice to use topical or oral ibuprofen for chronic knee pain in older people: randomised controlled trial and patient preference study. Brit. Med. J. 2008; 336(7636): 138-42

[44] Tugwell PS, Wells GA, Shainhouse JZ. Equivalence study of a topical diclofenac solution (pennsaid) compared with oral diclofenac in symptomatic treatment of osteoarthritis of the knee: A randomized controlled trial. J. Rheumatol. 2004; 31(10): 2002–12

[45] Simon LS, Grierson LM, Naseer Z, Bookman AA, Zev Shainhouse J. Efficacy and safety of topical diclofenac containing dimethyl sulfoxide (DMSO) compared with those of topical placebo. DMSO vehicle and oral diclofenac for knee osteoarthritis. Pain. 2009; 143(3): 238-45

[46] Makris UE, Kohler MJ, Fraenkel L. Adverse effects of topical non-steroidal anti-inflammatory drugs in older adults with osteoarthritis: a systematic literature review. J. Rheumatol. 2010; 3(6): 1236-43

[47] Baron R. Capsaicin and nociception: from basic mechanisms to novel drugs. Lancet. 2000; 356(9232): 785-7

[48] Nolano M, Simone DA, Wendelschafer-Crabb G, Johnson T, Hazen E, Kennedy WR. Topical capsaicin in humans: parallel loss of epidermal nerve fibres and pain sensation. Pain 1999; 81(1-2): 135-45

[49] Mason L, Moore RA, Derry S, Edwards JE, McQuay HJ. Systematic review of topical capsaicin for the treatment of chronic pain. Brit. Med. J. 2004; 328 (7446): 991-4

[50] Zhang W, Moskowitz RW, Nuki G, *et al.* OARSI recommendations for the management of hip and knee osteoarthritis, Part II: OARSI evidence-based, expert consensus guidelines. Osteoarthritis Cartilage. 2008; 16(2): 137–162

[51] Morton I, Hall J. The Royal Society of Medicine: Medicines. 6th Edition. London: Bloomsbury, 2002.

[52] Nilius B, Owsianik G, Voets T, Peters JA. Transient receptor potential cation channels in disease. Physiol. Rev. 2007; 87(1): 165–217

[53] Stanos SP. Topical agents for the management of musculoskeletal pain. J. Pain Symptom Management. 2007; 33(3): 342–55

[54] Matthews P, Derry S, Moore RA, McQuay HJ. Topical rubefacients for acute and chronic pain in adults. Cochrane Database Syst Rev. 2009 Jul 8; (3): CD007403

[55] Mason L, Moore RA, Edwards JE, McQuay HJ, Derry S, Wiffen PJ. Systematic review of efficacy of topical rubefacients containing salicylates for the treatment of acute and chronic pain. Brit. Med. J. 2004 Apr 24; 328(7446): 995

[56] Pyne D, Ioannou Y, Mootoo R, Bhanji A. Intra-articular steroids in knee osteoarthritis: a comparative study of triamcinolone hexacetonide and methylprednisolone acetate. Clin. Rheumatol. 2004; 23(2): 116-20

[57] Schumacher HR. Aspiration and injection therapies for joints. Arthritis Rheum. 2003; 49(3): 413-20

[58] Friedman DM & Moore ME. The efficacy of intra-articular steroids in osteoarthritis: a double blind study. J. Rheumatol. 1980; 7(6): 850-6

[59] Dieppe PA, Sathapatayavongs B, Jones HE, Bacon PA, Ring EF. Intra-articular steroids in osteoarthritis. Rheumatol. Rehab. 1980; 19(4): 212-17.

[60] Gaffney K, Ledingham J, Perry JD. Intra-articular triamcinolone hexacetonide in knee osteoarthritis: factors influencing the clinical response. Ann. Rheum. Dis. 1995; 54(5): 379-81

[61] Jones A & Doherty M. Intra-articular corticosteroids are effective in osteoarthritis but there are no clinical predictors of response. Ann Rheum Dis. 1996; 55(11): 829-32.

[62] Bellamy N, Campbell J, Robinson V, Gee T, Bourne R, Wells G. Intra-articular corticosteroids for osteoarthritis of the knee. Cochrane Database Syst. Rev. 2006 Apr 19; (2): CD005328.

[63] Flanagan J, Casale FF, Thomas TL, Desai KB. Intra-articular injection for pain relief in patients awaiting hip replacement. Ann. Roy. Coll. Surg. Engl. 1988; 70(3): 156-7

[64] Qvistgaard E, Christensen R, Torp-Pedersen S, Bliddal H. Intra-articular treatment of hip osteoarthritis: a randomized trial of hyaluronic acid, corticosteroid, and isotonic saline. Osteoarthritis Cartilage. 2006; 14(2): 163-70

[65] Meenagh GK, Patton J, Kynes C, Wright GD. A randomised controlled trial of intra-articular corticosteroid injection of the carpometacarpal joint of the thumb in osteoarthritis. Ann. Rheum. Dis. 2004; 63(10): 1260–3

[66] Day CS, Gelberman R, Patel AA, Vogt MT, Ditsios K, Boyer MI. Basal joint osteoarthritis of the thumb: a prospective trial of steroid injection and splinting. J. Hand. Surg. 2004; 29(2): 247–51

[67] Ayral X. Injections in the treatment of osteoarthritis. Best Pract. Res. Clin. Rheumatol. 2001; 15(4), 609-26

[68] Creamer P. Intra-articular corticosteroid treatment in osteoarthritis. Curr. Opin. Rheumatol. 1999; 11(5): 417-21

[69] Kumar N, Newman RJ. Complications of intra- and peri-articular steroid injections. Br. J. Gen. Pract. 1999; 49(443): 465-6

[70] Pattrick M, Doherty M. Facial flushing after intra-articular injection of bupivacaine and methylprednisolone. Brit. Med. J. 1987; 295(6610): 1380

[71] Habib GS. Systemic effects of intra-articular corticosteroids. Clin. Rheumatol. 2009 Jul;28(7):749-56

[72] Slotkoff A, Clauw D, Nashel D. Effect of soft tissue corticosteroid injection on glucose control in diabetics. Arthritis Rheum. 1994; 37(suppl 9): S347

[73] Papacrhistou G, Anagnostou S, Katsorhis T. The effect of intraarticular hydrocortisone injection on the articular cartilage of rabbits. Acta. Orthop. Scand. Suppl. 1997; 275: 132-4

[74] Raynauld JP, Buckland-Wright C, et al. Safety and efficacy of long-term intraarticular steroid injections in osteoarthritis of the knee: a randomized, double-blind, placebo-controlled trial. Arthritis Rheum. 2003; 48(2): 370-7

[75] National Institute for Health and Clinical Excellence. Osteoarthritis: national clinical guideline for care and management in adults London: NICE, 2008. www.nice.org.uk/ CG059

[76] Fife R. Osteoarthritis: A. Epidemiology, pathology and pathogenesis. In: Klippel JH, editor. Primer on the rheumatic diseases. 11th edition. Atlanta: The Arthritis Foundation; 1997. p. 216-7

[77] Bellamy N, Campbell J, Robinson V, Gee T, Bourne R, Wells G. Viscosupplementation for the treatment of osteoarthritis of the knee. Cochrane Database Syst. Rev. 2006 Apr 19; (2): CD005321

[78] Wobig M, Bach G, Beks P *et al.* The role of elastoviscosity in the efficacy of viscosup-
      plementaion for osteoarthritis of the knee: A comparison of hylan G-F 20 and a lower
      molecular weight hyaluronan. Clin. Ther. 1999; 21(9): 1549–62

[79] Qvistgaard E, Christensen R, Torp-Pedersen S, Bliddal H. Intra-articular treatment of
      hip osteoarthritis: a randomized trial of hyaluronic acid, corticosteroid, and isotonic
      saline. Osteoarthritis Cartilage. 2006; 14(2): 163-70

[80] Fuchs S, Mönikes R, Wohlmeiner A, Heyse T. Intra-articular hyaluronic acid com-
      pared with corticoid injections for the treatment of rhizarthrosis. Osteoarthritis Carti-
      lage. 2006; 14(1): 82-8

[81] Fox WW and Freed DLJ. Understanding arthritis. Macmillan, London, 1990.

[82] Steindler A and Luck JV. Differential diagnoses of pain in the low back. J. Amer.
      Med. Assoc. 1938; 110:106-113

[83] Travell JG, Simons DG (eds.) Myofascial Pain and Dysfunction: the Trigger Point
      Manual. Williams & Wilkins, Baltimore, MD, USA, 1983: 2-18

[84] Cailliet R. Chronic pain concept. In: Soft Tissue Pain and Disability. FA Davis, Phila-
      delphia, PA, USA, 1977: 25-40

[85] Kim PS. Role of injection therapy: review of indications for trigger point injections,
      regional blocks, facet joint injections, and intra-articular injections. Curr. Opin. Rheu-
      matol. 2002; 14(1): 52-7

[86] Scott NA, Guo B, Barton PM, Gerwin RD. Trigger point injections for chronic non-
      malignant musculoskeletal pain: a systematic review. Pain Med. 2009; 10(1): 54-69

[87] Yentür EA, Okcu G, Yegul I. The role of trigger point therapy in knee osteoarthritis.
      Pain Clinic 2003; 15: 385–90

[88] Sidel N and Abrams MI. Treatment of chronic arthritis; results of vaccine therapy
      with saline injections used as controls. J. Am. Med. Assoc. 1940; 11:1740-1742

[89] Traut EF, Passarelli EW. Study in the controlled therapy of degenerative arthritis.
      Arch. Intern. Med. 1956; 98(2): 181-186

[90] Frost FA, Jessen B, Siggaard-Andersen J. A controlled, double-blind comparison of
      mepivacaine versus saline injection for myofascial pain. Lancet. 1980; 1(8167):
      499-500

[91] Frost FA. Diclofenac versus lidocaine as injection therapy in myofascial pain. Scand.
      J. Rheumatol. 1986; 15: 153-156

[92] Byrn C, Olsson I, Falkheden L *et al.* Subcutaneous sterile water injections for chronic
      neck and shoulder pain following whiplash injuries. Lancet 1993; 341(8843): 449-52

[93]   Smith AS, Doré CJ, Dennis L, Julius A, Mackworth-Young CG. A randomised controlled trial of subcutaneous sodium salicylate therapy for osteoarthritis of the thumb. Postgrad. Med. J. 2010 Jun;86(1016):341-5

[94]   Kidd BL, Urban LA. Mechanisms of inflammatory pain. Br. J. Anaesth. 2001; 87(1): 3-11

[95]   Schaible HG, Ebersberger A, Von Banchet GS. Mechanisms of pain in arthritis. Ann. New. York. Acad. Sci. 2002; 966: 343-54

[96]   McCarthy GM, McCarty DJ Effect of topical capsaicin in the therapy of painful osteoarthritis of the hands. J. Rheumatol. 1992; 19: 604-607

[97]   C Witt, B Brinkhaus, S Jena, et al. Acupuncture in patients with osteoarthritis of the knee: a randomised trial. Lancet 2005; 366(9480): 136–43

[98]   Molsberger A, Böwing G, Jensen KU, Lorek M.[Accupuncture treatment for the relief of gonarthrosis pain-a controlled clinical trial]. Der Schmerz 1994; 8(1): 37–42 (German)

[99]   Petrou P, Winkler V, Genti G, Balint G. Double blind trial to evaluate the effect of acupuncture treatment on knee osteoarthritis. Scand. J. Acupunct. 1988; 3: 112–15

[100] Berman BM, Singh BB, Lao L, *et al.* A randomized trial of acupuncture as an adjunctive therapy in osteoarthritis of the knee. Rheumatology (Oxford). 1999; 38(4): 346–54

[101] Ezzo J, Hadhazy V, Birch S, Kaplan G, Hochberg M, Berman B. Acupuncture for osteoarthritis of the knee: a systematic review. Arthritis Rheum. 2001; 44(4): 819–25

[102] Melchart D, Weidenhammer W, Streng A Reitmayr S, Hoppe A, Ernst E, Linde K. Prospective investigation of adverse effects of acupuncture in 97733 patients. Arch. Intern. Med. 2004; 164(1): 104–5

[103] Berman BM, Lao L, Langenberg P, Lee WL, Gilpin AM, Hochberg MC. Effectiveness of Acupuncture as Adjunctive Therapy in Osteoarthritis of the Knee. Ann. Intern. Med. 2004; 141(12): 901-10

[104] Ernst E, White A. Acupuncture: safety first. Brit. Med. J. 1997; 314(7091): 1362.

[105] Warden SJ, Hinman RS, Watson MA Jr, Avin KG, Bialocerkowski AE, Crossley KM. Patellar taping and bracing for the treatment of chronic knee pain: a systematic review and meta-analysis. Arthritis Rheum. 2008; 59(1): 73–83

[106] Rannou F, Poiraudeau S, Beaudreuil J. Role of bracing in the management of knee osteoarthritis. Curr. Opin. Rheumatol. 2010; 22(2): 218-22

[107] Birmingham TB, Kramer JF, Kirkley A, Inglis JT, Spaulding SJ, Vandervoort AA. Knee bracing for medial compartment osteoarthritis: effects on proprioception and postural control. Rheumatology (Oxford). 2001; 40(3): 285–9

[108]   Ramsey DK, Briem K, Axe MJ, Snyder-Mackler L. A mechanical theory for the effectiveness of bracing for medial compartment osteoarthritis of the knee. J. Bone Joint Surg. Am. 2007; 89(11): 2398–407

[109]   Jordan KM, Arden NK, Doherty M, et al. EULAR Recommendations 2003: an evidence-based approach to the management of knee osteoarthritis: Report of a Task Force of the Standing Committee for International Clinical Studies Including Therapeutic Trials (ESCISIT). Ann. Rheum. Dis. 2003; 62(12): 1145–1155

[110]   Recommendations for the medical management of osteoarthritis of the hip and knee: 2000 update. American College of Rheumatology Subcommittee on Osteoarthritis Guidelines. Arthritis Rheum. 2000; 43(9): 1905–15

[111]   Kirkley A, Webster-Bogaert S, Litchfield R, Amendola A, MacDonald S, McCalden R, Fowler P. The effect of bracing on varus gonarthrosis. J. Bone Joint Surg. 1999; 81(4): 539–48

[112]   Brouwer RW, van Raaij TM, Verhaar JA,Coene LN, Bierma-Zeinstra SM. Brace treatment for osteoarthritis of the knee: a prospective randomized multicentre trial. Osteoarthritis Cartilage. 2006; 14(8): 777–83.

[113]   Beaudreuil J, Bendaya S, Faucher M, Coudeyre E, Ribinik P, Revel M, Rannou F. Clinical practice guidelines for rest orthosis, knee sleeves, and unloading knee braces in knee osteoarthritis. Joint Bone Spine. 2009; 76(6): 629-36

[114]   Pollo FE, Otis JC, Backus SI, Warren RF, Wickiewicz TL. Reduction of medial compartment loads with valgus bracing of the osteoarthritic knee. Am. J.Sports Med. 2002; 30 (3): 414–21

[115]   Giori NJ. Load-shifting brace treatment for osteoarthritis of the knee: a minimum 2 1/2-year follow-up study. J. Rehabil. Res. Dev. 2004; 41(2) : 187–94

[116]   Kristin Valdes and Tambra Marik. A Systematic Review of Conservative Interventions for Osteoarthritis of the Hand. J. Hand. Ther. 2010; 23(4): 334–50

[117]   Bijsterbosch J, Visser W, Kroon HM, Stamm T, Meulenbelt I, Huizinga TW, Kloppenburg M. Thumb base involvement in symptomatic hand osteoarthritis is associated with more pain and functional disability. Ann. Rheum. Dis. 2010; 69(3): 585–7

[118]   Rannou F, Dimet J, Boutron I, et al. Splint for base-of-thumb osteoarthritis: a randomized trial. Ann. Intern. Med. 2009; 150(10): 661-9

2

Cell-Based Therapy for Human Osteoarthritis

Rie Kurose and Takashi Sawai

1. Introduction

Articular cartilage has a function to smooth the movement of the joints and to decrease the coefficient of friction. Recently, it has been reported that "lubricin," a mucinous glycoprotein encoded by the *PRG4* gene, provides boundary lubrication in the articular joints [1]. Also, the articular cartilage has a role of shock absorber against an external force. The articular cartilage is hyaline cartilage composed of water (approximately 70%), cell (less than 3%), and abundant extracellular matrix (approximately 20%) such as type II collagen and proteoglycan. The articular cartilage is highly differentiated avascular tissue, and blood vessels, nerves, and lymphatic vessels are not present in the articular cartilage of adults. Based on the above, it is well known that damaged articular cartilage has a very limited capacity for self-repair. Even minor injuries may lead to progressive damage and result in osteoarthritic joint with significant pain and disability.

In 1989, it was reported that cartilage defect could be repaired with cultured chondrocytes in animal experiments in rabbits [2]. Based on this result, Brittberg et al. [3] performed clinical application for humans of autologous chondrocyte transplantation in 1994. However, some problems have been pointed out in this surgery. One was the possibility of dedifferentiated of cultured cells, which decreased matrix production ability because of monolayer culture. Another was the uneven distribution of injected chondrocytes caused in part by leak of the cell suspension from the periosteum covering the cartilage defect. To solve these problems, Ochi et al. [4] devised the use of atelocollagen as a scaffold: implantation of three-dimensional cartilage-like tissues using cultured autologous chondrocytes embedded in atelocollagen gel. This method has been currently used as a clinical application for osteochondritis dissecans since 2012 [5]. However, there is yet no clinically approved cell-based strategy for treatment of osteoarthritis (OA)-based cartilage lesions. Basic researchers and clinicians are focusing on alternative methods for cartilage repair, aiming to regenerate OA cartilage tissues. Cell-based therapy is an attractive biological method, and its studies have progressed in accordance with the development of tissue engineering.

2. Cell-based therapy for OA

Cell-based therapies using various cell types such as the chondrocytes or the bone marrow have been researched conventionally. Autologous chondrocytes are actually in clinical application for cartilage defects, and the surgical procedures such as marrow stimulation have also been performed for the purpose of cartilage repair. Although short-term results of these methods are good, there remains in doubt about long-term results. Mesenchymal stem cells (MSCs) are harvested from different sources such as the bone marrow, synovial tissue, and adipose tissue and have multilineage potentials. Recently, research in cartilage tissue engineering focuses on the use of MSCs as an alternative to autologous chondrocytes. Furthermore, induced pluripotent stem (iPS) cells or Muse cells might overcome the disadvantages of MSCs: insufficient number of cells, cell harvesting procedures with pain, and unstable differentiation potential of cells.

The regeneration of hyaline cartilage provides to improve the symptoms and ultimately prevent or delay progression to osteoarthritic joints. Cell-based therapies have been increasingly applied because they have the potential to regenerate the cartilage tissues.

2.1. Chondrocyte

2.1.1. Autologous chondrocyte implantation

Autologous chondrocyte implantation (ACI) was first reported in 1994 for treatment of focal cartilage defects in the tibiofemoral and patellofemoral compartments [3]. Since this report, chondrocyte-based therapy has become to be expected; a periosteal cover (first-generation ACI), a collagen-membrane cover (second -generation ACI), and a variety of three-dimensional scaffolds (third-generation ACI) are used for the methods of fixation. In these methods, arthrotomy and a two-stage surgical procedure are used. Long-term durability and success as long as 11 years of follow-up periods have been reported [6–13]. ACI is the first articular cartilage repair method using tissue engineering, but there is a problem that a sufficient number of cells cannot be secured by the case. Its usefulness is still under discussion.

2.1.2. Matrix-induced autologous chondrocyte implantation

A variation of the original periosteum membrane technique is matrix-induced autologous chondrocyte implantation (MACI). MACI membrane consists of a porcine type I/III collagen bilayer seeded with chondrocytes and MACI can promote hyaline-like cartilage repair. The technique of MACI procedure can eliminate many problems of first- or second-generation ACI, and the cell-seeded membrane can be implanted over a less inaccessible area or at osteochondral junctions because of its adhesive property [14]. Meyerkort et al. reported that both MACI and tibial tubercle transfer (TTT) using the Fulkerson technique were used to treat cartilage defects in the patellofemoral joints and provided a durable graft on 5-years resultant with clinical improvement [15–17].

2.2. Bone marrow

Marrow stimulation techniques such as abrasion arthroplasty, drilling, and microfracture penetrate the subchondral bone and induce the formation of fibrocartilage repair tissues [18]. Although these methods were performed traditionally, it has been shown recently that bleeding from the bone marrow resulted in the supply of cytokines, osteoprogenitor cells, and chondroprogenitor cells. Also, there have been many reports related to induction of MSCs by bone marrow stimulation techniques. Clinically, although excellent short-term outcomes have been reported after bone marrow stimulation, the durability of marrow-stimulated repair tissues has shown the tendency to functional decline with further follow-up.

2.2.1. Abrasion arthroplasty

In 1986, Johnson [19] reported about achievement of abrasion arthroplasty, removing dead bone superficially and providing vascularity tissues for blood clot attachment. According to this method, subsequent fibrocartilage formation was maintained integrity for up to 6 years. Sansone et al. [20] reported a 20-year follow-up of abrasion arthroplasty, with a positive functional outcome of 67.9%.

2.2.2. Multiple perforation (drilling)

In 1959, Pridie [21] reported about a method for multiple perforation to subchondral bone using a drill with a 6-mm diameter. After partial weight bearing for 6 weeks, holes drilled were filled with fibrocartilage. However, recent reports related to medial opening-wedge high tibial osteotomy suggest that subchondral drilling is not necessary because there is no significant difference in the formation of fibrocartilage with or without subchondral drilling [22].

2.2.3. Microfracture

Microfracture is common procedure for cartilage repair, which produces a small fracture of the subchondral bone using awls to penetrate eburnated bone to promote blood flow to the bony surface. There is a report that short-term results were good, but 38.1% proceeded to total knee arthroplasty (TKA) in a 6.8-year follow-up [23]. In other papers, the survival rate was 88.8% at a 5-year follow-up and decreased 67.9% at a 10-year follow-up [24, 25].

2.3. Mesenchymal stem cell

Nucleated cells in the bone marrow are mostly hematological cells, which float when they are cultured. However, some of the cells in the bone marrow adhere to culture dishes *in vitro*, proliferate itself, and form colonies. Thus, adherent cells are regarded as bone marrow mesenchymal cells (BMMCs). In 1974, Friedenstein et al. [26] reported that osteochondral progenitor cells were present in BMMCs, and in 1999, Pittenger et al. [27] reported about the pluripotency of BMMCs, named MSCs. Currently, it is well known that MSCs are adult stem cells and have the possibility of differentiating into multiple cell types, including adipocytes, chondrocytes, osteocytes, and cardiomyocytes [28].

2.3.1. Bone marrow MSC

Articular cartilage is insufficient for the capacity of cartilage repair, and the damaged cartilage tissues are not restored in complete hyaline cartilage in adults. We reasoned that the chondroprogenitor cells supplied to the cartilage defects are not sufficient. Then we have focused on the BMMCs, which might include MSCs, to supply sufficient chondroprogenitor cells to cartilage defects [29]. In our study in rabbits, BMMCs, which had a fibroblastic morphology and pluripotency for differentiation, were isolated from the bone marrow of the tibiae of rabbits, grown in monolayer culture. The autologous cells were then implanted into full-thickness articular cartilage defects in the knee joints of each rabbit. Advantages of this method included the use of autologous cells and absence of immunoreactivity. Furthermore, we investigated the efficiency of cartilage-derived morphogenetic protein 1 (CDMP1) gene-transfected autologous BMMCs for cartilage repair in a rabbit cartilage defect model [30]. CDMP1, a member of the transforming growth factor-β superfamily, is an essential molecule for the aggregation of mesenchymal cells and acceleration of chondrogenic differentiation. BMMCs were isolated from the bone marrow of the tibiae of rabbits, grown in monolayer culture, and transfected with the CDMP1 gene or a control gene (GFP) by a lipofection method. During *in vivo* repair of full-thickness articular cartilage defects, cartilage regeneration was enhanced by the implantation of CDMP1-transfected autologous BMMCs (Figure 1). The defects were filled with hyaline cartilage, and the deeper zone showed remodeling to subchondral bone over time. The repair and the reconstitution of zones of hyaline articular cartilage were superior to simple BMMC implantation. The histological score of the CDMP1-transfected BMMC group was significantly better than those of both control BMMC group and empty control group (Tables 1 and 2). Our studies suggest that the modulation of BMMCs by factors such as CDMP1 allows enhanced repair and remodeling compatible with hyaline articular cartilage.

2.3.2. Synovial MSC

Sekiya et al. [31] previously reported that MSCs in synovial fluid from anterior cruciate ligament injury, meniscus injury, or patients with OA were much more than those from healthy volunteers and increased according to postinjury period or severity. The MSCs in synovial fluid are considered to be derived from synovial tissue and are positive for CD44, CD73, and CD90, which are markers of MSCs, and negative for CD34 and CD45, which is a marker of hematopoietic stem cells and leukocyte progenitor cells, respectively. Intra-articular injection of the synovial MSCs promoted meniscus regeneration and protected articular cartilage by arthroscopic and histological observations in pig [32], rat [33], or porcine [34] massive meniscal defect models. We research for synovial fluid cells that are not accompanied by pain in the cell harvest and describe about its advantage in the latter part of this manuscript.

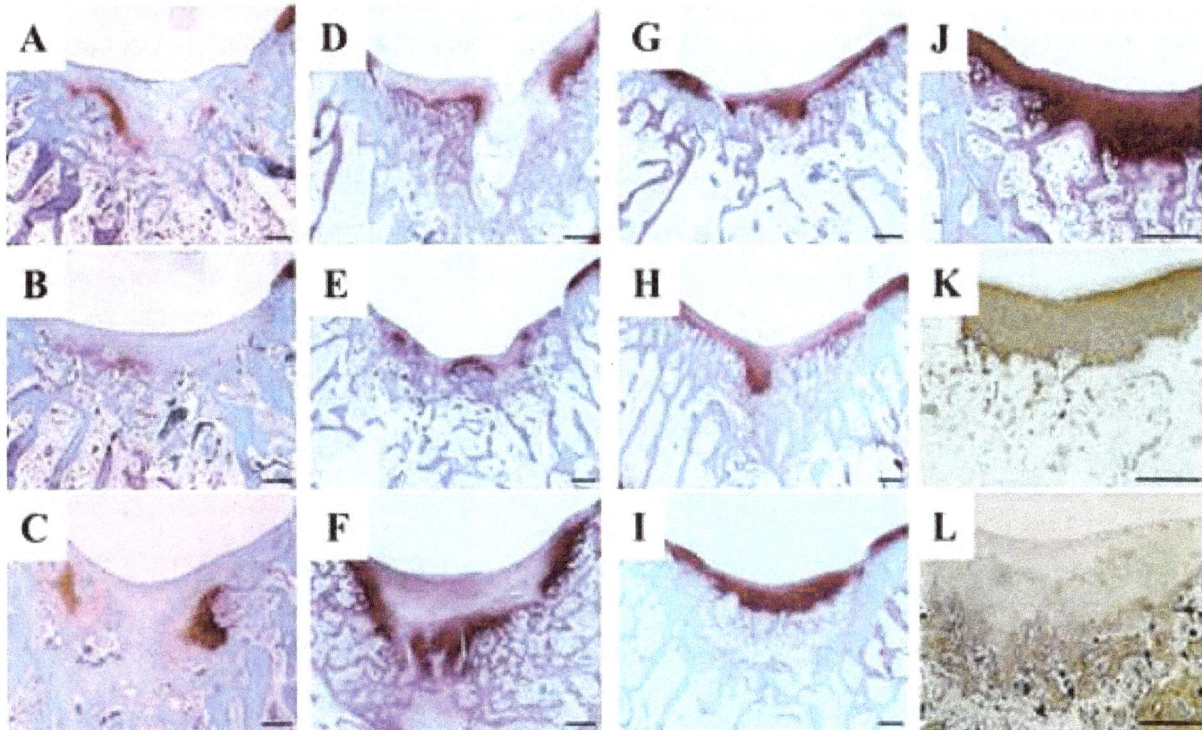

Figure 1. Representative histological appearance of the defects after 4 weeks. (A–J) Safranin-O/fast green staining. (A–C) Empty control group. (D–F) Left knees of GFP-transfected BMMC group. (G–I) Right knees of CDMP1-transfected BMMC group. (D and G, E and H, F and I) Bilateral knee specimens from the same rabbits. (J) Higher magnification of I. (K) Immunohistochemical staining specific for type II collagen. (L) Immunohistochemical staining specific for type I collagen. (A–L) Scale bar is 500 μm.

2.3.3. Adipose-derived MSC

Adipose tissues contain various cells such as blood cells, endothelial cells, and smooth muscle cells, in addition to adipocytes. Adipose tissues are also rich in microvasculature which adjoins with MSCs. Adipose-derived MSCs (ASCs) can be established by following method. Subcutaneous or visceral adipose tissues are minced and treated with type I collagenase. Then infranatant cells are centrifuged at low speed, and the cell pellet is placed in a flask. ASCs propagate themselves rapidly. Currently, two clinical trials for humans, which are the intra-articular injection for OA in France and the intravenous administration to rheumatoid arthritis in Spain, have been undergoing.

2.4. Induced pluripotent stem cells

iPS cells have pluripotency and the potential for self-renewal similar to ES cells. Recent study has made it possible to generate integration-free iPS cells and to differentiate iPS cells toward chondrocytes [35]. As an alternative approach, chondrocytic cells can be induced directly from dermal fibroblasts without going through the iPS cell stage. In 2011, Hiramatsu et al. [35] generated *in vitro* polygonal chondrogenic cells from adult dermal fibroblast cultures by ectopic expression of reprogramming factors (c-Myc and Klf4) and one chondrogenic factor

(SOX9). Namely, this approach could lead to the preparation of hyaline cartilage directly from skin without generating iPS cells. Recently, Yamashita et al. [36] reported that hyaline cartilage was generated from human iPS cells in immunodeficiency rats and immunosuppressed mini-pigs.

		Points
Category I		
A. Cell morphology	0	Hyaline cartilage
and Matrix staining	2	Mostly hyaline cartilage
	4	Moderately hyaline cartilage
	6	Partly hyaline cartilage
	8	Fibrous
B. Surface regularity[†]	0	Smooth (>3/4)
	1	Moderate (>1/2–3/4)
	2	Irregular (>1/4–1/2)
	3	Severely irregular (<1/4)
C. Integration of donor with	0	Both edges integrated
host adjacent cartilage	1	One edge integrated
	2	Neither edge integrated
		(Subtotal 13)
Category II		
D. Filling of defect	0	~100%
	1	~75%
	2	~50%
	3	~25%
	4	0%
E. Reconstitution of	0	Yes
subchondral bone and	1	Almost
osseous connection	2	Partly
	3	Not close
		(Subtotal 7)
Total maximum		20

*Modified from the scale described by Pineda et al. [46] and Wakitani et al. [47].

†Total smooth area of the reparative cartilage compared with the entire area of the cartilage defect.

Table 1. Histological grading scale for cartilage defect*

Interval until animals were killed (weeks)	No.	Grade (points)							
		A. Cell morphology and matrix staining	B. Surface regularity	C. Integration	Subtotal (A–C)	D. Filling of defect	E. Reconstitution of subchondral bone and osseous connection	Subtotal (D–E)	Total
CDMP1 transfected BMMCs									
2	10	6.2	0.7#	1.2	8.1#	0.8	2.6#	3.4#	11.5#
4	10	4.4	0.1#	0.7	5.2#	0.7	1.5	2.2	7.4#
8	10	4.6	0.3*,#	1.0	6.0*,#	0.7	1.1	1.8#	7.8*,#
GFP transfected BMMCs									
2	10	7.0	1.2	1.4	9.6	1.2	2.6	3.8	13.4
4	10	6.2	0.9	0.9	8.0	1.1	1.6	2.7	10.7
8	10	6.8	1.5	1.0	9.3	1.5	1.9	3.4	12.7
Empty control									
2	2	8.0	3.0	2.0	13.0	2.5	3.0	5.5	18.5
4	7	6.6	1.1	1.6	9.3	1.6	1.9	3.4	12.7
8	7	7.4	1.6	1.0	10.0	1.6	2.0	3.6	13.6

*$P < 0.05$, when compared to the GFP group at corresponding time (Mann–Whitney U-test).

#$P < 0.05$, when compared to the empty control at corresponding time (Scheffe test for multiple comparison).

Table 2. Results of the histological grading scale

2.5. Multilineage-differentiating stress enduring (Muse) cell

As a novel type of pluripotent stem cells, Muse cells were recently reported as adult human MSCs without introducing exogenous genes, and they are present in mesenchymal tissues such as the bone marrow, adipose tissue, dermis, and connective tissue of organs [37–40]. In particular, Muse cells have been detected more abundant in adipose tissues than in other organizations [41]. Also, Muse cells have a low tumor-forming ability compared with embryonic stem (ES) cells and a high efficiency of change to iPS cells by Yamanaka gene introduction [42]. They can migrate to damaged tissues by intravenous injection *in vivo*, spontaneously differentiate into cells compatible with the targeted tissue, and contribute to tissue repair. Thus, Muse cells will be expected to play important role in regenerative therapy by further studies.

3. MSCs in synovial fluid of human OA

In 2004, Jones et al. [43, 44] reported that the MSCs in synovial fluid in the inflammatory and degenerative arthritis, including OA, possessed high proliferative potential and could differentiate into several mesenchymal lineages. Aspiration of synovial fluid in the cases of hydrarthrosis caused by OA has the following great advantages: extremely simple technique, feasible during routine practice in outpatients, no need for local or general anesthesia for cell harvest, and effective usage of synovial fluid supposed to be discarded in the cases of hydrarthrosis.

3.1. Potential of chondrogenic differentiation of synovial fluid cells

We investigated the possibility of chondrogenic differentiation of the cells derived from synovial fluid and compared with the BMMCs previously performed in human OA [45]. Synovial fluid was aspirated from 26 knee joints of outpatients with OA and those of six patients just before skin incision at TKA. Bone marrow was obtained from the femur before the insertion of the femur rod at the time of TKA. Each aspirated fluid was diluted in α-modified Eagle's minimum essential medium (αMEM), and mononuclear cells using Ficoll-Paque PLUS (GE Healthcare) were harvested and cultured. Primary passage cells were used for flow cytometry assay and for chondrogenic assay, total RNA was prepared from each pellet of cultured cells, and pellets were used for immunohistochemical staining.

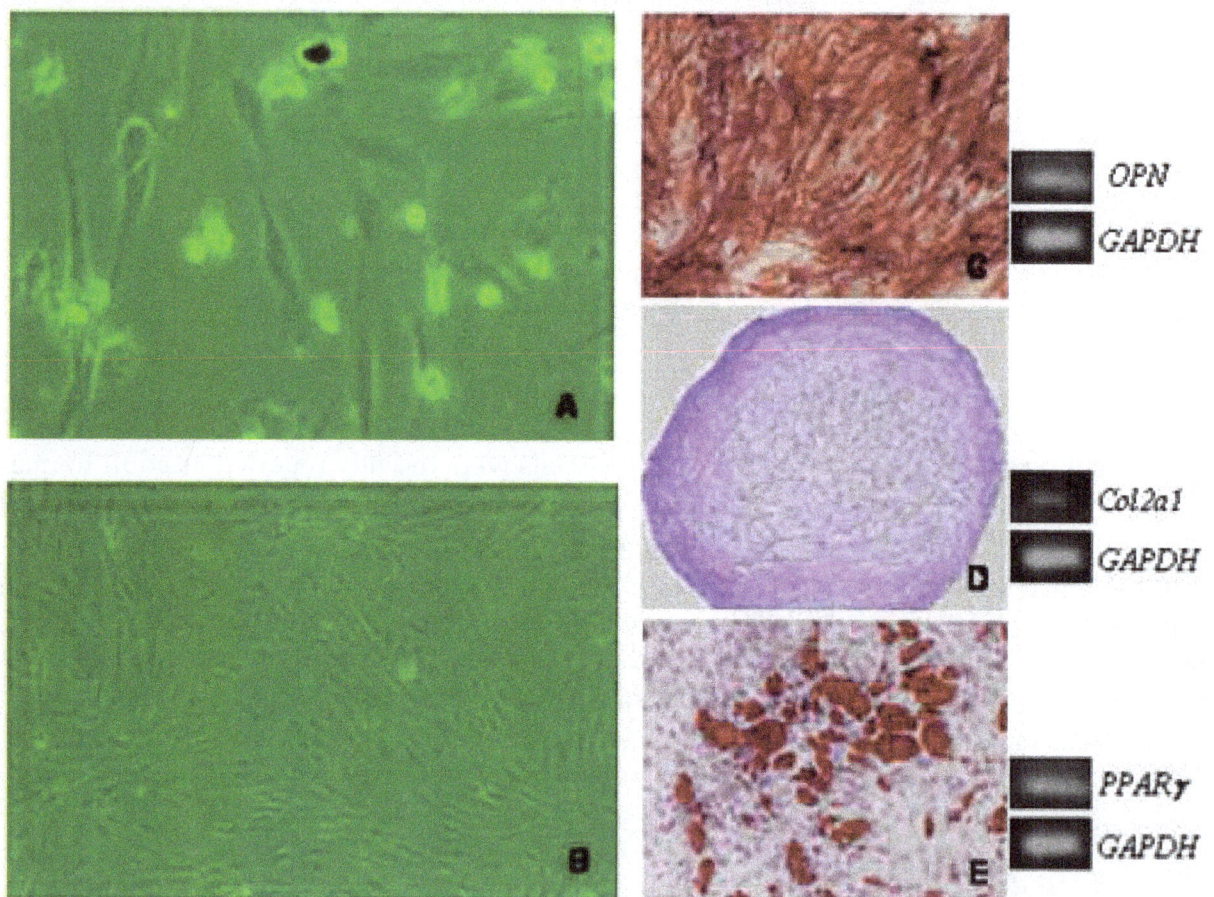

Figure 2. A, B) Phase-contrast photomicrographs of cultured synovial fluid cells on day 6 (A) and day 28 (B) showing fibroblast-like morphology. On day 28, the culture dish in subconfluency. (C–E) Multipotency of the cultured synovial fluid cells. (C) Osteogenesis was shown by alkaline phosphatase staining and the expression of osteopontin messenger (m) RNA (*OPN*). (D) Chondrogenesis was shown by toluidine blue staining and the expression of type II collagen mRNA (*Col2a1*). (E) Adipogenesis was shown by oil red-O staining and the expression of PPARγ mRNA (*PPARγ*).

In the results, the morphology of the cultured synovial fluid cells was fibroblastic, similar to that of BMMCs. Also, the synovial fluid cells had an ability to differentiate into osteoblasts, chondrocytes and adipocytes (Figure 2). The cultured synovial fluid cells strongly expressed

CD13, CD44, and CD105 but lacked CD10, CD14, and CD45 in flow cytometry analysis. Both mRNA expression of aggrecan and type II collagen had an increasing tendency at day 21 compared with day 7. Also, the cell pellets derived from synovial fluid showed intense toluidine blue staining, indicating chondrogenic differentiation.

3.2. Potential of cartilage regeneration of synovial fluid cells

Synovial fluid was aspirated from the OA knees before 1 month of TKA and cultured *in vitro*. Degenerative OA cartilage was obtained at the time of TKA. Approximately 5×10^5 autologous synovial fluid cells were labeled with Cell Tracker Green (CTG) (Invitrogen) in 200-µL αMEM and were transplanted gently on macroscopic degenerative tissues of OA cartilage. After10 min, medium was removed and changed into chondrogenic medium. One week later, the tissues were observed under a fluorescent microscope.

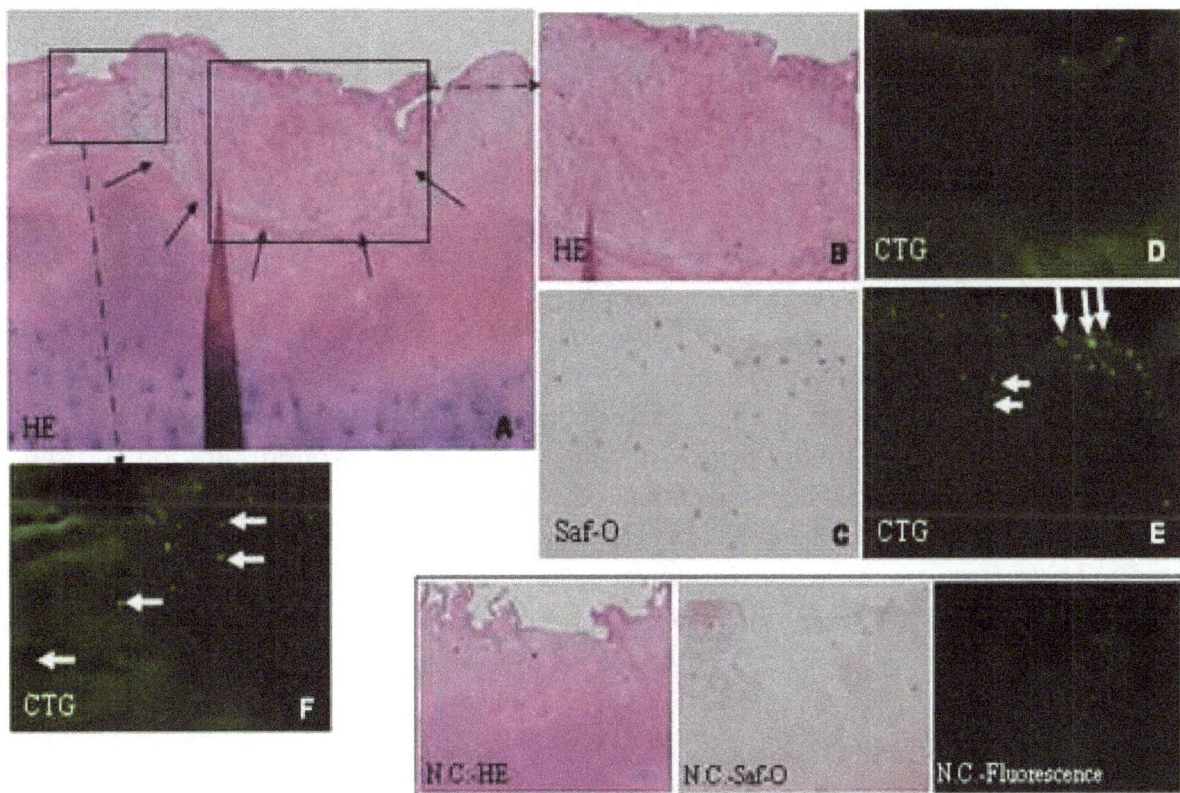

Figure 3. *Ex vivo* study using synovial fluid cells. (A) The formation of repaired tissue was shown by hematoxylin and eosin (HE) staining (Black arrows). (B) Magnified feature of A. (C) Repaired tissues and the surroundings of CTG-stained cells were weakly positive by safranin-O staining. (D) Fluorescent microscopy showed that CTG-labeled synovial fluid cells existed in repaired cartilage. (E) Magnified feature of D. (F) CTG-positive cells had a tendency to infiltrate into the original degenerative cartilage (White arrows). N.C.: Negative Control without CTG-labeled cells.

Histopathologically, degenerative tissues with transplanted CTG-labeled cells were weakly positive by safranin-O staining, which indicated that they were toward cartilage tissues (Figure 3). Fluorescent microscopy showed that CTG-labeled synovial fluid cells existed in the repaired tissues, which indicated that the tissues were constructed of autologous transplanted cells and the synovial fluid cells had a tendency to adhere to the degenerative cartilage. Furthermore, they seemed to infiltrate into the original degenerative cartilage of OA.

3.3. Cell-based therapy using synovial fluid cells

From previous and our current study, it has been recognized that synovial fluid in OA knee joints contain the adherent cells, and these cells have a potential of cell proliferation and chondrogenic differentiation *in vitro*. The primary culture of the human synovial fluid cells showed the formation of colonies of fibroblast-like cells, similar to those of BMMCs in both flow cytometry and real-time PCR analysis [34]. The infiltration of synovial fluid cells into the degenerative cartilage indicates that the possibility of attachment to OA cartilage in humans may promote the production of extracellular matrix and regeneration of hyaline cartilage. Further studies are need, but we expect the benefits of synovial fluid cells on OA cartilage tissues.

4. Conclusions

Many studies using various cell types for OA treatment are being performed. These short-term results appear mostly satisfactory, but there remains a problem that repaired tissues become fibrocartilage thereafter. Fibrocartilage leads to different biomechanical characteristics compared with hyaline cartilage and progresses to OA. MSCs based on self-repair and multilineage potentials provide to hyaline cartilage regeneration. In particular, bone marrow-derived MSCs are the most commonly used cell type for cartilage regeneration, but harvesting of the bone marrow is a painful procedure and has the risk of wound infection and sepsis. Alternatively, synovial fluid cells have great advantages and cartilage regeneration potential similar to bone marrow-derived MSCs. Naturally, long-term studies are needed whether repaired tissues are durable within the joint, but the use of synovial fluid cells may be expected to cartilage regeneration for OA therapy.

Author details

Rie Kurose[1*] and Takashi Sawai[2]

*Address all correspondence to: riekuro@hirosaki-u.ac.jp

1 Department of Orthopaedic Surgery, Hirosaki University Graduate School of Medicine, Hirosaki, Japan

2 Department of Histopathology, Tohoku University Graduate School of Medicine, Sendai, Japan

References

[1] Kimberly AW, Ling XZ, Khaled AE, Braden CF, Matthew LW, Gregory DJ. Role of lubricin and boundary lubrication in the prevention of chondrocyte apoptosis. Proc Natl Acad Sci USA 2013; 110 (15): 5852–5857.

[2] Grande DA, Pitman MI, Peterson L, Menche D, Klein M. The repair of experimentally produced defects in rabbit articular cartilage by autologous chondrocyte transplantation. J Orthop Res 1989; 7(2): 208–218.

[3] Brittberg M, Lindahl A, Nilsson A, Ohlsson C, Isaksson O, Peterson L. Treatment of deep cartilage defects in the knee with autologous chondrocyte transplantation. N Engl J Med 1994; 331(14): 889–895.

[4] Ochi M, Uchio Y, Kawasaki K, Wakitani S, Iwasa J. Transplantation of cartilage-like tissue made by tissue engineering in the treatment of cartilage defects of the knee. J Bone Joint Surg Br 2002; 84(4): 571–578.

[5] Takazawa K, Adachi N, Deie M, Kamei G, Uchio Y, Iwasa J, Kumahashi N, Tadenuma T, Kuwata S, Yasuda K, Tohyama H, Minami A, Muneta T, Takahashi S, Ochi M. Evaluation of magnetic resonance imaging and clinical outcome after tissue-engineered cartilage implantation: prospective 6-year follow-up study. J Orthop Sci 2012; 17(4): 413–424.

[6] Peterson L, Minas T, Brittberg M, Lidahl A. Treatment of osteochondritis dissecans of the knee with autologous chondrocyte transplantation: results at two to ten years. J Bone Joint Surg Am 2003; 85: 17–24.

[7] Peterson L, Vasiliadis HS, Brittberg M, Lindahl A. Autologous chondrocyte implantation: a long-term follow-up. Am J Sports Med 2010; 38: 1117–1124.

[8] Knutsen G, Drogset JO, Engebretsen L, Grøntvedt T, Isaksen V, Ludvigsen TC, Roberts S, Solheim E, Strand T, Johansen O. A randomized trial comparing autologous chondrocyte implantation with microfracture. Findings at five years. J Bone Joint Surg Am 2007; 89: 2105–2112.

[9] Knutsen G, Engebretsen L, Ludvigsen TC, Drogset JO, Grøntvedt T, Solheim E, Strand T, Roberts S, Isaksen V, Johansen O. Autologous chondrocyte implantation compared with microfracture in the knee. A randomized trial. J Bone Joint Surg Am 2004; 86: 455–464.

[10] Wood JJ, Malek MA, Frassica FJ, Polder JA, Mohan AK, Bloom ET, Braun MM, Coté TR. Autologous cultured chondrocytes: adverse events reported to the United States Food and Drug Administration. J Bone Joint Surg Am 2006; 88: 503–507.

[11] Henderson I, Tuy B, Oakes B. Reoperation after autologous chondrocyte implantation. Indications and findings. J Bone Joint Surg Br 2004; 86: 205–211.

[12] Gobbi A, Kon E, Berruto M, Filardo G, Delcogliano M, Boldrini L, Bathan L, Marcacci M. Patellofemoral full-thickness chondral defects treated with second-generation autologous chondrocyte implantation: results at 5 years' follow-up. Am J Sports Med 2009; 37: 1083–1092.

[13] Harris JD, Siston RA, Pan X, Flanigan DC. Autologous chondrocyte implantation: a systematic review. J Bone Joint Surg Am 2010: 92(12); 2220–2233.

[14] Goyal D, Keyhani S, Goyal A, Lee EH, Hui JHP, Vaziri AS. Evidence-based status of second- and third-generation autologous chondrocyte implantation over first generation: a systematic review of level I and II studies. Arthroscopy 2013; 29: 1872–1878.

[15] Meyerkort D, Ebert JR, Ackland TR, Robertson WB, Fallon M, Zheng MH, Wood DJ. Matrix-induced autologous chondrocyte implantation (MACI). Knee Surg Sports Traumatol Arthrosc 2014; Epub ahead of print.

[16] Bartlett W, Skinner JA, Gooding CR, Carrington RW, Flanagan AM, Briggs TW, Bentley G. Autologous chondrocyte implantation versus matrix-induced autologous chondrocyte implantation for osteochondral defects of the knee: a prospective, randomised study. J Bone Joint Surg Br 2005; 87: 640–645.

[17] Zeifang F, Oberle D, Nierhoff C, Richter W, Moradi B, Schmitt H. Autologous chondrocyte implantation using the original periosteum-cover technique versus matrix-associated autologous chondrocyte implantation: a randomized clinical trial. Am J Sports Med 2010; 38: 924–933.

[18] Steadman JR, Rodkey WG, Briggs KK. Microfracture to treat full-thickness chondral defects: surgical technique, rehabilitation, and outcomes. J Knee Surg 2002; 15: 170–176.

[19] Johnson LL. Arthroscopic abrasion arthroplasty historical and pathologic perspective: present status. Arthroscopy 1986; 2(1): 54–69.

[20] Sansone V, Girolamo L, Pascale W, Melato M, Pascale V. Long-term results of abrasion arthroplasty for full-thickness cartilage lesions of the medial femoral condyle. Arthroscopy 2015; 31: 396–403.

[21] Pridie KH. A method of resurfacing osteoarthritic knee joints. J Bone Joint Surg 1959; 41-B: 618–619.

[22] Jung WH, Takeuchi R, Chun CW, Lee JS, Jeong JH. Comparison of results of medial opening-wedge high tibial osteotomy with and without subchondral drilling. Arthroscopy 2015; 26: Epub ahead of print.

[23] Bert JM. Abandoning microfracture of the knee: has the time come? Arthroscopy 2015; 31: 501–505.

[24] Lubowitz JH. Arthroscopic microfracture may not be superior to arthroscopic debridement, but abrasion arthroplasty results are good, although not great. Arthroscopy 2015; 31: 506.

[25] Bae DK, Song SJ, Yoon KH, Heo DB, Kim TJ. Survival analysis of microfracture in the osteoarthritic knee—minimum 10-year follow-up. Arthroscopy 2015; 29: 244–250.

[26] Friedenstein AJ, Chailakhyan RK, Latsinik NV, Panasyuk AF, Keiliss-Borok IV. Stromal cells responsible for transferring the microenvironment of the hemopoietic tissues. Cloning in vitro and retransplantation in vivo. Transplantation 1974; 17(4): 331–340.

[27] Pittenger MF1, Mackay AM, Beck SC, Jaiswal RK, Douglas R, Mosca JD, Moorman MA, Simonetti DW, Craig S, Marshak DR. Multilineage potential of adult human mesenchymal stem cells. Science 1999; 284(5411): 143–147.

[28] Mazor M, Lespessailles E, Coursier R, Daniellou R, Best TM, Toumi H. Mesenchymal stem-cell potential in cartilage repair: an update. J Cell Mol Med 2014; 18: 2340–2350.

[29] Wakitani S, Imoto K, Yamamoto T, Saito M, Murata N, Yoneda M. Human autologous culture expanded bone marrow mesenchymal cell transplantation for repair of cartilage defects in osteoarthritic knees. Osteoarthritis Cartilage 2002; 10: 199–206.

[30] Katayama R, Wakitani S, Tsumaki N, Morita Y, Matsushita I, Gejo R, Kimura T. Repair of articular cartilage defects in rabbits using CDMP1 gene-transfected autologous mesenchymal cells derived from bone marrow. Rheumatology (Oxford) 2004; 43: 980–985.

[31] Sekiya I, Ojima M, Suzuki S, Yamaga M, Horie M, Koga H, Tsuji K, Miyaguchi K, Ogishima S, Tanaka H, Muneta T. Human mesenchymal stem cells in synovial fluid increase in the knee with degenerated cartilage and osteoarthritis. J Orthop Res 2012; 30(6): 943–949.

[32] Nakamura T, Sekiya I, Muneta T, Kobayashi E. Articular cartilage regenerative therapy with synovial mesenchymal stem cells in a pig model. Clin Calcium 2013; 23(12): 1741–1749.

[33] Katagiri H, Muneta T, Tsuji K, Horie M, Koga H, Ozeki N, Kobayashi E, Sekiya I. Transplantation of aggregates of synovial mesenchymal stem cells regenerates meniscus more effectively in a rat massive meniscal defect. Biochem Biophys Res Commun 2013; 14: 435(4) 603–609.

[34] Hatsushika D, Muneta T, Nakamura T, Horie M, Koga H, Nakagawa Y, Tsuji K, Hishikawa S, Kobayashi E, Sekiya I. Repetitive allogeneic intraarticular injections of synovial mesenchymal stem cells promote meniscus regeneration in a porcine massive meniscus defect model. Osteoarthritis Cartilage 2014; 22(7): 941–950.

[35] Hiramatsu K, Sasagawa S, Outani H, Nakagawa K, Yoshikawa H, Tsumaki N. Generation of hyaline cartilaginous tissue from mouse adult dermal fibroblast culture by defined factors. J Clin Invest 2011; 121(2): 640–657.

[36] Yamashita A, Morioka M, Yahara Y, Okada M, Kobayashi T, Kuriyama S, Matsuda S, Tsumaki N. Generation of scaffoldless hyaline cartilaginous tissue from human iPSCs. Stem Cell Reports 2015; 4(3): 404–418.

[37] Wakao S, Akashi H, Kushida Y, Dezawa M. Muse cells, a novel type of non-tumorigenic pluripotent stem cells, reside in human mesenchymal tissues. Pathol Int 2014; 64(1): 1–9.

[38] Kuroda Y, Wakao S, Kitada M, Murakami T, Nojima M, Dezawa M. Isolation, culture and evaluation of multilineage-differentiating stress enduring (Muse) cells. Nat Protoc 2013; 8(7): 1391–1415.

[39] Wakao S, Kuroda Y, Ogura F, Shigemoto T, Dezawa M. Regenerative effects of mesenchymal stem cells: contribution of muse cells, a novel pluripotent stem cell type that resides in mesenchymal cells. Cells 2012; 1: 1045–1060.

[40] Wakao S, Kitada M, Kuroda Y, Shigemoto T, Matsuse D, Akashi H, Tanimura Y, Tsuchiyama K, Kikuchi T, Goda M, Nakahata T, Fujiyoshi Y, Dezawa M. Multilineage-differentiating stress-enduring (Muse) cells are a primary source of induced pluripotent stem cells in human fibroblasts. Proc Natl Acad Sci USA 2011; 108(24): 9875–9880.

[41] Kuroda Y, Kitada M, WakaoS, Nishikawa K, Tanimura Y, Makinoshima H, Goda M, Akashi H, Inutsuka A, Niwa A, Shigemoto T, Nabeshima Y, Nakahata T, Nabeshima Y, Fujiyoshi Y, Dezawa M. Unique multipotent cells in adult human mesenchymal cell populations. Proc Natl Acad Sci USA 2010; 107: 8639–8643.

[42] Takahashi K, Tanabe K, Ohnuki M, Narita M, Ichisaka T, Tomoda K, Yamanaka S. Induction of pluripotent stem cells from adult human fibroblasts by defined factors. Cell 2007; 131: 861–872.

[43] Jones EA, English A, Henshaw K, Kinsey SE, Markham AF, Emery P, McGonagle D. Enumeration and phenotypic characterization of synovial fluid multipotential mesenchymal progenitor cells in inflammatory and degenerative arthritis. Arthritis Rheum 2004; 50: 817–827.

[44] Jones EA, Crawford A, English A, Henshaw K, Mundy J, Corscadden D, Chapman T, Emery P, Hatton P, McGonagle D. Synovial fluid mesenchymal stem cells in health and early osteoarthritis: detection and functional evaluation at the single cell level. Arthritis Rheum 2008; 58: 1731–1740.

[45] Kurose R, Ichinohe S, Tajima G, Horiuchi S, Kurose A, Sawai T, Shimamura T. Characterization of human synovial fluid cells of 26 patients with osteoarthritis knee for cartilage repair therapy. Int J Rheum Dis 2010; 13(1): 68–74.

[46] Pineda A, Pollack A, Stevenson S, Goldberg V, Caplan A. A semiquantitative scale for histologic grading of articular cartilage repair. Acta Anat 1992; 143: 335–340.

[47] Wakitani S, Goto T, Pineda SJ, Young RG, Mansour JM, Caplan AI, Goldberg VM. Mesenchymal cell-based repair of large, full-thickness defects of articular cartilage. J Bone Joint Surg Am 1994; 76: 579–592.

3

The Cholinergic System in Relation to Osteoarthritis

Sture Forsgren

1. Introduction

The cholinergic system is of interest for the synovial tissue of joints and for arthritic processes, including in osteoarthritis (OA). One aspect is that stimulation via the vagal nerve leads to hampering of arthritic processes. Another is that there is evidence of local acetylcholine (ACh) production within the synovial tissue of human joints, including joints in OA and rheumatoid arthritis. There is furthermore a marked presence of the nicotinic acetylcholine receptor AChRα7 (α7nAChR) in the synovial tissue. Influences on this receptor are known to have anti-inflammatory and healing effects. Overall, the concept of a "cholinergic anti-inflammatory pathway" has emerged for various parts of the body. That includes the situation in arthritis. This means that released ACh can have anti-inflammatory effects, in parallel with other favourable effects including wound-healing effects, implying that increased ACh effects might be of value in situations with arthritis. However, focus should further be made on the fact that there is not only evidence of ACh production but also ACh degradation within the synovial tissue. This is related to expressions of acetylcholinesterase (AChE). Of interest in this respect is that reductions of AChE activity via use of AChE inhibitor drugs are used in other situations (e.g. Alzheimer's disease). The aspects concerning ACh production/degradation in the synovial tissue, the fact that vagal stimulation decreases arthritic processes and the known presence of the potent AChRα7 receptor in synovial tissue should be further considered concerning arthritis in the future. That includes the situation in OA.

2. Why focus on the cholinergic system when discussing osteoarthritis

It can seem far-fetched to consider aspects related to the cholinergic system when discussing arthritis, including osteoarthritis. It is thus namely well-known that there is no cholinergic innervation of the joints. They are on the other hand well-equipped with sensory and sympathetic innervations. Nevertheless, as will be discussed below, cholinergic stimulations (via the vagal nerve) have been shown to have effects for joints. It has actually also been shown that the bones of mice are functionally innervated by the vagus nerve [1]. On the whole, it is well-known that the vagus nerve plays an anti-inflammatory role in various other parts of the body [2].

Another aspect concerning joint synovial tissue and the cholinergic system has evolved. That is related to the existence of a so-called non-neuronal cholinergic system. Such a system is nowadays well-known for different parts of the body [3]. New information on this system is gradually attained. We have noticed the existence of a non-neuronal cholinergic system in the synovial tissue of the knee joint of humans [4]. We have thus observed that immunoactive cells as well as fibroblasts in the synovial tissue of patients suffering from severe arthritis [rheumatoid arthritis (RA) as well as osteoarthritis (OA)] show expressions of the acetylcholine (ACh)-synthesizing enzyme choline acetyltransferase (ChAT) at both mRNA and protein levels [4]. This observation suggests that there is a local ACh production in the synovial tissue. There is only little information on the other aspect of ACh metabolism, namely ACh degradation. This will be discussed below.

Another noteworthy aspect is the finding that there are marked expressions of the nicotinic alpha7nACh receptor (α7nAChR) in the synovial tissue of arthritic patients. These observations have been made in studies in our laboratory [5] and in studies by other researchers [6,7]. That includes patients with osteoarthritis and is related to α7nAChR expressions for the fibroblast-like and inflammatory cells within the synovial tissue as well as for the synovial lining [5,8]. This receptor is known to be involved in inflammatory and remodulation processes, most notably having anti-inflammatory effects [9,10]. The findings have lead to suggestions that increased functions of ACh via effects on the α7nAChR can be positive for the arthritic processes [8,11].

Based on the aspects described above, further considerations on the cholinergic system for arthritis are here focused on. These relate to considerations on vagal effects for joint function, possible interference of the ACh-degrading enzyme acetylcholinesterase (AChE) and the possibility that increased ACh influences on the α7nAChR might be a promising strategy.

3. The vagus nerve in relation to arthritis

It has since several years been considered that effects via the vagal nerve can be of functional importance for the synovial tissue, not least in situations with arthritis. Thus, stimulatory effects on the vagal nerve have been show to be hampering for experimentally-induced arthritic processes [6] and paw inflammation [12]. There is on the other hand an exacerbation of the experimental arthritis after vagotomy [6,13]. The findings concerning the vagus nerve and vagotomy are unexpected as there is no vagal, nor other cholinergic, innervation in synovial tissue. One possibility that is discussed is that the effects are indirect, namely via vagal effects on other sites such as the region of the spleen [14] (see also [6]). It is well known that there are communications between the vagal nerve and the splenic nerve via the celiac and superior mesenteric ganglia (for a review, see [15,16]).

It is known that signaling via the vagus nerve that is leading to anti-inflammatory effects is initiated in the brainstem nuclei of the vagus nerve, secondarily leading to effects on the peripheral ganglia referred to above. This is part of the so-called inflammatory reflex whereby peripheral afferent nerves are primarily sensed, secondarily leading to efferent effects [17], in this case via the efferent part of the vagus nerve. It is well-known that the vagus nerve is a main component in the neuro-endocrine homeostasis via effects through its afferent and efferent neurons (for a review, see [2]).

From a functional point of view, it is of interest to note that ACh released from cholinergic nerves like the vagus nerve has immunomodulatory effects. These effects are considered to be anti-inflammatory [9,12]. The concept of a "cholinergic anti-inflammatory pathway" has hereby emerged [10,18], including for the synovial tissue [11]. In accordance with this, it is shown that electrical stimulation of the vagus nerve leads to an attenuation in macrophage activation [19].

It has been shown that subdiaphragmatic vagotomy in mice leads to reduced bone mass, bearing in mind that the mouse skeleton normally has a vagal innervation [1]. In a recent sudy it was shown that the severity of collagen-induced arthritis was reduced by electrical vagus nerve stimulation using a cuff electrode [20]. The cuff electrode that was used is analogous to the one used in treatment of drug-resistant epilepsy [21]. It was suggested that electrical neurostimulation via use of implanted vagus nerve stimulation cuff electrodes can be useful in treatment tests for various immune-mediated inflammatory disorders in man [20].

4. The α7nAChR in relation to arthritis

The α7nAChR is considered to be much involved in the obtaining of anti-inflammatory effects of ACh in various situations [3,22]. It is namely shown that this receptor contributes to anti-inflammatory effects of ACh in several models [12,23]. α7nAChR agonists are shown to suppress the production of various cytokines such as TNF alpha [12,22].

Based on what is described above, it is of great interest to note that the α7nAChR is present in the synovial tissue. That has been shown for the synovial tissue of patients with OA [5,8], RA [7,11] and psoriatic arthritis [7]. The findings concerning the α7nAChR have led to suggestions that interference with this receptor in clinical situations with arthritis might be useful [24,25]. α7nAChR agonists are not least suggested to be candidates as treatments for RA [26]. In accordance with such a proposal are the findings that synovial fibroblasts respond in vitro to cholinergic stimulation, via the α7nAChR, leading to a potent inhibition of proinflammatory cytokines [27]. Studies on the healing of skin wounds do also suggest that the α7nAChR is involved in the repair processes that occur for these wounds [28]. It is also shown that the α7nAChR is involved in the repair of wounds of respiratory epithelium [29].

5. AChE in relation to arthritis

The main ACh-degrading enzyme is acetylcholinesterase (AChE). The bulk of AChE of the neurons is in the axons and AChE is known to be associated with the membrane of this [30]. AChE is shown to be functional in embryonic muscle before it is accumulated at the sites of nerve-muscle contact [31]. AChE activity is also shown for a large number of non-neuronal cell types. That includes T-cells [32], fibroblasts of various locations [33], cells in lung tissue [34], cells of human gingival and esophageal epithelia [35] and embryonic stem cells [36]. AChE is also typically confined to the membranes of red blood cells [37]. Other components of the cholinergic system are also present in these cell types.

It is of relevance to notice that interference with AChE activity can be performed and that treatments for which this is done are used clinically. That includes the situations in myastenia gravis and Alzheimer's disease. In the case of myastenia gravis, where there is an occurrence of few receptors, the treatment is of value in order to extend the effects of ACh [38]. The AChE inhibitor drugs donepezil, galantamine and rivastigmine are being tried for patients with Alzheimer's disease [39]. In this case, where there is a reduced concentration of ACh, the point with the AChE inhibitors is to increase the concentration of the transmitter. A cholinergic deficiency is a feature that can be important for the development of the cognitive decline that occurs in Alzheimer's disease. There are also other fields of usage of AChE inhibitors; they are e.g. used in insecticides and nerve gases.

There is very little information on the patterns of AChE activity for synovial tissue. Nevertheless, AChE activity, in parallel with other components of cholinergic function, has been clearly detected in the knee joint synovial tissue of patients with RA and OA in a study using RT-PCR methods [40]. In our laboratory, existence of AChE activity in human knee joint synovial tissue has also been observed histochemically (unpublished observations).

The most well known function of AChE is to terminate neurotransmission at the cholinergic synapses via splitting of ACh. ACh is hereby hydrolyzed into choline and acetate. The degradation is rapid. However, AChE is also known to exhibit several non-classical roles, features that are of importance when considering both the neuronal and non-neuronal cholinergic systems [41]. That includes effects on cell differentiation and synaptogenesis along the nervous system, hydrolysis of neuropeptides, and effects in heart morphogenesis (for a review, see [42]). One cell type for which AChE is highly expressed is re-epithelialising epidermal keratinocytes during in vivo healing of mouse skin [43].

The exact functions of AChE in relation to the regulations of the non-neuronal cholinergic system at its various locations in the body are somewhat unclear [3]. It may be that the magnitude of ACh degrading activity is low in tissues like airway epithelium [44,45], and in cells of the placenta [33]. How the situation is for synovial tissue remains to be defined. Nevertheless, as there indeed is an occurrence of AChE in the synovial tissue it is likely that the function of the ACh that is produced in synovial tissue is limited to the precise area where it is produced. It may well be so that up- and down-regulations of production and release of ACh in the synovial tissue are parallelled by up- and down-regulations of AChE activity. In line with such a proposal is the finding that the immunological stimulation that leads to T-cell activation and upregulation of ACh synthesis and ACh receptor expression also leads to a marked ACh degradation [46].

Further studies on the importance and function of AChE for synovial tissue are needed in order to reveal the possible usefulness of interference with the effects of the enzyme in arthritis.

6. Concluding remarks

This review shows three aspects of the cholinergic system in relation to arthritis. It is obvious that stimulation of the vagal nerve has effects, that there is a non-neuronal cholinergic system in the synovial tissue and that there in parallel with expressions favouring ACh production also are expressions favouring ACh degradation in the synovial tissue. Although a lot of the information is related to the situation in RA, the various features of the cholinergic system are also related to the situation in OA. All these features concerning the cholinergic system highlight the relevance of further studies on the functional importance of this system for joint function, including the situation in OA.

Acknowledgements

Financial support for the studies performed at Department has been provided by the Faculty of Medicine.

Author details

Sture Forsgren[*]

Address all correspondence to: Sture.Forsgren@anatomy.umu.se

Department of Integrative Medical Biology Anatomy Section Umeå University Umeå, Sweden

References

[1] Bajayo A, Bar A, Denes A, Bachar M, Kram V, Attar-Namdar M, Zallone A, Kovacs KJ, Yirmiya R, Bab I. (2012). Skeletal parasympatheitic innervation communicates central IL-1 signals regulating bone mass accrural. Proc Natl Acad Sci USA. Vol 109, pp15455-15460

[2] Bonaz B, Pico C, Sinniger V, Mayol JF, Clarencon D. (2013). Vagus nerve stimulation: from epilepsy to the cholinergic anti-inflammatory pathway. Neurogastroenterology and Motility. Vol 25, pp. 208-221

[3] Kawashima K, Fujii T. (2008).Basic and clinical aspects of non-neuronal acetylcholine: Overview of non-neuronal cholinergic systems and their biological significance. Journal of Pharmacological Sciences. Vol 106, pp. 167-173

[4] Grimsholm O, Rantapää-Dahlqvist S, Dalén T, Forsgren S. (2008). Unexpected findings of a marked non-neuronal cholinergic system in human knee joint synovial tissue. Neuroscience Letters. Vol. 442, pp. 128-133

[5] Forsgren S. The cholinergic system can be of unexpected importance in osteoarthritis. (2011). In: Rotschild BM, editor. Osteoarthritis, In Tech – Open Access Publisher

[6] van Maanen, MA, Lebre MC, van der Poll T, LaRosa GJ, Elbaum D, Vervoordeldonk MJ, Tak PP. (2009). Stimulation of nicotinic acetylcholine receptors attenuates collagen-induced arthritis in mice. Arthritis and Rheumatism, Vol.60, pp. 114-122

[7] Westman, M.; Engström, M.; Catrina, AI., Lampa, J. (2009). Cell specific synovial expression of nicotinic alpha 7 acetylcholine receptor in rheumatoid arthritis and psoriatic arthritis. Scandinavian Journal of Immunology, Vol.70, pp. 136-140

[8] Waldburger, JM.; Boyle, DL.; Pavlov, VA.; Tracey, KJ., Firestein, GS. (2008). Acetylcholine regulation of synoviocyte expression by the alpha7 nicotinic receptor. Arthritis and Rheumatism, Vol.58, pp. 3439-3449

[9] de Jonge WJ, Ulloa L. (2007). The α7 nicotinic acetylcholine receptor as a pharmalogical target for inflammation. British Journal of Pharmacology. Vol. 151, pp. 915-929

[10] Tracey, KJ. (2007). Physiology and immunology of the cholinergic antiinflammatory pathway. Journal of Clinical Investigation Vol.117, pp. 289-296

[11] Van Maanen MA, Stoof S, LaRosa G, Vervoordeldonk M, Tak PP. (2010). Role of the cholinergic system in rheumatoid arthritis: aggravation of arthritis in nicotinic acetylcholine receptor α7 subunit gene knockout mice. Annals of Rheumatic Disease. Vol. 69, pp. 1717-1723

[12] Borovikova LV, Ivanova S, Zhang M, Yang H, Botchina GI, Watkins LR, Wang H, Abumrad N, Eaton JW, Tracey KJ. (2000). Vagus nerve stimulation attenuates the systemic inflammatory response to endotoxin. Vol. 405, pp. 458-462

[13] Li T, Zuo X, Wang Y, Zhuang H, Zhang L, Zhang H, Xiao X. (2010). The vagus nerve and nicotinic receptors involve inhibition of HMGB1 release and early pro-inflammatory cytokines function in collagen-induced arthritis. Journal of Clinical Immunology. Vol. 30, pp. 213-220

[14] Huston JM, Ochani M, Rosas-Ballina M, Liao H, Ochani K, Pavlov VA, Gallawitsch-Puerta, Ashok M, Czura CJ, Foxwell B, Tracey KJ, Ulloa L. (2006). Splenectomy inac-

tivates the cholinergic antiinflammatory pathway during lethal endotoxemia and polymicrobial sepsis. Journal of Experimental Medicine. Vol. 203, pp. 1623-1628

[15] Koopman FA, Stoof SP, Straub RH, van Maanen MA, Vervoordeldonk MJ, Tak PP. (2011). Restoring the balance of the autonomic nervous system as an innovative approach to the treatment of rheumatoid arthritis. Molecular Medicine. Vol. 17, pp. 937-948

[16] Rosas-Ballina M, Olofsson PS, Ochani M, Valdes-Ferrer SI, Levine YA, Reardon C, Tusche MW, Pavlov VA, Andersson U, Chavan S, Mak TW, Tracey KJ. (2011). Acetylcholine-synthesizing T cells relay neural signals in a vagus nerve circuit. Science. Vol 334, pp. 98-101

[17] Andersson U, Tracey KJ. (2012). Reflex principles of immunological homeostasis. Annual Reviews of Immunology. Vol 30, pp. 313-335

[18] Pavlov, VA., Tracey, KJ. (2005). The cholinergic anti-inflammatory pathway. Brain Behaviour Immunology, Vol.19, pp. 493-499

[19] de Jonge, W, van der Zanden E, The FO, Bijlsma MF, van Westerloo DJ, Bennink RJ, Barthoud HR, Uematsau S, Akira S, van den Wijngaard RM, Boeckxstaens GE. (2005). Stimulation of the vagus nerve attenuates macrophage activation by activating the Jak2-STAT3 signaling pathway. Nature Immunology, Vol.6, pp. 844-851

[20] Levine Y, Koopman F, Faltys M, Caravaca A, Bendele A, Zitnik R, Vervoordeldonk M, Tak PP. (2014). Neurostimulation of the cholinergic anti-inflammatory pathway ameliorates disease in rat collagen-induced arthritis. Plos ONE 9(8): e104530. doi: 10.1371

[21] Beekwilder JP, Beems T. (2010). Overview of the clinical applications of vagus nerve stimulation. Journal of Clinical Neurophysiology. Vol 27, pp. 130-138

[22] Wang H, Yu M, Ochani M, Amella CA, Tanovic M, Susarla S, Li JH, Wang H, Yang H, Ulloa L, Al-Abed Y, Czura CJ, Tracey KJ. (2003). Nicotinic acetylcholine receptor alpha7 subunit is an essential regulator of inflammation. Nature. Vol. 42, pp. 384-388

[23] Ulloa, L. (2005). The vagus nerve and the nicotinic anti-inflammatory pathway. Nature Review of Drug Discovery, Vol.4, pp. 673-784

[24] Pan, XH.; Zhang, J.; Yu, X.; Qin, L.; Kang, L., Zhang, P. (2010). New therapeutic approaches for the treatment of rheumatoid arthritis may rise from the cholinergic anti-inflammatory pathway and antinociceptive pathway. ScientificWorldJournal, Vol.10, pp. 2248-2253

[25] Zhang, P.; Qin, L., Zhang, G. (2010). The potential application of nicotinic acetylcholine receptor agonists for the treatment of rheumatoid arthritis. Inflammation Research, publ online 2010, 59(6):415-7, DOI 10.1007/s00011-010-0160-1

[26] Bruchfeld A, Goldstein RS, Chavan S, Patel NB, Rosas-Ballina M, Kohn N, Qureshi AR, Tracey KJ. (2010). Whole blood cytokine attenuation by cholinergic agionists ex

vivo and relationship to vagus nerve activity in rheumatoid arthritis. Journal of Internal Medicine. Vol. 268, pp. 94-101

[27] Das UN. (2011). Can vagus nerve stimulation halt or ameliorate rheumatoid arthritis and lupus? Lipids Health Disease. Vol 10: 19

[28] Fan YY, Yu TS, Wang T, Liu WW, Zhao R, Zhang ST, Ma WX, Zheng JL, Guan DW. (2011). Nicotinic acetylcholine receptor alpha7 subunit is time-dependently expressed in distinct cell types during skin wound healing in mice. Histochemistry and Cell Biology, publ online, 135(4): 375-87 DOI: 10.1007/s00418-001-0798-y

[29] Tournier JM, Maoche K, Coraux C, Zahm JM, Cloez-Tayarani I, Nawrocki-Raby B, Bonnomet A, Burlet H, Lebargy F, Polette M, Birembaut P. (2006). Alpha3alpha5beta2-nicotinic acetylcholine receptor contributes to the wound repair of the respiratory epithelium by modulating intracellular calcium in migrating cells. American Journal of Pathology, Vol.168, pp. 55-68.

[30] Papp M, Bozsik G. (1966). Comparison of the cholinesterase activity in the reticular formation of the lower brain stem of cat & rabbit. Journal of Neurochemistry. Vol. 12, pp. 697-703

[31] Ziskind-Conhaim L, Inestrosa N, Hall Z. (1984). Acetylcholinesterase is functional in embryonic rat muscle before its accumulation at the sites of nerve-muscle contact. Developmental Biology. Vol. 103, pp. 369-377

[32] Szelenyi J, Baratha E, Hollan S. (1982). Acetylcholinesterase activity of lymphocytes: an enzyme characteristic of T-cells. British Journal of Haematology. Vol. 150, pp. 241-245

[33] Sastry BV, Sadavongvivad C. (1979). Cholinergic systems in non-nervous tissues. Pharmacological Review. Vol. 30, pp. 65-132

[34] Adler M, Reutter SA, Moore DH, Filbert MG. (1991). Regulation of acetylcholine hydrolysis in canine tracheal smooth muscle. European Journal of Pharmacology. Vol. 205, pp. 73-79

[35] Nguyen VT, Hall LL, Gallacher G, Ndoye A, Jolkovsky DL, Webber RJ, Buchli R, Grando SA. (2000). Choline acetyltransferase, acetylcholinesterase, and nicotinic acetylcholine receptors of human gingival and esophageal epithelia. Journal of Dental Research. Vol. 79, pp. 939-949

[36] Paraoanu LE, Steinert G, Koehler A, Wessler I, Layer PG. (2007). Expression and possible functions of the cholinergic system in a murine embryonic stem cell line. Life Sciences. Vol. 80, pp. 2375-2379

[37] Bartels CF, Zelinski T, Lockridge O. (1993). Mutation at codon 322 in the human acetylcholinesterase (ACHE) gene accounts for YT blood group polymorphism. American Journal of Human Genetics. Vol. 52, pp. 928-936

[38] Taylor P. (1996). Anticholinesterase agents. In "The Pharmalogical Basis of Therapeutics". Eds; Hardman JG, Limbird LE, Molinoff PB, Ruddon RW, Gilman AG. New York, McGraw-Hill, pp. 161-176

[39] Pohanka. (2011). Alzheimers disease and related neurodegenerative disorders: implication and counteracting of melatonin. Journal of Applied Biomedicine. Vol. 9, pp. 185-196

[40] Schubert J, Beckmann J, Hartmann S, Morhenn H-G, Szalay G, Heiss C, Schnettler R, Lips KS. (2012). Expression of the non-neuronal cholinergic system in human knee synovial tissue from patients with rheumatoid arthritis and osteoarthritis. Life Sciences. Vol. 91, pp. 1048-1052

[41] Silman I, Sussman JL. (2005). Acetylcholinesterase: classical and non-classical functions and pharmacology. Current Opinion in Pharmacology. Vol. 5, pp. 293-302

[42] Tripathi A, Srivastava UC. (2008). Acetylcholinesterase: A versatile enzyme of nervous system. Annals of Neuroscience. Vol. 15, no 4

[43] Anderson A, Ushakov D, Ferenczi M, Mori R, Martin P, Saffell J. (2008). Morphoregulation by acetylcholinesterase in fibroblasts and astrocytes. Journal of Cellular Physiology. Vol. 215, pp. 82-100

[44] Degano B, Prevost MC, Berger P, Molimard M, Pontier S, Rami J, Escamilla R. (2001). Estradiol increases the acetylcholine-elicited airway reactivity in ovariectomized rats through an increase in epithelial acetylcholinesterase activity. American Journal of Respiration and Critical Care Medicine. Vol. 16, pp. 1849-1854

[45] Kummer W, Lips KS, Pfeil U. (2008). The epithelial cholinergic system of airways. Histochemistry and Cell Biology. Vol. 130, pp. 219-234

[46] Kawashima K, Fujii T, Moriwaki Y, Misawa H. (2012). Critical roles of acetylcholine and the muscarinic and nicotinic acetylcholine receptors in the regulation of immune function. Life Sciences. Vol. 91, pp. 1027-1032

4

Validation of Mechanical Hypothesis of hip Arthritis Development by HIPSTRESS Method

Veronika Kralj-Iglič

1. Introduction

Hip joint connects the upper part of the body to the lower limb. As in human (a bipodal) the motion derives from periodical extension of lower limbs, the one-limb support is a common body position attained in everyday life. Keeping the body in balance and performing the required activities by means of attaining particular body positions or motions and by activating particular muscles is the main function of the hip joint. When the load is transmitted to the supporting leg, the hip bears the body weight (aside from the weight of the supporting leg). Besides the weight the joint is affected also by forces exerted by the surrounding tissues (e.g. muscles, tendons, ligaments and fluids). As the human body is subject to laws of physics, it is therefore indicated that mechanical parameters such as forces and stresses can be connected to physiological and patophysiological processes in the hip joint.

Understanding of causes of the effects on development of the body was dramatically accelerated by the discovery of X-rays in 1895, which enabled imaging of inner body structures without cutting them. It was found that the lateral coverage of the femoral head with the acetabulum is an important parameter in predicting the development of hip cartilage degeneration and hip osteoarthritis [1]. Besides providing new diagnostic technologies, physical methods contributed also to revealing mechanisms of disease development. According to the mechanical hypothesis, too high load of the hip was empirically considered as a cause for deterioration of the hip joint.

2. Hip stress as a relevant biomechanical parameter

Poor lateral coverage of the femoral head by the acetabulum was connected to smaller load bearing area and therefore larger contact stress on the hip cartilage and bones. To increase the load bearing area and prevent early hip osteoarthritis, various operative techniques were suggested [2-9]. In these operations the load bearing area was increased by increasing the lateral coverage of the femoral head by the acetabular roof. However, proof for the mechanical hypothesis stating that unfavorable distribution of stress in the hip is connected to early hip osteoarthritis, requires a method for assessment of hip stress.

Hip stress was measured in vitro and in vivo by using different techniques (e.g. pressure sensitive film and instrumented prothesis) [10]. After a thorough study involving development of a special Austin Moore partial endoprothesis and its validation in vitro, a specimen was implanted into a patient [11]. Contact hip stress was recorded by electromagnetic signal deriving from piezoelectric transducers on the head of the prothesis. The signal was recorded by a coil placed arround the patient's thigh. The location of the particular transducer was distinguished by the frequency of the signal. The patient was followed during the rehabilitation and in different activities for several years. Measurements recorded nonuniform distribution of hip stress over the load bearing area. Peak stresses as high as 15 MPa were recorded in everyday activities (e.g. standing up from a cca 25 cm chair).

To assess biomechanical parameters, theoretical models were developed. Finite element method was used to predict stresses within hip bones [12]. According to this method the hip is imagined as composed of small elements which act one upon another according to laws of elastomechanics. Two dimensional and three dimensional models were elaborated. Taking into account the materials elastic constants, the relevant constraints and the load on the hip the values of stress subject to each element can be calculated. Calculation requires solving large systems of equations which became possible by development of powerful computers. Important general knowledge was obtained by this method as for example the effect of the bone stiffening and cartilage elastic modulus on the stress values and distribution. Dynamic effects were studied by measurements of the effect of the movement on the piezoelectric force plate and by recording the motion of the subject by the video camera in combination with mathematical model [13]. In the model, the body was divided into segments connected by joints. Muscle and tendon mechanics was taken into account. Resultant joint forces were calculated from intersegmental forces by solving the inverse dynamics problem.

However, these methods were not appropriate for clinical studies where large number of hips should be assessed within reasonable time and possibilities. Also, the elastic constants of the material composing hip and pelvis for a particular person are largely unknown. For clinical studies of disease specificity, analytically or almost analytically solvable models based on the individual hip geometry were found more appropriate [14-16]. The strength of these methods lies in appropriate abstractions and choices of a small number of relevant features that render the model simple enough to be transparent with respect to the effect of the parameters. Development of such methods enabled analysis of large populations of hips with different pathologies. The mechanical hypothesis claiming that elevated contact hip stress is a possible cause of hip osteoarthritis was tested on a large cohort of hips with idiopathic osteoarthrosis and compared to a population of »normal« hips [16]. It was found that »compressive stress is of minor importance with respect to the etiology of idiopathic osteoarthrosis of the hip joint«. The results of this thorough study seemed decisive and discouraging for further questioning the mechanical hypotehsis as regards osteoarthritis, but the effect of stress was further investigated by determination of stress in patients with congenital dislocation of te hip [17,18]. It was found that an integral of stress over time statistically significantly correlated with clinical status [18] and that the values of stress beyond a threshold of 2MPa and integrated stress beyond threshold of 10MPa-years were connected to poor clinical outcome [17].

3. Method HIPSTRESS

Method HIPSTRESS was intended for analyses of large populations of hips. Its use is simple enough to be used by medical doctors and it requires some minutes to assess biomechanical parameters if the geometrical parameters of hips are known. The method consists of two mathematical models, one for determination of the resultant hip force in one legged stance [19] and the other for determination of contact hip stress distribution [20]. Both methods introduced some improvements with respect to previously developed models.

3.1. Model HIPSTRESS for resultant hip force

The model for the resultant hip force [19] considers the body to be composed of two segments: the lower segment (the loaded leg) and the upper segment (the rest of the body). The static equilibrium requires that the resultant of all external forces acting on each segment is zero and that the resultant of all external torques acting on each segment is zero. For the upper segment this requirement is

$$\left(\mathbf{W_B} - \mathbf{W_L}\right) + \sum \mathbf{F}_i - \mathbf{R} = 0, \tag{1}$$

$$\mathbf{a} \times \left(\mathbf{W_B} - \mathbf{W_L}\right) + \sum \mathbf{r}_i \times \mathbf{F}_i = 0, \tag{2}$$

where $\mathbf{W_L}$ is the weight of the loaded leg, $\mathbf{W_B}$ is the body weight, $\mathbf{F}_i$ are forces of muscles that are active in the one-legged stance, $\mathbf{R}$ is the resultant hip force, $\mathbf{a}$ is the vector to the center of the mass of the body without the loaded leg and $\mathbf{r}_i$ are vectors to the origins of the muscle forces. The coordinate system for the upper body segment was chosen at the origin of the resultant hip force (the center of the feomral head) and therefore the torque due to this force is 0. The index i runs over all included muscles.

For the upper body segment, forces of 9 effective muscles are taken into account. Muscle forces are considered to act in straight lines between the muscle attachment points. The muscles that attach in larger areas were represented by several effective muscles. The effective muscles included in the model are gluteus minimus anterior, gluteus minimus middle, gluteus minimus posterior, gluteus medius anterior, gluteus medius middle, gluteus medius posterior, tensor fasciae lateae, piriformis and rectus femoris. The force of each muscle $\mathbf{F}_i$ was considered proportional to the muscle cross section area A_i and average tension in the muscle f_i,

$$\mathbf{F}_i = f_i A_i \left(\mathbf{r}_i - \mathbf{r}'_i \right) \big/ \left\| \left(\mathbf{r}_i - \mathbf{r}'_i \right) \right\|, \; i = 1, 2, 3, \ldots, 9. \tag{3}$$

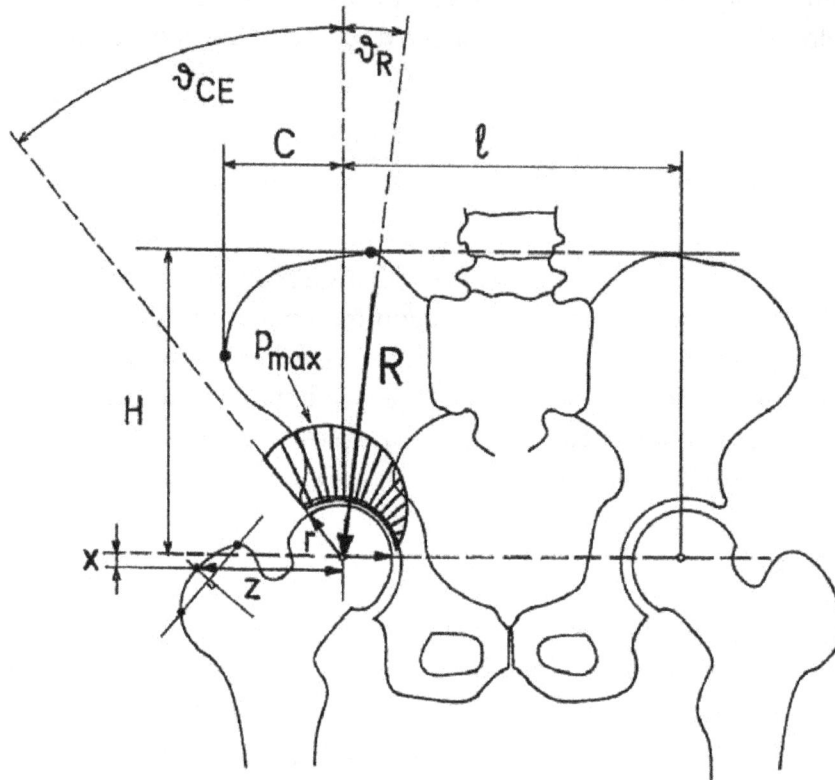

Figure 1. Geometrical parameters of the hip and pelvis for the HIPSTRESS method, resultant hip force and hip stress distribution. From [23].

The forces and the torques have three dimensions, therefore the model consists of six equations (3 for equilibrium of forces and 3 for equilibrium of torques). For known origin and insertion points of the muscles, and known cross section areas the unknown quantities are the muscle tensions and three components of the resultant hip force **R**. Since there are 9 effective muscles and 3 components of the force **R**, there are 12 unknowns and 6 equations. To solve this problem, a simplification was introduced by dividing the muscles into three groups (anterior, middle, posterior) with respect to the position. It was assumed that the muscles in the same group have the same tension. This reduced the number of unknowns to 6 as required for solution of the complex of 6 equations. The muscle origin and insertion points and the muscle cross-section were taken from [21] and [22], respectively. The geometry of the individual patient was taken into account by correction of muscle attachment points according to the geometrical parameters obtained from the standard anteroposterior radiograph (the interhip distance (l), the height (H) and the width (C) of the pelvis, and the position on the greater trochanter relative to the centre of the femoral head (x,z)).

Results obtained with the HIPSTRESS model for resultant hip force showed that the force lies almost in the frontal plane of the body through both femoral heads. To further simplify the calculations it was assumed in most studies that the force lies in the frontal plane and is represented by its magnitude R and its inclination with respect to the vertical ϑ_R.

3.2. Model HIPSTRESS for contact hip stress

Model for contact hip stress was thoroughly described in a previous contribution [24] and will be only briefly described here. Femoral head is represented by a part of the sphere and acetabulum is represented by a part of the spherical shell. Articular sphere represents both, the acetabular sphere and the femoral head sphere. When unloaded, both representative spheres have the same origin. Between the spheres there is an elastic continuum representing cartilage. The cartilage is subject to Hooke's law. When loaded, the origin of the femoral head sphere is slightly displaced with respect to the acetabular sphere and the cartilage is squeezed. It is assumed that stress is proportional to displacement. Some points on the femoral head are moved closer to the acetabulum and some points are moved away from the acetabulum. The stress pole is the point on the articular sphere that corresponds to the closest approach of the femoral head and the acetabulum spheres. It is assumed that there is no friction in the tangential direction to the spherical surface, so the normal stress is the only relevant stress acting in the hip.

The base of the mathematical model is the cosine dependence of contact stress on the space angle between the position of the stress pole and the chosen point on the articular surface γ [16],

$$p = p_0 \cos \gamma \, , \tag{4}$$

where p_0 is the value of stress at the pole. The essential contribution of the HIPSTRESS model for stress is the elaboration of the load bearing area. The choice of the coordinate system and the definition of the borders of the load bearing area renders the elaborated load bearing area always symmetric, regardless of the direction of the resultant hip force. The lateral boundary of the load bearing area is defined by intersection of the articular sphere and the plane which is inclined with respect to the sagittal plane for ϑ_{CE} (the centre-edge angle of Wiberg). On the medial side the border is defined by the condition that the stress vanishes, i.e. the medial border is for the angle $\pi/2$ allienated from the stress pole. The connection between the resultant hip force and the hip stress distribution

$$\mathbf{R} = \int p \, \mathbf{dA} \, , \tag{5}$$

where the integration is performed over the load bearing area, yields three equations for three unknowns: the angles defining the position of the hip stress pole (Θ and Φ) and the value of stress at the pole p_0 [20,24]

$$\Phi = 0, \, \pi \, , \tag{6}$$

$$\tan\left(\vartheta_R + \Theta\right) = \cos^2\left(\vartheta_{CE} - \Theta\right)\Big/\left(\pi/2 + \vartheta_{CE} - \Theta + \sin\left(2(\vartheta_{CE} - \Theta)\right)/2\right), \qquad (7)$$

$$p_0 = 3R\sin\left(\vartheta_R + \Theta\right)\Big/2r^2\cos^2\left(\vartheta_{CE} - \Theta\right), \qquad (8)$$

where Φ is the azimuth coordinate of the stress pole on the articular surface. To determine stress at any point of the load bearing area, the solution of the nonlinear equation for the coordinate of the pole Θ Eq. (4) should be found. Re-arranging Eq.(7) by substitution [25]

$$\Theta = x - \left(\vartheta_R - \vartheta_{CE}\right)/2 \qquad (9)$$

transforms the nonlinear equation (7) into

$$\tan\left(\left(\vartheta_R + \vartheta_{CE}\right)/2 + x\right) =$$
$$= \cos^2\left(\left(\vartheta_R + \vartheta_{CE}\right)/2 - x\right)\Big/\left(\pi/2 + \left(\vartheta_R + \vartheta_{CE}\right)/2 - x + \sin\left(2\left(\left(\vartheta_R + \vartheta_{CE}\right)/2 - x\right)\right)/2\right). \qquad (10)$$

It follows from Eq. (10) that the solution of Eq. (7) (i.e. the position of the stress pole depends solely on $(\vartheta_R + \vartheta_{CE})$).

The integration of Eq.(5) is performed over the load bearing area. Stress is unevenly distributed over the load bearing area. It decreases towards the medial border while on the lateral side there are two possibilities, depending on the position of the hip stress pole. If the pole lies within the load bearing area, stress increases in the medial direction, reaches maximum and then decreases. The pole, being an abstract quantity that reflects the extent and the direction of the relative movement of the femoral head and the acetabulum upon loading, may however lie outside the load bearing area. In this case, stress monotonously decreases towards the medial border. The contact hip stress distribution is represented by the peak value of hip stress on the load bearing area (p_{max}). If the pole lies in the weight bearing area the peak stress is equal to its value at the pole ($p_{max} = p_0$). If the stress pole lies outside the load bearing area, the peak stress is equal to the value of stress at the point of the load bearing area which is closest to the pole. Other parameters that represent stress distribution are the index of the stress gradient at the lateral acetabular rim (G_p)

$$G_p = -p_0/r \cos\vartheta_F \qquad (11)$$

where ϑ_F is the functional angle of the load bearing,

$$\vartheta_F = \pi/2 + \vartheta_{CE} - \Theta \qquad (12)$$

and the load bearing A_F

$$A_F = 2r^2 \vartheta_F \ . \tag{13}$$

An example of the stress distribution calculated by HIPSTRESS method is shown in Figure 2. The green line denotes the magnitude of the contact hip stress p in the frontal plane through centres of both articular spheres. The left hip has normal shape. The right hip is considerably deformed as the patient underwent in the childhood the Perthes disease. In the normal (left) hip the stress increases in the medial direction, reaches maximum and then decreases. The functional angle and the load bearing area are large. The pole lies within the load bearing area and the index of hip stress gradient is negative. In the deformed (right) hip the stress monotonously decreases in the medial direction. The functional angle is small. The pole lies outside of the load bearing area and the index of hip stress gradient is positive. However, the load bearing area is not small in the deformed hip as the smaller functional angle is compensated by the larger radius of the articular sphere (Eq. (13)). Consequnetly, the peak stress is almost equal in both hips.

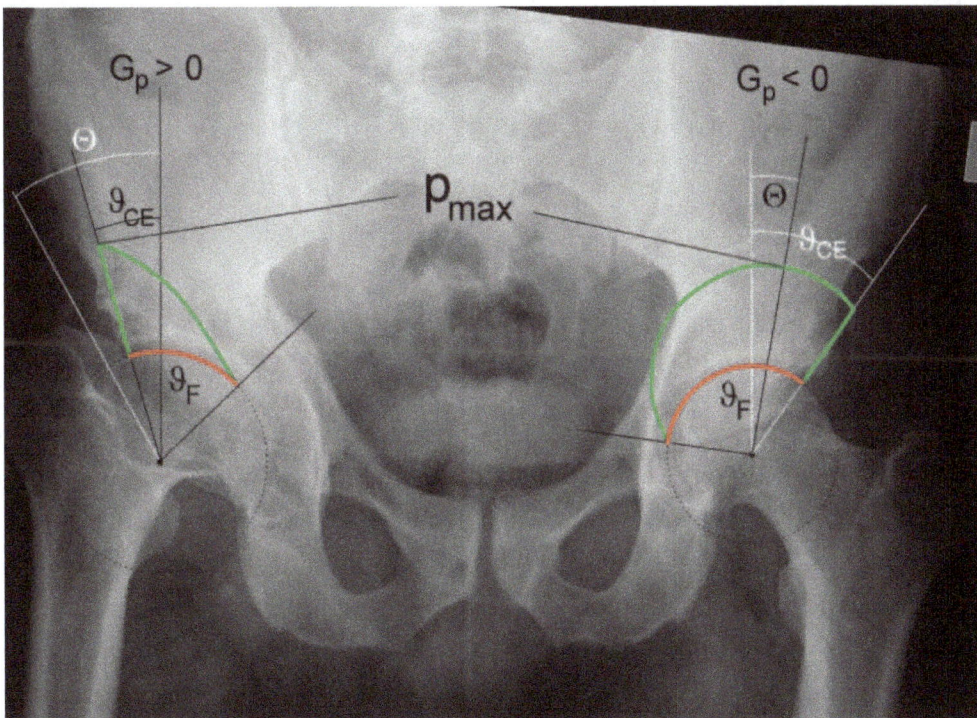

Figure 2. Distribution of hip stress on the load bearing area of a normal hip (left) and a hip after Legg-Calve-Perthes disease (right). The green line represents the magnitude of stress in the frontal plane through the centers of the femoral heads. The red line indicates the functional angle determining the load bearing area. From [26].

Figure 3 shows the peak hip stress (A) and the coordinate of the stress pole (B) in dependence on the sum of the angles $(\vartheta_{CE} + \vartheta_R)$. As this sum implies the solution of the system of equations representing the vector equation (5), the two angles can compensate each other. Smaller centre-

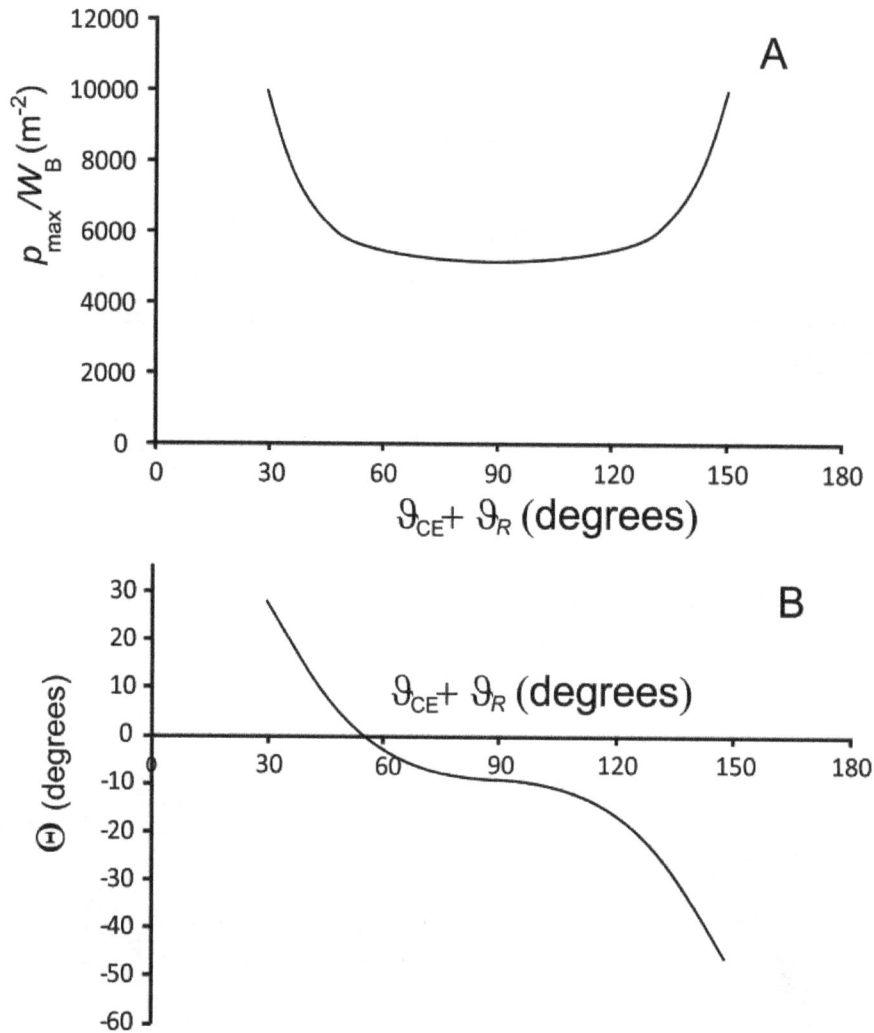

Figure 3. A: Peak contact stress as a function of the parameter ($\vartheta_{CE} + \vartheta_R$). B: position of the stress pole as a function of the parameter ($\vartheta_{CE} + \vartheta_R$). Lines were for a hypothetical hip with $R/W_B = 2.6$ and $r = 1.6$ cm. Adapted from [25].

edge angle can be complemented by larger inclination of the resultant hip force to assure favorably large enough functional angle and load bearing area. It is expected that large centre-edge angle means larger load bearing area and lower stress, but Figure 3 shows that for very large centre-edge angles combined with large inclinations of the resultant hip force, stress increases. Such situation would take place for large centre-edge angles (larger than 70 degrees) since the resultant hip force in the one-legged stance is usually smaller than 20 degrees. The above described model of resultant hip force describes the one-legged stance. The model for stress is general with respect to body position and enables calculation of hip stress distribution if the resultant hip force and some additional geometrical parameters of the hip are known. To obtain stress with the HIPSTRESS model for stress it is therefore not necessary that the resultant hip force is calculated by the HIPSTRESS model for the resultant hip force. The force can also be determined experimentally. However, it is necessary to know additional geometrical parameters such as the centre-edge angle ϑ_{CE} and the radius of the articular sphere r (Figure 1).

4. Computer program and nomograms for determination of the resultant hip force and peak contact stress in the HIPSTRESS method

Computer program was developed to calculate the force **R** (its magnitude and inclination with respect to the vertical direction), the peak hip stress p_{max} and the coordinate Θ of the pole. The program is available at http://physics.fe.uni-lj.si/projects/orthopaedic.htm Also, the nomograms were elaborated [27] for those who do not have a possibility to use the computer. They prove useful also as the rapid development of computer science requires compatibility of the program with hardware and other software which is not always available. The input data of the program HIPSTRESS are the geometrical parameters of the hip and pelvis that can be assessed from images of the hip and pelvis geometry (e.g. X-rays or magnetic resonance) (Figure 1): the interhip distance (l), the pelvic width (C), the pelvic height (H), the coordinates of the effective muscle attachment point on the greater trochanter in the coordinate system of the femur (z and x), the femoral head radius (r) and the centre-edge angle ϑ_{CE}. To determine the resultant hip force and the contact hip stress distribution also the magnitude of the body weight W_B should be known. However, besides the force and the stress, also the parameters normalized with respect to body weight are of interest, R/W_B, p_{max}/W_B and G_p/W_B. These normalized parameters reflect the effect of the hip and pelvis geometry on the force and the stress.

Below we present nomograms for determination of resultant hip force and peak hip stress. The nomograms were calculated by using the computer programs. As there are many parameters that define the model it was not appropriate to consider all possible combinations of parameters but only those that yield the largest effect. The vertical position of the effective muscle attachment point on the greater trochanter was therefore not taken into account. Determination of the force is performed in two steps: determination of the inclination of the resultant hip force and determination of the magnitude of the resultant hip force. In determination of the magnitude, the effect of the pelvic width and height was disregarded as these parameters proved less important than the lateral extension of the greater trochanter and the interhip distance. To assess stress from the nomograms, we choose the $R/W_B(l/2)$ curve (Figure 4) pertaining to the combination of z and $l/2$ closest to the measured values and determine R/W_B. Then we choose the $\vartheta_R(l/2)$ diagram (Figure 5) pertaining to the combination of z, H and C closest to the measured values and determine ϑ_R. Using thus determined R/W_B and ϑ_R, and the measured values of ϑ_{CE} and r we choose the $p_{max}r^2/W_B(\vartheta_{CE}+\vartheta_R)$ diagram pertaining to the relevant interval of $(\vartheta_{CE}+\vartheta_R)$ (Figure 6) and determine $p_{max}r^2/W_B$. To assess p_{max}/W_B we divide the obtained value by r^2. To obtain p_{max} we multiply the obtained value with body weight W_B.

For example, let us determine the resultant hip force and peak hip stress in a hip with parameters $l/2$=9.8 cm, C=5.6 cm, H=15.0 cm, x=1.0 cm, z=6.1 cm, r=2.3 cm, ϑ_{CE}=32 degrees and W_B=750 N. To assess R/W_B we chose in Figure 4 the curve pertaining to z=6 cm and obtain for $l/2$=10 cm the value R/W_B=2.7 (see dotted lines in Figure 4). Then we assess ϑ_R. The closest values of the parameters $l/2$, H and z are $l/2$=10cm, H=16cm and z=6 cm while the value of C is between 5

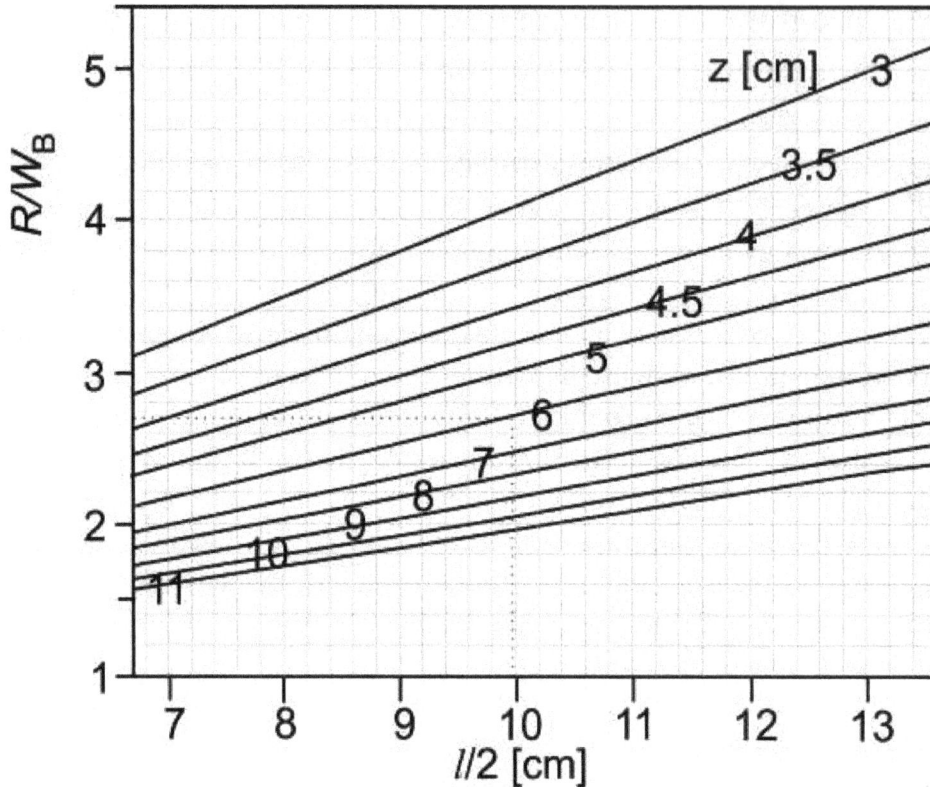

Figure 4. Nomograms for determination of the magnitude of the resultant hip force. The dependence of the magnitude of the force R on half of the interhip distance $l/2$ for different lateral extensions of the greater trochanter z. Adapted from [27].

and 6 cm, therefore we can assess ϑ_R from panels h and k (Figure 5). The value of ϑ_R obtained from panel h (pertaining to $C = 5$ cm) is 8 degrees and the value of ϑ_R obtained from panel k (pertaining to $C = 6$cm) is 7 degrees (dotted lines in Figure 5). For $C = 5.6$ cm we can estimate that $\vartheta_R = 7.5$ cm. Using the obtained values $\vartheta_R = 7.5$ degrees, $R/W_B = 2.7$ and the geometrical parameters $r = 2.3$ cm and $\vartheta_{CE} = 32$ degrees we assess $p_{max}r^2/W_B$ from Figure 6 (see dotted lines in Figure 6). The sum $(\vartheta_{CE}+\vartheta_R)$ is $(32+7.5 \cong 40)$ degrees, therefore we chose panel c and the curve pertaining to $z = 6$ cm. The obtained value of $p_{max}r^2/W_B$ is 1.75. Dividing this value by $r = 2.3$ cm yields $p_{max}/W_B = 3300$ m^{-2}. For $W_B = 750$N the peak stress is finally $p_{max} = 2.47$ MPa.

It can be seen from the nomograms that smaller C and smaller H are biomechanically favorable as they yield larger ϑ_R. As regards ϑ_R, for large z smaller interhip distance is favorable and for smaller z larger interhip distance is more favorable, however, the dependencies are weak. Smaller lateral extension of the greater trochanter z and larger interhip distance l increase the magnitude of resultant hip force R/W_B. Peak hip stress decreases with decreasing $(\vartheta_{CE} + \vartheta_R)$ up to $(\vartheta_{CE} + \vartheta_R = \pi/2)$ and increases with increasing R/W_B [25]. For low hip stress $(\vartheta_{CE} + \vartheta_R)$ is large enough that the curve $p_{max}r^2/W_B(\vartheta_{CE}+\vartheta_R)$ is almost flat, mostly on the account of large ϑ_{CE}. Thus, the most favorable hip geometry has small interhip distance, large lateral extension of the grater trochanter, small pelvic width and height, large radius of the femoral head and large (but within limits) centre edge angle.

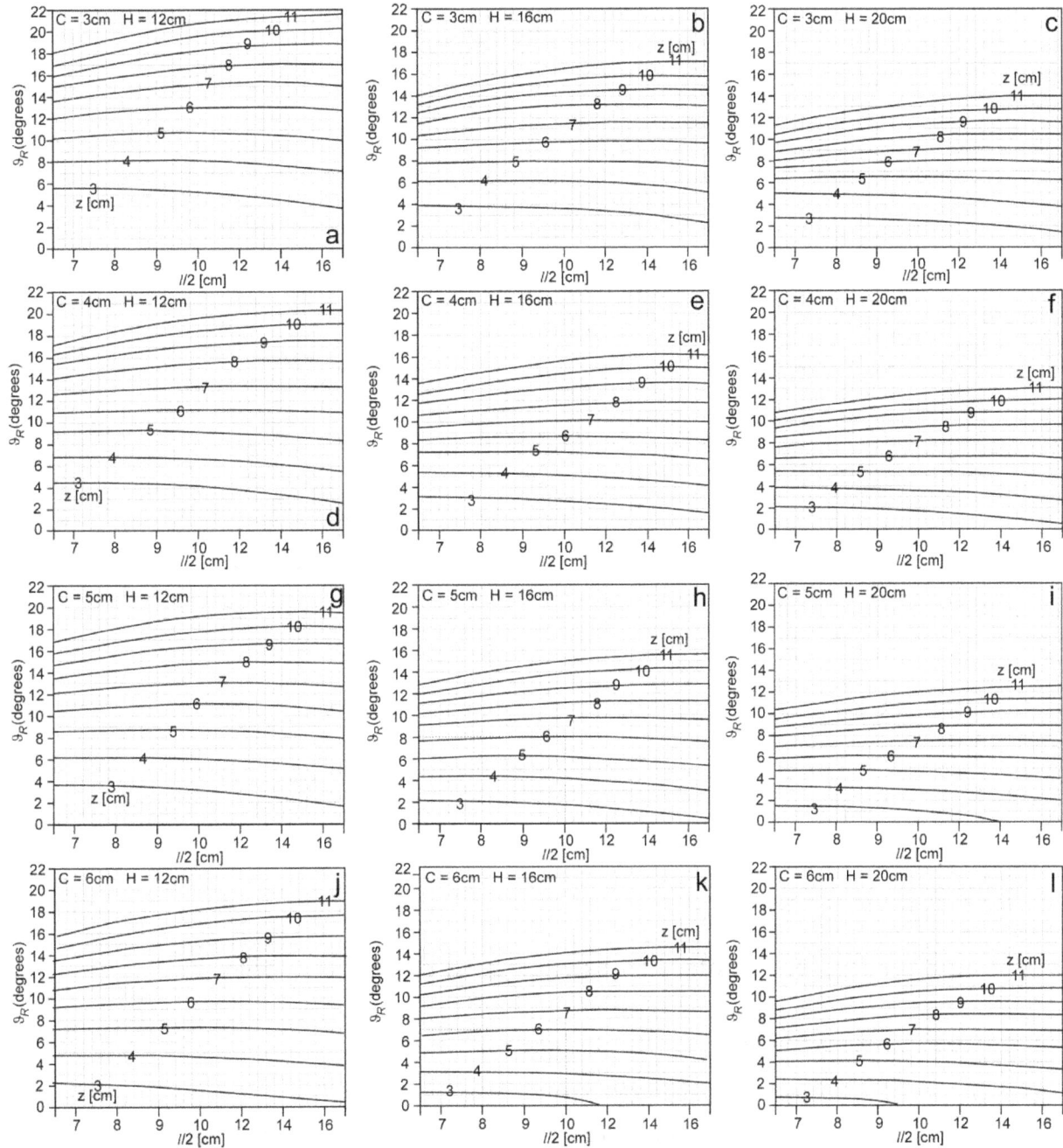

Figure 5. Nomograms for determination of the inclination of the resultant hip force. The dependence of the inclination of the force ϑ_R on half of the interhip distance $l/2$ for different lateral extensions of the greater trochanter z. a: C=3cm, H=12 cm, b: C=3cm, H=16cm, c: C=3cm, H=20 cm, d: C=4cm, H=12 cm, e: C=4 cm, H=16 cm, f: C=4 cm, H=20 cm, g: C=5 cm, H=12 cm, h: C=5 cm, H=16 cm, i: C=5cm, H=20 cm, j: C=6 cm, H=12 cm, k: C=6 cm, H=16 cm, l: C=6 cm, H=20 cm. Adapted from [27].

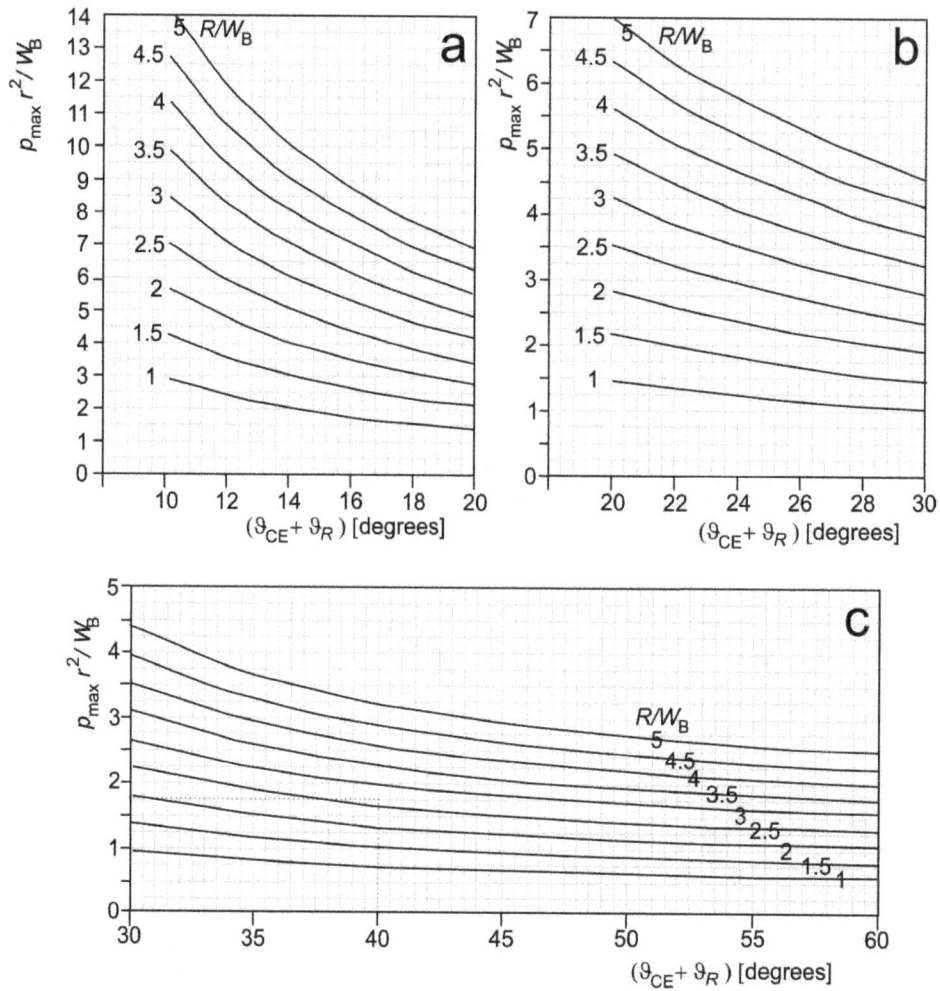

Figure 6. Nomograms for determination of the peak hip stress. The dependence of $p_{max}r^2/W_B$ on the sum of the angles $(\vartheta_{CE}+\vartheta_R)$ for different values of the resultant hip force R/W_B. Due to large variation of the values with $(\vartheta_{CE}+\vartheta_R)$ panel a pertains to the range of $(\vartheta_{CE}+\vartheta_R)$ between 10 and 20 degrees, panel b pertains to the range between 20 and 30 degrees and panel c pertains to the range between 30 and 60 degrees. Adapted from [27].

5. Biomechanical parameters in normal and dysplastic hips

5.1. Comparison between »normal« female and male hips

The early population studies by the HIPSTRESS method considered »normal« hips. Geometrical parameters were assessed from standard anteroposterior radiograms retrieved from the archives. The pictures that showed no abnormalities in the hip region were included in the analysis; the patients had the pictures taken due to back pain. The exclusion criteria for participation in the study were clinical or radiographic signs of hip pathology, insufficient technical quality of the radiograph and incomplete presentation of pelvis on the radiograph. The first clinical study addressed differences between female and male hips [28]. Study of relevant geometrical parameters showed differences between 79 female and 21 male hips (Table 1). Female subjects had considerable and statistically significantly larger interhip distance and smaller femoral heads than male subjects, which is biomechanically unfavorable as it increases the magnitude of the peak stress. It was suggested that less favorable hip and pelvis geometry as regards hip stress »could be one of the reasons for the increased incidence of arthritis in women« [28]. However, stress was not actually calculated in that study.

	Female (79)	Male (21)	Difference (%)	p
w(cm)	14.05	12.94	8	10^{-4}
H(cm)	15.13	15.42	-2	0.11
C(cm)	6.12	5.47	11	0.07
r(cm)	2.38	2.68	-12	10^{-4}
ϑ_{CE}	37	36.5	1	0.31

Table 1. Median values of the geometrical parameters of 79 female and 21 male »normal« hips as determined in the first HIPSTRESS population study. Parameter w is the distance between the medial acetabular rims.

The differences between parameters (e.g., x) were calculated with respect to the mean value $(x_{female} + x_{male})/2$. The statistical significance of the difference (the probability p) was calculated by using Mann-Whitney test. Instead of the interhip distance l the study considered the distance between the medial acetabular rims w as to avoid the effect of the femoral head size on the interhip distance. Adapted from [28].

5.2. Comparison between »normal« and dysplastic hips

Stress was assessed in a population of dysplastic hips to test the hypothesis that it is higher than in »normal« hips and at the same time test the models [29]. The diagnosis of dysplasia was made on the basis of standard clinical and radiographic evaluation [29]. As it was found in the previous study [28] that female and male hips have considerably different geometrical and biomechanical parameters, the groups of female and male hips were considered separately, however the group of male hips was too small to allow for gender-matched comparison with »normal« hips, therefore the male hips were excluded from the analysis. 47 dysplastic female hips were included in the final analysis. The sample consisted of 20 right and 27 left hips, and the age of the subjects ranged from 18 to 52 years with a median of 33 years. The gender- and age-matched control group consisted of subjects who had had a radiograph taken of the pelvic region for reasons other than degenerative hip disease and in whom the pelvic radiograph had shown no signs of hip pathology. This group consisted of 36 hips, 18 right and 18 left, and the age of the subjects ranged from 18 to 41 years with a median age of 33 years. The results showed considerable and statistically very significant differences in most of geometrical parameters relevant for the HIPSTRESS model, in particular in resultant hip force and in peak contact stress (Table 2). The largest difference (80%) was in the centre-edge angle (Table 2). There was a 65% difference in contact hip stress; small centre-edge angle in dysplastic hips was to some extent compensated by larger radius of the femoral head and more favorable shape of the pelvis (smaller width and height). This study [28] was the first one that clearly showed on a relatively large cohort that contact hip stress is considerably higher (for about twice) in dysplastic female hips than in »normal« female hips. Also, it provided the first estimate of »normal« stress, i.e. the average value 3100 m^{-2}. It was therefore suggested that the peak contact stress is a suitable parameter to assess risk for development of early arthritis of the hip.

	Dysplastic (47)	Normal (36)	Difference(%)	p
$(l \pm SD)$ (cm)	20.8±1.2	19.5±0.9	6	<0.001
$(C \pm SD)$ (cm)	4.7±1.0	5.6±1.1	-17	<0.001
$(H \pm SD)$ (cm)	14.4±1.3	15.0±1.0	4	0.024
$(x \pm SD)$ (cm)	1.4±0.6	1.0±0.5	33	<0.001
$(z \pm SD)$ (cm)	5.6±0.6	6.1±0.6	8	<0.001
$(r \pm SD)$ (cm)	2.6±0.2	2.3±0.1	12	<0.001
$(\vartheta_{CE}\pm SD)$ (degrees)	13±8	31±6	80	<0.001
$R/W_B\pm SD$	3.1±0.3	2.7±0.1	14	<0.001
$(\vartheta_R \pm SD)$ (degrees)	8±2	8±1	0	0.60
$(p_{max}/W_B \pm SD)$ (m^{-2})	7100±3500	3500±900	65	<0.001

SD: standard deviation. Adapted from [29].

Table 2. Average values of geometrical and biomechanical parameters of 47 dysplastic and 36 »normal« female hips.

It seems reasonable that in hips that were assigned dysplastic, mostly due to poor coverage of the femoral head by the acetabulum the area that bears resultant hip force is smaller. So it could be concluded that in these hips the reasons for development of arthritis are mechanical in a sense that too high stress causes degeneration of the tissues and inflammation of hip joint. In other words, hip arthritis in these cases is secondary to increased contact hip stress that reflects unfavorable geometry of the hips and pelvis.

It can be seen from Table 2 that the parameters for the above example assessed from nomograms were the average parameters of the »normal« hips. The peak stress obtained by using the nomograms (3300 m^{-2}) differs from the average hip stress calculated by the computer program 3500±900 m^{-2} (Table 2) for about 6%. Yet it should be considered that the value 3500 m^{-2} was not obtained by calculating stress from the average parameters presented in Table 2 but by averaging stresses of hips included in the study.

5.3. »Normal« hips

Secondary arthritis caused by hip dysplasia represents a minor part in the population of hip arthritis, so the question was posed whether the hips with diagnosis »dysplasia coxae« are in fact the extreme subpopulation of hips with too high hip stress and that a considerable number of hips with diagnosis »idiopathic hip arthritis« are in fact poorly described hips with too high hip stress. This question has already been addressed previously and the negative answer given by the thorough study of large cohort [16] brought evidence against the mechanical hypothesis.

However, decisive and transparent description of dysplastic hips by the HIPSTRESS method was an indication to reconsider the validity of the mechanical hypothesis also in idiopathic osteoarthritis.

As it was expected that the differences between the diseased and »normal« hips would in the population considering hips with idiopathic osteoarthritis be smaller, another question was rised, i.e. which hips can be considered »normal«. To better define the »normal« hips, a more thorough study was performed considering asymptomatic hips [30]. The population considered in the previous study [27] was expanded to 164 female and 42 male »normal« hips. In the female group the subjects' age ranged from 18 to 86, median 54. In the male group the subjects' age ranged from 23 to 82, median 54.

Figure 7 shows the dependence of the peak hip stress on the age of the subject. It can be seen that in the female and in the male population the values of peak stress were scattered over a large interval (between 2000 and 6000 m^{-2} in the female population and between 1500 and 4000 m^{-2} in the male population). With increasing age, the lower bound of the peak stress values remained more or less the same while the upper bound diminished. There were no »normal« old subjects with high hip stress. The average value of peak hip stress decreased with age. It was interpreted that hips that seem »normal« at young age (are asymptomatic) but have high peak stress are removed from the population of »normal« hips in the middle or old age due to development of early hip arthritis, thereby leaving in the »normal« population only hips with low peak stress. With aims at healthy ageing and higher lifespan it would be more appropriate to consider hip as »normal« only if it is asymptomatic at old age. According to the results presented in Figure 7, the appropriate value for »healthy« hips asymptomatic at 80 years would be about 2000 m^{-2} in both sexes. Most importantly, it was concluded that when comparing populations, special care should be taken with regard to the age of the subjects. In the study of Brinckmann et al. (1981) [16] the subjects in the group of »normal« hips were on the average younger than the subjects in the group of hips with arthritis, so some hips that were regarded as »normal« could have at the mathching age pertained to the group of hips with arthritis. These arguments encouraged reconsideration of validation of the mechanical hypotehsis also for hips with idiopathic arthritis.

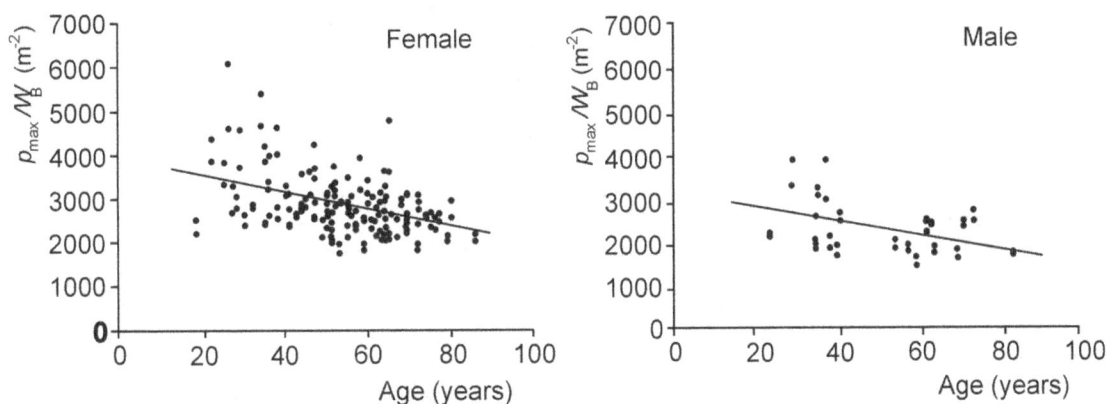

Figure 7. Peak contact hip stress in the population of »normal« hips in dependence on subject's age. Adapted from [30].

6. Comparison of »normal« hips and hips with idiopathic arthritis

The mechanical hypothesis for the primary hip arthritis was validated by considering a group of 431 female patients who underwent total hip replacement [31]. Patients for whom secondary causes for hip arthritis were known were excluded (90 patients with rheumatoid or psoriatic arthritis, avascular necrosis, slipped capital femoral epiphysis, dysplasia of the hip or lower extremity fracture). Radiograms of hips and pelvis of 92 of the patients that were taken years before the operation for various reasons (back pain, discrete pain in the hips or minor injury to the pelvis) were retrieved from the archives, 65 of these radiograms were of required quality and showed hips without considerable joint space narrowing (mean width 3 mm), large osteophytes, subchondral cysts or acetabular protrusion. Three of these patients could not be located and one did not consent to participate in the study while two patients reported a fracture of the lower extremity during childhood. The final analysis was performed on 59 radiograms of hips with no or only initial stage of hip arthritis. The side of arthritis that developed later was determined from medical records on arthroplasty. Geometrical and biomechanical parameters were assessed. There were 22 female patients with unilateral hip arthritis (aged 45 to 79 years, median 69 years) and 37 female patients with bilateral disease (aged 50 to 80 years, median 68 years). In the population with unilateral disease, the parameters of the hips with arthritis were compared to the respective parameters of the contralateral hips with no sign of degenerative process. In the population with bilateral disease, the parameters of hips with earlier implantation of hip endoprosthesis were compared to the respective parameters of contralateral hips with later implementation of hip endoprosthesis.

	Hips with arthritis (22)	Normal hips (36)	Difference (%)	p
$(C \pm SD)$ (cm)	6.4±1.1	6.5±1.0	-2	0.50
$(H \pm SD)$ (cm)	15.7±0.8	15.8±0.8	-1	0.18
$(x \pm SD)$ (cm)	1.1±0.9	1.2±0.9	-9	0.41
$(z \pm SD)$ (cm)	6.7±0.6	6.8±0.5	-1	0.07
$(r \pm SD)$ (cm)	2.6±1.5	2.6±1.4	0	
$(\vartheta_{CE} \pm SD)$ (degrees)	33.5±7.1	35.2±7.3	5	0.03
$R/W_B \pm SD$	2.61±0.21	2.58±0.21	1	0.21
$(\vartheta_R \pm SD)$ (degrees)	7.8±1.3	7.9±1.1	-1	0.47
$(p_{max}/W_B \pm SD)$ (m^{-2})	2440±490	2320±210	5	<0.001

SD: standard deviation. Adapted from [31].

Table 3. Average values of geometrical and biomechanical parameters of 22 female hips with arthritis and 22 contralateral »normal« hips.

	Hips with earlier arthritis (37)	Contralateral hips with later arthritis (37)	Difference (%)	p
$(C \pm SD)$ (cm)	6.5±10.9	6.5±0.9	0	0.65
$(H \pm SD)$ (cm)	15.4±0.8	15.4±0.9	0	0.22
$(x \pm SD)$ (cm)	1.4±0.7	1.1±0.8	23	0.05
$(z \pm SD)$ (cm)	6.5±0.5	6.7±0.5	3	0.01
$(r \pm SD)$ (cm)	2.6±1.8	2.6±1.7	0	0.09
$(\vartheta_{CE} \pm SD)$ (degrees)	35.1±8.3	36.7±8.5	-4	0.005
$R/W_B \pm SD$	2.59±0.17	2.54±0.17	2	0.005
$(\vartheta_R \pm SD)$ (degrees)	7.8±1.3	7.9±1.1	-1	0.016
$(p_{max}/W_B \pm SD)$ (m^{-2})	2540±550	2350±490	81	<0.001

SD: standard deviation. Adapted from [31].

Table 4. Average values of geometrical and biomechanical parameters of 37 female hips with bilateral arthritis. The hips in which arthritis developed earlier were compared with the hips in which arthritis developed later.

These results provided evidence in favor of the mechanical hypothesis by showing that hips with idiopathic arthritis had statistically significantly higher peak hip stress than contralateral asymptomatic hips (Table 3) and that higher peak hip stress meant clinically worse result (Table 4). As it is clear that hips with small centre-edge angle (smaller than 20 degrees) have very high peak stress and that hips with rather large centre-edge angle (larger than 35 degrees) have low hip stress, in hips in between these values the other geometrical parameters can importantly influence the stress. In standard procedures which are often based on the centre-edge angle and the shape of the femoral head, these hips are not recognized as dysplastic, however, a combination of high and wide pelvis, laterally small extension of the greater trochanter and small radius of the femoral head may result in high hip stress. It is therefore indicated that rough estimation of stress on the basis of the visual experience should be supported by actually calculating stress.

7. Hip stress gradient index as a relevant biomechanical parameter

It was suggested [23] that hip stress gradient index is an appropriate parameter to assess hip dysplasia. As described above, the hip stress gradient index describes the derivative of the hip stress with respect to medial direction, at the lateral acetabular rim. If the hip stress increases in the medial direction at the lateral rim, G_p is negative, while if it decreases, it is positive.

A population of hips diagnosed with hip dysplasia according to standard criteria and a group of »normal« hips were examined for the hip stress gradient index [23]. The respective populations consisted of 56 dysplastic hips (9 male and 47 female) and 146 »normal« hips. Figure

3 shows a dependence of hip stress gradient index on the centre-edge angle for both populations of hips. It can be seen that for small centre edge angles G_p is positive, but it diminishes with increasing centre-edge angle. The parameter G_p changes sign at the centre-edge angle approximately equal 20 degrees. The scattering of G_p shows that parameters besides the centre-edge angle are also important; the scattering is larger for smaller centre-edge angles. The difference between the average values of G_p pertaining to the group of dysplastic hips ($1.48.10^5$ m^{-3}) and to the group of normal hips ($-0.44.\ 10^5$ m^{-3}) as assessed by the t-test was statistically significant ($p<0.001$).

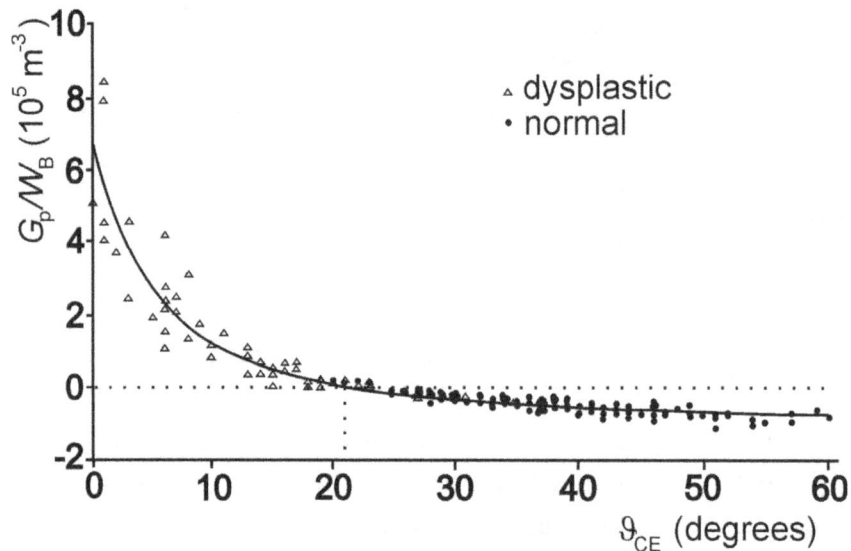

Figure 8. Hip stress gradient index in dependence on centre-edge angle for dysplastic and for »normal« hips. Adapted from [23].

An independent group of 45 dysplastic and »normal« hips was assessed by the Harris hip score for pain, performance and mobility [23]. A statistically significant correlation was found between the Harris hip score and the hip stress gradient index ($\varrho = -0.426$, $p<0.01$). Hip stress gradient index was tested as a criterion for hip dysplasia in these hips. The hips were divided into two groups. The group with positive G_p (16 hips) and the group with negative G_p (29 hips). For comparison, the method for estimating hip dysplasia based on the centre-edge angle was used; the hips with centre-edge angle smaller than 20 degrees were considered dysplastic. There were 10 such hips and 35 hips with centre-edge angle larger than 20 degrees. The difference in Harris hip score between the corresponding groups of dysplastic and »normal« hips were estimated by a non-parametrical statistical test (Kolmogorov-Smirnov test). By considering G_p as the criterion, the difference between the two groups was found statistically significant ($p = 0.031$) while by considering the centre-edge angle as a criterion, the difference was not statistically significant ($p=0.233$). In this group of hips the hip stress gradient index proved a better parameter to predict the Harris hip score than the centre-edge angle [23]. As the hip stress gradient index reflects the distribution of stress over the weight bearing area, it was suggested due to these results that G_p may prove complementary or even more important than he peak stress in assessment of the risk for hip arthritis development.

8. Hip stress gradient index as a relevant biomechanical parameter in hips that were in childhood subjected to Legg-Calve-Perthes disease

Legg-Calve-Perthes disease may considerably affect the development of the hip resulting in deformed femur and acetabulum (Figure 1, right hip). As the risk for arthritis development is increased in hips that were in the childhood subjected to Legg-Calve-Perthes disease, it was of interest to determine biomechanical parameters in these hips and compare them with the corresponding parameters of »normal« hips. The group of contralateral asymptomatic hips with no aparent deformities were considered as the group of »normal« hips. 259 patients were initially considered in the study [26]. 167 patients (64.5%) attended a control examination which included measurement of height and weight of the patient. 3 patients were omitted for missing X-ray pictures from the time of the disease, 19 patients were omitted due to bilateral disease, 3 patients were omitted due to absence of radiograms at the follow-up, 5 patients were omitted due to inadequate X-ray pictures and 2 patients were omitted as they already had a hip prosthesis implanted due to hip arthritis. The final cohort included 135 patients. 24 hips were female (17.8%) and 111 hips were male (82.2%). The mean age at follow-up was 32.5 (20.6 – 47.6) years and the mean body mass index (BMI) at follow-up was 26.7 (18 – 38) kg/m^2.The mean time interval between treatment and follow up was 25.6 (14.5 – 34.5) years. As the body weight was measured at the control examination it was possible to determine both, the normalized biomechanical parameters and the »whole« parameters.

Average±SD	Hips subjected to Legg-Calve-Perthes disease in childhood	Normal (contralateral asymptomatic) hips	Approximate difference (%)	p	Statistical power (1-β)
ϑ_{CE}(degrees)	24.1±9.7	32.9±6.5	-31	$<10^{-8}$	1.00
r (cm)	2.84±0.49	2.43±0.22	15	$<10^{-8}$	1.00
R (N)	2099±474	2100±472	0	0.936	< 0.20
R/W_B	2.59±0.23	2.59±0.20	0	0.797	< 0.20
θ (degrees)	24.3±13.9	13.9±7.0	55	$<10^{-8}$	1.00
p_{max} (MPa)	2.30±0.88	2.28±0.64	0	0.647	0.27
p_{max}/W_B (m^{-2})	2932±945	2911±773	0	0.762	< 0.20
G_p(MPa/m)	4.46±43.55	-29.45±29.69	>100	$<10^{-8}$	1.00
G_p/W_B (m^{-3})	4334±51011	-37959±35848	>100	$<10^{-8}$	1.00
A_F (cm^2)	12.2±3.0	11.3±2.4	7	2.10^{-4}	0.94
ϑ_F (degrees)	90.2±22.7	108.7±13.5	-18	$<10^{-8}$	1.00

Table 5. Average values of geometrical and biomechanical parameters of hips that were in the childhood subjected to Legg-Calve-Perthes disease and "normal" (contralateral) hips. The probabilities (p-value) were calculated with the two-tailed paired t-test and post-hoc statistical power (1-β) calculated for α = 0.05 and sample size N = 135. Statistical power was 1 also for α = 10^{-8} for the variables that yielded differences with statistical significance p <10^{-8}. Adapted from [26].

It can be seen in Table 5 that there were no statistically significant differences between the two groups in resultant hip force and peak contact hip stres (normalized and »whole«). The centre-edge angle was considerably and statistically significantly more favorable in »normal« hips, however, the hips that were in the childhood subjected to the disease had developed a considerably and statistically significantly larger femoral head which compensated the effect of the smaller centre-edge angle. Figure 9 shows that in the group of »normal« hips (red dots) the radii were smaller and uniformly distributed over the interval of centre-edge angles. The lower bound of this interval was approximately 20 degrees as previously acknowledged to be a criterion for hip dysplasia. The test group extended also below this interval, but here the radii were considerably larger. This effect overcompensated the load bearing area which was (statistically significantly) larger in the test group although the centre-edge angle was smaller (Table 5).

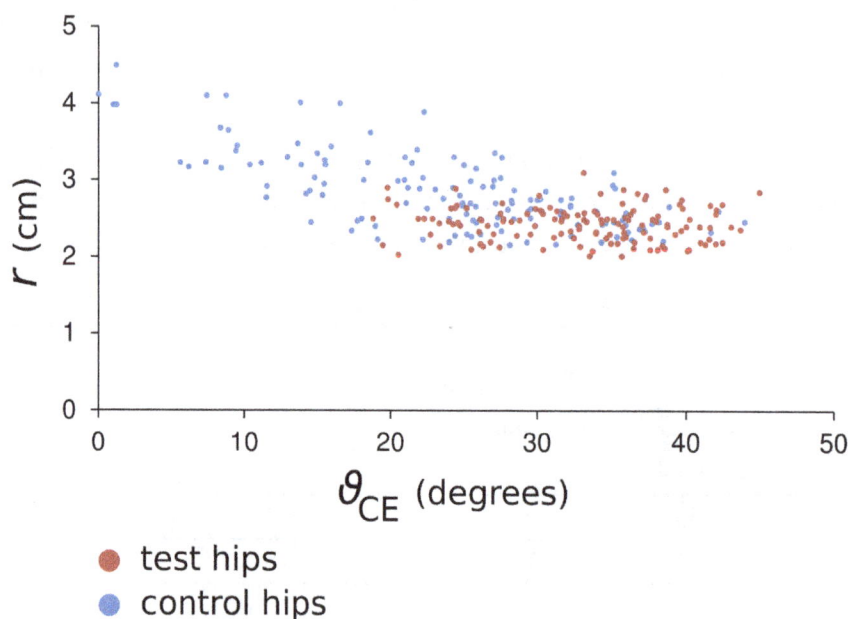

Figure 9. Interdependence between the radius of the femoral head and the centre-edge angle in hips that were in childhood subjected to Legg-Calve-Perthes disease (test group) and contralateral "normal" hips (control group). From [26].

In the hips that were in childhood subjected to Legg-Calve-Perthes disease the resultant hip force and the peak stress did not show differences while the load bearing area was more favorable, however, the stress pole was located considerably and statistically significantly more laterally than in the control group which was reflected also in the difference in the functional angle (Table 5). Most importantly, the biomechanical parameter that showed the difference between the two groups in favor of »normal« hips was the hip stress gradient index. The respective differences in the normalized and the »whole« parameter were considerable (larger than 100%) and statistically very significant (Table 5). The cohort was large enough (with high statistical power at very small probabilities) to render the above results decisive.

Figure 10 shows dependence of hip stress gradient index on the centre-edge angle (A) and on the radius of the femoral head (B). Almost all »normal« hips are confined within the boundaries of radii smaller than 3 cm, centre-edge angles larger than 20 degrees and negative hip stress gradient indexes while the hips that were in childhood subjected to Legg-Calve-Perthes disease extended beyond these boundaries (to larger radii, smaller centre-edge angles and positive hip stress gradient indexes). But there were also many hips from the test group that fitted well within the group of »normal« hips showing successful recovery from the disease in the childhood.

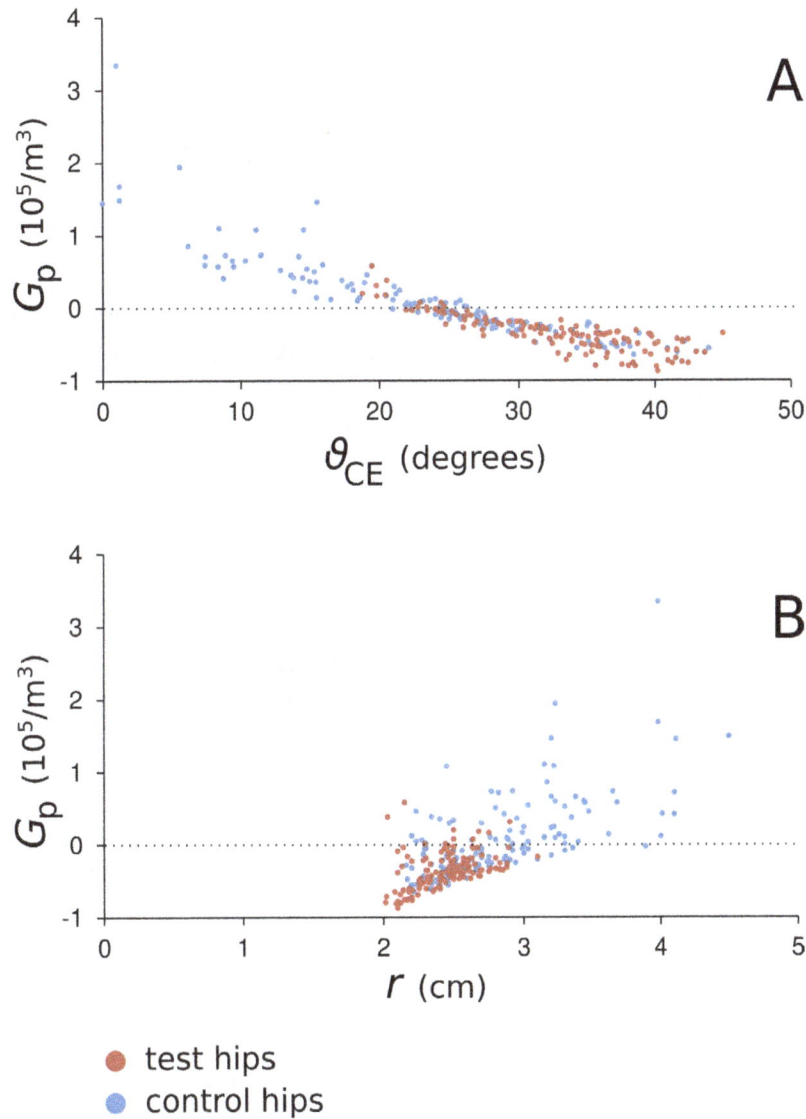

Figure 10. Dependence of the hip stress gradient index on the centre-edge angle (A) and on the radius of the femoral head (B) in hips that were in childhood subjected to Legg-Calve-Perthes disease (test group) and contralateral "normal" hips (control group). From [26].

9. Conclusion

Method HIPSTRESS proved useful in contributing evidence in favor of mechanical hypothesis stating that long lasting unfavorable stress distribution is an etiological factor in development of hip arthritis. The mathematical model for resultant hip force contains the relevant choice of muscles and appropriate scaling of their attachment points that emphasize the individual geometry. The mathematical model is not simple in its derivation, however, it is expressed by transparent and almost analytical solution. The computer program and nomograms enable medical doctors and students to use the mathematical models without extensive mathematical skills. Knowing the geometrical parameters the resultant hip force and the peak stress can be determined within minutes. It is shown above that peak hip stress showed differences between dysplastic and normal hips and between hips with idiopathic arthritis and normal hips. However in dysplastic hips also the hip stress gradient index was less favorable (larger), so it is unclear which of these parameters is the most relevant to estimate the risk for development of hip arthritis. The role of hip stress gradient index is emphasized also by the study of hips that were in childhood subjected to Legg-Calve-Perthes disease since in these hips the resultant hip force and the peak stress were not elevated. Further studies are needed to obtain answer to this question. The method could be supported by using improved imaging of hips (three dimensional data on muscle attachment points) and refined by considering particularities of diseases (such as nonsphericity of femoral head after the Legg-Calve-Perthes disease). Most importantly, the hypothesis involving macroscopic hip stress distribution should be connected to molecular mechanisms underlaying cartilage deterioration and onset and spreading of inflammation.

The criteria for biomechanical measures suggested by R.A. Brand [32] are that they (a) should be accurate and reproducible, (b) the measuring technique must not significantly alter the function it is measuring, (c) it should exhibit reasonable stability, (d) the measure should not be directly observable by the skilled clinician, (e) it should be independent of mood, motivation or pain, (f) it must clearly distinguish between normal and abnormal, (g) it should be reported in a form analogous to some accepted clinical concept, (h) it should be cost-effective and (i) it must be appropriately validated. As a method based on physical laws the HIPSTRESS method completely fulfills the criteria (b), (c), (d), (e), (g) and (h). As for criterion (a) it is reproducible, but its accuarcy is limited by the model assumptions and by the accuracy of measurement of geometrical parameters. Further improvements should be made in these directions. Criterion (f) adresses »normal« and »abnormal«. A clear criterion can be given within the HIPSTRESS method (i.e. threshold values of biomechanical parameters such as $G_p=0$), however, these are based on correspondence of the parameters with clinical assessment which is also not always clear. The criterion (i) was implemented by validation of the HIPSTRESS method by studies of the effect of different operations on biomechanical and clinical outcome and related problems [32-57]. The strongest point of the method is low invasiveness (it uses data that were obtained for therapeutic purposes). Also, the development of the method and its use required no experiments on laboratory animals or any other material that would require burden on patients, volunteers or animals.

Author details

Veronika Kralj-Iglič*

Address all correspondence to: veronika.kralj-iglic@fe.uni-lj.si

Laboratory of Clinical Biophysics, Faculty of Health Sciences, University of Ljubljana, Ljubljana, Slovenia

References

[1] Wiberg G. Studies on dysplastic acetabula and congenital subluxation of the hip joint: with special reference to the complication of osteoarthritis. Acta Chir Scand Suppl. 1939; 58:7-135.

[2] Chiari K. Pelvic osteotomy in hip arthroplasty. Wien Med Wochenschr. 1953;103(38): 707–709.

[3] Salter RB. Innominate osteotomy in the treatment of congenital dislocation and subluxation of the hip. J Bone Joint Surg Br. 1961; 43(3):518–539.

[4] Pemberton PA. Pericapsular osteotomy of the ileum for treatment of congenital subluxation and dislocation of the hip. J Bone Joint Surg Am. 1965; 47(1):65–86.

[5] Chiari K. Medial displacement osteotomy of the pelvis. Clin Orthop Relat Res. 1974; 98:55–71.

[6] Salter RB, Hansson G, Thompson GH. Innominate osteotomy in the management of residual congenital subluxation of the hip in young adults. Clin Orthop Relat Res. 1984; 182:53–68.

[7] Steel HH. Triple osteotomy of the innominate bone. J Bone Joint Surg Am. 1973; 55(2):343–350.

[8] Ganz R, Klaue K, Vinh TS, Mast JW. A new periacetabular osteotomy for the treatment of hip dysplasias. Technique and preliminary results. Clin Orthop Relat Res. 1988; 232:26–36.

[9] Tonnis D. Surgical treatment of congenital dislocation of the hip. Clin Orthop Relat Res.1990; (258):33–40.

[10] Brand RA, Iglic A, Kralj-Iglic V. Contact stresses in human hip: implications for disease and treatment. Hip Int. 2001; 11:117-126.

[11] Hodge WA, Fijan RS, Carlson KL, Burgess RG, Harris WH, Mann RW. Contact pressures in the human hip joint measured in vivo. Proc Natl Acad Sci USA.1986; 83 (9): 2879-2883.

[12] Brown TD, DiGioia AM 3rd. A contact-coupled finite element analysis of the natural adult hip. J Biomech. 1984; 17(6):437-448.

[13] Crowninshield RD, Johnston RC, Andrews JG, Brand RA. A biomechanical investigation of the human hip. J Biomech. 1968; 11:75-77.

[14] Pauwels F. Biomechanics of the normal and diseased hip: Theoretical foundations, technique, and results of treatment, 276. Berlin: Springer-Verlag; 1976.

[15] Legal H, Reinecke M, Ruder H. Zur biostatischen analyse des hüftgelenks III. Z Orthop Ihre Grenzgeb. 1980; 118(5):804-15.

[16] Brinckmann P, Frobin W, Hierholzer E. Stress on the articular surface of the hip joint in healthy adults and persons with idiopathic osteoarthrosis of the hip joint. J Biomech. 1981; 14:149–156.

[17] Hadley NA, Brown TD, Weinstein SL. The effects of contact pressure elevations and aseptic necrosis on the long-term outcome of congenital hip dislocation. J Orthop Res. 1990; 8:504-513.

[18] Maxian TA, Brown TD, Weinstein SL. Chronic stress tolerance levels for human articular cartilage: Two nonuniform contact models applied to long-term follow-up of CDH. J Biomech. 1995; 28:159-166.

[19] Iglic A, Srakar F, Antolic V, Kralj Iglic V, Batagelj V. Mathematical analysis of Chiari osteotomy. Acta Orthop Iugosl. 1990; 20:35-39.

[20] Ipavec M, Brand RA, Pedersen DR, Mavcic B, Kralj-Iglic V, Iglic A. Mathematical modelling of stress in the hip during gait. J Biomech. 1999; 32:1229-1235.

[21] Dostal WF, Andrews JG. A three dimensional biomechanical model of hip musculature. J. Biomehanics. 1981; 14:803-812.

[22] Johnston RC, Brand RA, Crowninshield RD. Reconstruction of the Hip. J. Bone and Joint Surg. 1979; 61A:639-652.

[23] Pompe B, Daniel M, Sochor M, Vengust R, Kralj-Iglic V, Iglic A. Gradient of contact stress in normal and dysplastic human hips. Med Eng Phys. 2003; 25:379-385.

[24] Kralj-Iglic V, Dolinar D, Ivanovski M, List I, Daniel M. Role of biomechanical parameters in hip osteoarthritis and avascular necrosis of femoral head. Applied Biological Engineering - Principles and Practice, Naik GR (Ed.), InTech, DOI: 10.5772/30159; 2012.

[25] Rijavec B, Kosak R, Daniel M, Kralj-Iglic V, Dolinar D. Effect of cup inclination on predicted stress-induced volumetric wear in total hip replacement. Comput Meth Biomech Biomed Eng. 2014; DOI: 10.5772/30159.

[26] Kocjancic B, Molicnik A, Antolic V, Mavcic B, Kralj-Iglic V, Vengust R. Unfavorable hip stress distribution after Legg-Calve-Perthes syndrome: a 25-year follow-up of 135 hips. J Orthop Res. 2014; 32:8-16.

[27] Daniel M, Antolic V, Iglic A, Kralj Iglic V. Determination of contact hip stress from nomograms based on mathematical model. Med Eng Phys. 2001; 23:347-357.

[28] Kersnic B, Iglic A, Kralj-Iglic V, Srakar F, Antolic V. Increased incidence of arthrosis in female population could be related to femoral and pelvic shape. Arch Orthop Trauma Surg. 1997; 116:345-347.

[29] Mavcic B, Pompe B, Antolic V, Daniel M, Iglic A, Kralj-Iglic V. Mathematical estimation of stress distribution in normal and dysplastic human hips. J Orthop Res. 2002; 20:1025-1030.

[30] Mavcic B, Slivnik T, Antolic V, Iglic A, Kralj-Iglic V. High contact hip stress is related to the development of hip pathology with increasing age. Clin Biomech. 2004; 19:939-943.

[31] Recnik G, Kralj-Iglic V, Iglic A, Antolic V, Kranberger S, Vengust R. Higher peak contact hip stress predetermines the side of hip involved in idiopathic osteoarthritis. Clin Biomech. 2007; 22:1119–1124.

[32] Brand RA. Can biomechanics contribute to clinical orthopaedic assessments? Iowa Orthop J 1989; 9:61-64.

[33] Pompe B, Antolic V, Mavcic B, Iglic A, Kralj-Iglic V. Hip joint contact stress as an additional parameter for determining hip dysplasia in adults: Comparison with severin's classification. Med Sci Monit. 2007; 13:CR215-219.

[34] Kristan A, Mavcic B, Cimerman M, Iglic A, Tonin M, Slivnik T, Kralj-Iglic V, Daniel M. Acetabular Loading in Active Abduction. IEEE T Rehabil Eng. 2007; 15:252-275.

[35] Daniel M, Dolinar D, Herman S, Sochor M, Iglic A, Kralj-Iglic V. Contact stress in hips with osteonecrosis of the femoral head. Clin Orhop Rel Res. 2006; 447:92-99.

[36] Kralj M, Mavcic B, Antolic V, Iglic A, Kralj-Iglic V. The Bernese periacetabular osteotomy: clinical, radiographic and biomechanical 7-15 year follow-up in 26 hips. Acta Orthop. 2005; 76:833-840.

[37] Daniel M, Iglic A, Kralj-Iglic V. The shape of acetabular cartilage optimizes hip contact stress distribution. J Anat. 2005; 207:85–91.

[38] Daniel M, Iglic A, Kralj-Iglic V, Konvickova S. Computer system for definition of the quantitative geometry of musculature from CT images. Comput Methods Biomech Biomed Engin. 2005; 1:25-29.

[39] Kosak R, Antolic V, Pavlovcic V, Kralj-Iglic V, Milosev I, Vidmar G, Iglic A. Polyethylene wear in total hip prostheses: the influence of direction of linear wear on

volumetric wear determined from radiographic data. Skeletal Radiol. 2003; 23: 679-686.

[40]   Dolinar D, Antolic V, Herman S, Iglic A, Kralj-Iglic V, Pavlovcic V. Influence of contact hip stress on the outcome of surgical treatment of hips affected by avascular necrosis, Arch Orthop Trauma Surg. 2003; 123:509-513.

[41]   Daniel M, Sochor M, Iglic A, Kralj-Iglic V. Hypothesis of regulation of hip joint cartilage activity by mechanical loading. Med Hypotheses. 2003; 60: 936-937.

[42]   Herman S, Jaklic A, Herman S, Iglic A, Kralj-Iglic V. Hip stress reduction after Chiari osteotomy. Med Biol Eng Comput. 2002; 40: 369-375.

[43]   Iglic A, Kralj-Iglic V, Daniel M, Macek-Lebar A. Computer determination of contact stress distribution and size of weight bearing area in the human hip joint. Comp Methods Biomed. Eng. 2002; 5: 185-192.

[44]   Vengust R, Daniel M, Antolic V, Zupanc O, Iglic A, Kralj-Iglic V. Biomechanical evaluation of hip joint after Salter innominate osteotomy: a long-term follow-up study. Arch Orthop Trauma Surg. 2001; 121: 511-516.

[45]   Iglic A, Daniel M, Kralj-Iglic V, Antolic V, Jaklic A. Peak hip-joint contact stress in male and female populations. J Musculoskeletal Res. 2001; 5: 17-21.

[46]   Zupanc O, Antolic V, Iglic A, Jaklic A, Kralj-Iglic V, Stare J, Vengust R. The assessment of contact stress in the hip joint after operative treatment for severe slipped capital femoral epiphysis. Int Orthop. 2001; 25:9-12.

[47]   Antolic V, Srakar F, Iglic A, Kralj-Iglic V, Zaletel-Kragelj L, Macek-Lebar A. Changes in configuration of the hip due to Chiari osteotomy. Int Orthop. 1996; 4:183-186.

[48]   Iglic A, Antolic V, Srakar F, Kralj-Iglic V, Macek-Lebar A, Brajnik D. Biomechanical study of various greater trochanter positions. Arch Orthop Trauma Surg. 1995; 114:76-78.

[49]   Antolic V, Iglic A, Herman S, Srakar F, Kralj-Iglic V, Macek-Lebar A, Stanic U. The required and the available abductor force after operative changes in pelvic geometry. Acta Orthop Belg. 1994; 60:374-377.

[50]   Iglic A, Kralj-Iglic V, Antolic V. Reducing of stress in the articular surface of the hip joint after shifting the upper part of the body towards the painful hip. Acta Chir Orthop Traum Cech. 1994; 61:268-270.

[51]   Iglic A, Kralj-Iglic V, Antolic V, Srakar F, Stanic U. Effect of the periacetabular osteotomy on the stress on the human hip joint articular surgace. IEEE Trans Rehab Engr. 1993; 1:207-212.

[52]   Iglic A, Antolic V, Srakar F. Biomechanical analysis of various operative hip joint rotation center shifts. Arch Orthop Trauma Surg. 1993; 112:124-126.

[53] Iglic A, Srakar F, Antolic V. The influence of the pelvic shape on the biomechanical status of the hip. Clin Biomech. 1993; 8:223-224.

[54] Srakar F, Iglic A, Antolic V, Herman S. Computer simulation of the periacetabular osteotomy. Acta Orthop Scand. 1992; 63:411-412.

[55] Kosak R, Kralj-Iglic V, Iglic A, Daniel M. Polyethylene wear is related to patient-specific contact stress in THA. Clin Orthop Rel Res. 2011; 469:3415-3422.

[56] Mavcic B, Daniel M, Antolic V, Iglic A, Kralj-Iglic V. Contact hip stress measurements in orthopaedic clinical practice. In: Biomechanics: Principles, Trends and Applications. Ed: Levy JH. Nova Science Publishers; (2010). p281-294.

[57] Debevec H, Pedersen DR, Iglic A, Daniel M. One-legged stance as a representative static body position for calculation of hip contact stress distribution in clinical studies. J Appl Biomech. 2010; 26:522-525.

5

The Conservative Management of Osteoarthritis — Hyaluronic Acid, Platelet Rich Plasma or the Combination?

Michele Abate, Isabel Andia and Vincenzo Salini

1. Introduction

Osteoarthritis (OA) is a progressively degenerating joint disease. The prevailing paradigm suggests that OA results from an impaired regeneration ability of the damaged cartilage due to biomechanical and biochemical changes. There is an increasing recognition that OA is a disease of the joint as an organ involving all intraarticular tissue i..e. subchondral bone, synovium, cartilage, menisci, ligaments. Therefore, changes as increased metabolism and sclerosis of the subchondral bone, chondrocyte death and extracellular matrix (ECM) catabolism, as well as primary or secondary changes in the synovium (including endothelial cell proliferation, macrophage infiltration and inflammation) will induce alterations in the molecular composition of the synovial fluid. The clinical signs associated with these changes include pain, rigidity and decreased functionality, which may compromise overall health and quality of life [1].

The prevalence of OA is very high, expected to affect more than 50 million subjects in the US by 2020, and will increase with the ageing of the population [2]. According to the American College of Rheumatology, nearly 70% of people over age 70 have X-ray evidence of OA, although only half ever develop symptoms [3].

The barriers to treatment development include the insufficient understanding of the pathology and the fact that the OA physiopathology may not be identical for all patients. Several pharmaceutical approaches (analgesics, non steroidal anti-inflammatory drugs, COX-2 inhibitors and steroids) have been proposed, with the aim of reducing pain and maintaining and/or improving function [4]. However, none of these options has shown to delay the progression of the disease or reverse joint damage. In addition, the incidence of adverse reactions to these drugs increases with age. Data from epidemiological studies consistently show that the risk of cardio-vascular and gastro-intestinal complications is very high and largely dose-dependent [5]. It is well known that non steroidal anti-inflammatory drugs, as well as selective COX-2 inhibitors, may cause renal failure, hypertension and water retention and have a thrombotic potential, especially for high doses and long term treatments [6]. On the other hand, corticosteroids are burdened with relevant side effects, when given systemically, and therefore are usually administered by intra-articular (IA) injection in patients who fail to respond to other conservative measures; in particular, patients with joint effusions and local tenderness may have greater benefit from this option. Although it has been established that corticosteroid injections are relatively safe, there are concerns regarding their possible adverse events following repeated treatments. These effects include local tissue atrophy, particularly when small joints are injected, long-term joint damage, due to reduced bone formation, and risk of infection, due to suppression of adrenocortical function [7].

Considering the limits of therapies at present available, drugs with minimal side effects, and which can stop the progression of the disease, are therefore warranted. Research in Regenerative Medicine in the last decades, has shaped new investigational biological preparations that can be injected within the joints. These include mesenchymal stem cells (BMSCs [Bone Marrow Mesenchymal Stem Cells] and AdSCs [Adipose Mesenchymal Stem Cells]). The initial idea of MSC therapies was to replace damaged or death cells but moved towards using MSCs as a tool to modify the tissue environment. The concept is based on the paracrine actions of MSCs, hence major biological mechanisms to be targeted by these therapies are inflammation, angiogenesis or modifications of the catabolic environment. Injectable MSCs therapies are not capable of structurally modifying the OA joint. Due to the costs, and lack of evidences of the regenerative potential of these cellular therapies, other less expensive and easier to implement approaches are being investigated. These include Platelet Rich Plasma (PRP) injections or combination products such as PRP + Hyaluronic acid (HA).

Both PRP and HA have been extensively used to improve lubrication, modulate inflammation and modify the catabolic micro-environment. In doing so, these conservative treatments not only aim to reduce clinical symptoms, but interfere with OA progression.

In this article we seek to summarize the current pre-clinical and clinical knowledge on this topic, reporting comparative studies between HA and PRP injections, and suggesting the possibility of the combined use of these therapeutic agents.

2. Hyaluronic acid

2.1. Basic concepts and experimental research

Hyaluronan is a polyanionic, unbranched glycosaminoglycan polymer composed of disaccharide subunits of N-acetyl-D-glucosamine and D-glucuronic acid. It was isolated for the first time in 1934 by Karl Meyer and John Palmer from the vitreous of bovine eyes [8]. These scientists proposed the name "hyaluronic acid" from hyaloid (vitreous) and uronic acid.

Although the term HA is often used in the literature, the correct name reflecting the configuration of this molecule in vivo is hyaluronan. Indeed, *in vivo*, at physiological pH, it exists as a polyanion and not in the protonated acid form [9,10]. In this chapter, for convenience, we will use the term HA all through the text. HA is present in many tissues, but the larger amount of hyaluronan resides in the dermis and epidermis. It is also an essential component of the hyaline cartilage (1mg/g wet weight) where it organizes the ECM by creating specific interactions with aggrecan, a large chondroitin sulfate proteoglycan, present at higher concentration (25-50 mg/g wet weight). Aggrecan and type II collagen are the main macromolecules in the cartilage ECM. The spatial configuration of aggrecan and type II collagen are responsible of mechanical properties of the hyaline articular cartilage.

High molecular weight (HMW) HA is also the main component of synovial fluid; it is synthesized and extruded within the synovial fluid by the lining fibroblastic cells of the joint capsule named type B synoviocytes [10]. The volume of synovial fluid in the knee is 3-4 ml. Its role, in addition to lubrication, is to provide nutrients to the hyaline cartilage and create a hypoxic environment on the cartilage surface.

The physiologic turnover (i.e. catabolism balanced by production) of HA within the joint is very dynamic; the half-life of HA is estimated in 12 hours [11]. Importantly, HA turnover, in both the cartilage ECM and the synovial fluid, is fundamental in the maintenance of joint homeostasis. Reticulo-endothelial cells lining the lymphatic vessels actively remove about 90% of the HA. HA catabolism can occur through hyalurodinase actions and/or peroxidative cleavage. It has been hypothesized that peroxidative cleavage, a process that consumes O_2 and helps to maintain the hypoxic environment within the joint, is required for normal synovial function and joint homeostasis [12].

HA polymers are synthesized by three different synthases termed HAS (HAS-1, -2 and -3). HMW HA has anti-inflammatory, anti-angiogenic and anti-immunogenic properties [13-16]. The high viscosity of HMW HA grants viscoelastic properties to the fluid, and along with lubricin contributes to the boundary lubrication that is necessary for low friction levels on the articular surface [17]. Thus, it has a shielding effect on cartilage surfaces and other joint components.

Beside HA role in viscosupplementation and major functions in the biophysical and homeostatic conditions of the joint, an important aspect of HA biology to be considered is its influence on cell behavior.

Basic research, performed in OA models in animals (rats, rabbits, dogs and sheep), has shown that HA has several pleiotropic signaling properties (biosupplementation), such as immunosuppressive, anti-inflammatory, anti-apoptotic, anti-angiogenic and anti-fibrotic effects, with normalization of endogenous HA synthesis, and chondroprotection [16]. Actually, HA binds to a number of cell membrane receptors termed hyaladherins. The predominant and more widely expressed is CD44, a membrane glycoprotein made of ten stable exons and ten variable exons inserted in different combinations at a particular extra-membrane site [16].

HA can be pro-inflammatory, however immune cells only bind HA when activated by an inflammatory agent. Actually, CD44 is expressed in the membrane of immune cells, therefore

HA can participate in the recruitment of neutrophils, macrophages and lymphocytes [13]. Indeed, CD44 decrease in articular cartilage is related to progression of knee OA [16].

Paradoxically, HA-CD44 binding is involved in the resolution of inflammation. Besides, both CD44 and RHAMM (CD168) (the HA receptor for HA-mediated motility) are involved in the regulation of growth factor (GF) signaling.

A recent study has been performed in an experimental model of murine OA (TGF-β1 injection and treadmill running), which displays many OA-like changes, including synovial activation. HA injection, 24 hours after TGF-β1 injection, hinders neovascularization and fibrosis of the synovium, and keeps in good condition articular cartilage in wild-type, but not in CD44 knockout mice. This finding suggests that the injected HA enhances the synthesis of chondrogenic proteins, and blocks that of fibrogenic/degradative proteins in both the cartilage and subchondral bone [18].

A further research, performed in patients with knee or hip OA, has demonstrated the presence of activated T cells in the synovial fluid, so confirming that OA is a disease with a immunological/inflammatory involvement. In these patients, HA injections decreased the levels of activated T cells, and so regulated the articular milieu [19].

The analgesic properties of HA, besides to the activities previously described, could be also attributed to a specific activity on opioid receptors [20]. Pain in OA is likely to have multiple sources, including subchondral bone marrow lesions, synovium and the periostium as well as soft tissues surrounding the joint, including extra-articular bursae and fat pad. Pain in OA is classified as nociceptive, based on the presence of opioid receptors in the synovial lining and sublining cells. Various molecules present in extracellular space modulate nociceptor sensitivity by targeting different receptor types. The biological mechanisms responsible for HA analgesic activity have been partially elucidated by Zavan et al. [20] in experiments performed with Chinese Hamster Ovary cells that express a panel of opioid receptors. The results demonstrated that HA stimulates the k receptor (KOP), also expressed on fibroblast-like synoviocytes, in a concentration dependent manner, but not the DOP, MOP and NOP receptors. This selective activity could be due to the singular conformational structures of HA compared to morphine, more closely related to dynorphin organization. The pain threshold also increases, due to the direct analgesia through inhibition of pain receptors, and by a direct action on synovial nerve endings and stimulation of synovial lining cells.

At present, HA compounds with different molecular weight (MW) are commercially available. The enhanced diffusion of LMW preparations (0.5-1.5 millions Dalton) through the ECM of the synovium makes possible the interaction with synovial cells [21]. However, because of the modest elastoviscosity of these compounds, compared to native hyaluronan in the synovial fluid, HA preparations with HMW (6-7 millions Dalton), have been developed. These formulations retain higher amounts of fluid in the articular space using their hydrophilic properties, and also have a greater anti-inflammatory activity, as shown by reduced prostaglandin E 2 and bradykinin concentration attributed to a reduced migration of inflammatory cells [22].

Currently, many types of particulate carriers have been investigated aiming to increase the retention time of the therapeutic agents within the joint capsule. Among them, cationic polymeric nanoparticles form ionically connected filamentous arrangements ("ionically cross-linked hydrogels") linked with local hyaluronan [23]. After intra-articular (IA) injection in rat knees about 70% of these hydrogels are retained into the joint for 1 week. Thus, cationic polymeric nanoparticles increase HA retention into joints and are suitable for therapeutic use. Another medical device combines chondroitin sulphate and HA [24]. The role of chondroitin sulfate is twofold: a) to create specific interactions designed to optimize HA rheological behavior; and b) to regulate cartilage metabolism by performing as a substrate for polysulphated glycosaminoglycans synthesis, as well as inhibiting the synthesis of catabolic cytokines and metalloproteinases.

To ameliorate OA treatment while avoiding adverse effects, a mixture of celecoxib-loaded liposomes embedded in HA gel has been formulated [25]. Celecoxib is a COX-2 selective inhibitor with analgesic and anti-inflammatory properties. Liposomes are good candidates for local delivery of therapeutic agents because they are derived from naturally occurring biodegradable and nontoxic lipids. The combination of the two drugs, both efficient in the treatment of OA, but with different mechanisms, injected into the joints, is expected to have synergistic effect. Indeed, in a rabbit knee OA model, the liposomal combination was more effective than a single drug in pain control and cartilage protection, as shown by histopathological studies [26].

Preliminary studies suggest positive results using an innovative viscosupplement (SynolisV-A) produced from high a concentration of HA, combined with a high concentration of sorbitol as a free radical scavenger (single injection of 4 ml in total), in subjects with symptomatic hip OA [27].

These pharmaceutical studies taken together show how intense is nowadays the research aiming to ameliorate the therapeutic efficacy of HA. Open-label, non controlled studies have proven the clinical efficacy of some of these products. However, high quality clinical studies proving their superiority towards the available preparations of HA are still lacking.

2.2. Clinical trials

2.2.1. Knee

Viscosupplementation with HA in knee OA has been approved by the FDA and is recommended by OARSI for non-severe OA. Guidelines are based on a meta-analysis of randomized saline-controlled trials, including a total of 29 studies representing 4866 unique subjects (IA HA: 2673; IA saline: 2193) [28].

Prospective single or double-blind trials have been done using different types of HA. The number of injections varied from 3 to 5 weekly, with a maximum of 11 in 23 weeks, the doses ranged from 15 to 60 mg, and follow-up periods ranged from 4 weeks to 18 months. Pain outcomes were followed using the Visual Analogic Scale (VAS) and Western Ontario and McMaster Universities Osteoarthritis Index (WOMAC). A minor number of studies evaluated the functional outcomes (WOMAC, Lequesne Index, Range of motion [ROM]), the subjective global assessment and the quality of life of the patients.

HA injection resulted in very large treatment effects between 4 and 26 weeks for knee pain and function compared to pre-injection values. Compared to saline controls, standardized mean difference values with IA HA ranged from -0.38-0.43 for knee pain and +0.32-0.34 for knee function. Clinical changes were similar in the trials where LMW or HMW HA was used. However, the number of injections was lower for HMW preparations, and this is an important advantage for the patients and the clinician. There were no statistically significant differences between IA HA and saline controls in any safety outcomes, including serious adverse events, and study withdrawal. The authors concluded that IA HA injections are safe and effective in patients with symptomatic knee OA [28].

Another meta-analysis [29], comparing the time course of symptoms (the "therapeutic trajectory") in HA and corticosteroid treated patients, highlights that, from baseline to week 4, IA corticosteroids were more effective than HA. By week 4, the two approaches had equal efficacy, but beyond week 8 HA was superior.

It must be noted that, in all trials, some of the patients were non-responders to therapy. Currently, the characteristics of responders have not been clearly identified, but a greater benefit was observed in patients with low grade OA (Kellgren and Lawrence [KL] grade I-II) [9]. This is indirectly confirmed by changes of the serum levels of specific OA biomarkers (Coll2-1 and Coll2-1 NO2) after viscosupplementation. The serum concentrations of these biomarkers were significantly higher in KL grade III/IV patients compared to KL grade I/II patients, and were significantly lower at baseline in responders than in non-responders [30]. Therefore, a rapid decrease of type II collagen degradation and joint inflammation after HA injection supports the utility of serum biomarkers as predictive factors for response to treatment. The role of age in predicting the therapeutic response is debated: some authors report no significant difference among subjects of different ages, whereas others claim that IA joint HA injections are effective in both young and old patients with regard to pain and functional status over a short-term period, but that, in the long term (12 months), the benefit declines rapidly in the elderly subjects [15]. Essentially, advanced OA may be a non-return back irreversible condition.

2.2.2. Hip

The number of studies about viscosupplementation of hip OA is limited when compared with knee OA. The reasons can be the deeper localization of this joint, and the proximity of femoral vessels and nerves, which makes mandatory performing the injections under imaging control [31]. Moreover, the level of evidence for most of these trials is low, because they are cohort studies and lack of a reference group [9].

In these studies, several HA compounds were used. The number of injections ranged from 1 to 3 for each patients, and only in few cases 4 or 5 injections were performed. In general, the injections number was lower for HMW preparations. The length of treatments and the outcome measures were similar to those used in knee randomized controlled trials. All the trials have shown a reduction of pain, which, in general, becomes evident within 3 months and persists in the following 6, 12 and 18 months. Besides the reduction of pain, also the articular function (Harris Hip Score, WOMAC score, Lequesne Index, and American Academy of Orthopaedic

Association Lower Limb Core Scale) was improved [9,15]. Moreover, an improvement of kinematic and kinetic parameters in walking pattern at 6 months (higher cadence, stride length, significant increase for the pelvic tilt at heel contact and for hip flexion-extension moment at loading response sub-phases of gait cycle) has been shown by a recent study [32]. Interestingly, the IA injection of both LMW and HMW HA has been proven efficacious in delaying the total hip replacement in patients affected by symptomatic hip OA [33,34].

A further observation, which confirms the previous data, is the reduction of non steroidal anti-inflammatory drugs consumption [35].

2.2.3. Ankle

In the few studies performed in ankle OA, patients suffering from post-traumatic KL grade II-IV ankle OA were enrolled. Different HA preparations were used, and patients received 1 up to 5 injections. Clinical benefit was evaluated by means of different scales (VAS, Ankle Osteoarthritis Scale, American Orthopaedic Foot and Ankle Society, Short Form-12, Short Form-36, WOMAC), and the follow-up period varied from 6 to 18 months [36].

An improvement in all the outcome measures was reported, with the effect lasting for 18 months. However, it is not clear from reports whether the pain reduction was clinically significant, or could be ascribed only to a placebo effect. In addition, the lack of controls does not allow definitive conclusions on the efficacy of HA.

The level 1 evidence studies are more qualified to assess the therapeutic efficacy, but also these trials show several limitations (e.g., no information on the actual number of potential patients, no clear randomization, imbalance of baseline characteristics between intervention and control groups, statistical weakness), and therefore have to be considered as low quality. The patients treated with HA showed a significant decrease in pain and disability at 6 months, with the effects lasting 12-13 months [37, 38].

Besides the reduction of these parameters, an improvement in ankle sagittal ROMs, and gait quality was observed. However, it must be noted that in any study the authors found difference between HA and controls groups. In particular, in the studies performed by Salk [38], Cohen [39] and DeGroot [37], the patients, treated with a 1-2.5 ml phosphate-buffered saline solution injection, reported a similar improvement in all parameters evaluated. Analogously, positive results were observed in patients, who followed a 6 weeks exercise therapy (muscle strengthening and ankle ROM exercises) [40], and after arthroscopic lavage of OA ankle joint [41].

Recent observations aimed to identify the baseline prognostic factors of outcome have shown that early stage disease and duration of pain less than 1 year are independent predictors associated with higher satisfaction at 3 and 6 months after treatment [42]. However, this assumption has been challenged by Lucas et al. [43], who have observed that viscosupplementation had a significant positive effect after a very long observation period (45.5 months), and that neither etiology nor severity of OA was predictive of the response.

On the basis of these observations, the efficacy of HA in reducing pain and improving function in ankle OA is still debated. Several factors can explain these discrepancies. Ankle joint, anatomically and functionally, is more complex than other joints, which are usually treated with positive results with HA (hip, knee) [36].

Finally, it must be considered that the majority of studies has been performed blindly and only few under imaging guidance [36]. This can be a valid explanation of several unsatisfactory results, because there is evidence that about one third of IA injections are not delivered into the IA cavity, when performed without a visual aid [44]. At this regard, ankle joint presents many technical difficulties of injecting IA, due to its complex anatomy, further complicated from the OA joint changes.

2.2.4. Shoulder

HA is effective and well tolerated for the treatment of OA and persistent shoulder pain refractory to other standard non operative interventions. Both 3 and 5 weekly IA injections of LMW HA provide significant improvement in terms of shoulder pain (VAS score on movement), with the effects lasting 7-26 weeks [9].

Similarly, in a 6 months follow-up study, a significant reduction in VAS pain score was also provided with 3 weekly IA HMW HA (Hylan G-F 20) injections [45]. In addition, most of the patients experienced an improvement in the shoulder function scores (Oxford Shoulder Score and Constant-Murley Score) and in the activities of daily living.

Studies comparing Hylan G-F 20 *versus* 6 methylprednisolone acetate [46] or versus physiotherapy [45] show that HA is effective in reducing pain for up to 6 months, whereas the positive results observed after corticosteroid or physiotherapy have a shorter efficacy and decline after 1 or 2 months. However, these positive results are challenged by a double-blind, randomized, controlled multicenter trial, where patients who received 3 weekly HA injections did not report any significant difference in term of pain reduction at 26 weeks when compared with placebo [47].

2.2.5. Other joints

The efficacy of HA has been investigated in the treatment of carpo-metacarpal OA, and positive results have been reported by most of the authors [9]. In particular, an early improvement in VAS score was observed after 2 weeks post treatment, with the effects lasting until 1-3 months. The long term effects of HA were demonstrated only in few studies, in which the pain relief was reported at 6 months [48]. Beside pain reduction, also grip strength improved significantly, although this effect was achieved slowly, with better results observed at 6 months. Moreover, the local inflammation measured by means of Power Doppler exam significantly decreased after 2 weeks of treatment [49].

Similar positive results have been reported in the treatment of temporo-mandibular OA (with or without effusion). The superiority of HA injections (associated or not with arthrocentesis) was shown only against placebo saline injections, whereas outcomes were comparable with those achieved with corticosteroid injections [50-53]. Interestingly, in an experimental model of arthropatic temporo-mandibular joint, El-Hakim and Elyamani [54] found, after repeated

IA injections, an increase in the thickness of the cartilagineous layer, suggesting that HA can inhibit the progression of OA changes. A recent study, aiming to identify predictors for treatment efficacy, has shown that only unilateral temporo-mandibular joint OA predicts better the benefit [55], while sex, age, pain duration are not provided of predictive power.

In the treatment of elbow OA the results are inconclusive [9,15]. Positive effects have been observed only in two small studies, while, in a larger study (18 patients), IA HA was not effective in the treatment of post-traumatic OA of the elbow.

Controversial results have been observed also in the treatment of spine OA. Fuchs et al. [56] reported significant pain relief and improved quality of life, also in the long term, in patients affected from facet joints OA with chronic non-radicular pain in the lumbar spine. However, these results are not in agreement with a recent study by Cleary et al. [57], who have not shown any benefit of viscosupplementation in the management of symptomatic lumbar facet OA.

Finally, it is worth of note that the side effects of HA are negligible. In quite all the clinical trials, no general side effects were observed, and only few patients reported a sensation of heaviness and pain in their joint after injection [9]. These effects were more frequent in studies performed in blind conditions compared to those performed under imaging guidance. No differences were observed in relation to HA preparation used or to the number of injections [9]. Side effects usually disappeared after 2-7 days without any therapeutic intervention and did not limit basic or instrumental activities of daily living. Vascular or nervous complications were never reported, neither gout, chondrocalcinosis, sometimes observed after viscosupplementation of the knee [15]. Septic arthritis or aseptic synovial effusion occurred in a very limited number of cases [58].

3. Platelet rich plasma

Assuming that tissue repair involves the sequential signaling of multiple factors, and therefore the delivery of a single type of molecule is insufficient, the use of PRP is gaining ground focusing on the concept that the co-delivery of various proteins can break the vicious circle based on failure of the repair process that progressively leads to OA.

Indeed, the PRP therapeutic activity is to release a collection of signaling proteins, including growth factors (GFs) and chemokines, among other proteins, to the joint environment, thereby inducing tissue regeneration mechanisms [59-61]. Briefly, regulatory proteins released from PRP must be capable of interfering with the catabolic microenvironment in OA joints while modulating the inflammatory response, inducing cell migration and proliferation, and regulating angiogenesis and cell differentiation. Since PRPs can have a broad range of functions, it is difficult to decide which function or aspect is the most relevant for OA outcome. A full description of signaling proteins released from PRP and their role in modulating inflammation and vascular pathology have been recently appraised in a personal review [59]. Here we focus on describing the properties of PRP on mechanisms that help in building the rationale for creating a combined HA/PRP treatment.

3.1. Precursor cell migration, proliferation and differentiation

Precursor cell migration, proliferation and differentiation are intended biological effects theoretically related to the PRP clinical response. Cartilage is composed of post-mitotic cells incapable of proliferation. Therefore, regeneration may be based on migration of mitotic stem cells or their progeny (precursor cells) to the cartilage surface, followed by differentiation and the synthesis of ECM components. However, avascular nature of cartilage hinders migration of circulating stem cells, thus precursor cells identified in other joint tissues such as the synovium or the Hoffa fat, although with distinct differentiation potency, are candidates to repair cartilage defects; alternatively cells can home cartilage lesions by migrating from the subchondral bone when arthroscopic drilling is performed [62].

3.1.1. Cell migration

PRP exploits the ability of cells to migrate. Actually, by inducing changes in the cell microenvironment, PRP facilitates the motility of BMSCs, Adipose-Derived Stem Cells (ADSCs) and chondrocytes. The ability of PRP to create gradients of GFs and chemokines is based on three central features: first, on the kinetics of release of chemokines from α-granules in platelets, second on the structural and chemical properties of the fibrin scaffold, and finally on the plasmin degradation of the fibrin [63,64].

Platelets release upon activation a huge repertoire of chemokines, GFs and other cytokines prestored in their α-granules. In parallel upon PRP activation, a specialized provisional fibrin network is formed. Fibrin binds several plasma proteins including vitronectin, fibronectin, Von Willebrand factor (vWF), and thrombospondin. Recent research has identified fibronectin as a major factor in human serum to recruit subchondral progenitor cells [65]. Additionally, these proteins within the fibrin bind GFs and form molecular complexes that can dramatically enhance the potency of GFs.

Besides these effects PRP stimulates HA synthesis, as shown by *in vitro* experiments performed on synovial fibroblasts isolated from the synovium of patients with OA undergoing prosthetic surgery, and the newly synthesized HA may help to improve cell motility [66,67].

3.1.2. Cell proliferation

PRP also supports other mechanisms necessary for cartilage repair (i.e. proliferation) [68]. In fact, PRP has been deeply tested and shown to be a safe and suitable supplement to achieve large scale expansion of MSCs for cell therapy purposes. Moreover, PRP not only supports MSCs proliferation, but it is safer and more effective than fetal bovine serum (the typical serum supplement used to expand cells). However, there is no consensus on which PRP formulation is more proliferative: the PRP releasate or the platelet lysate. The former is the supernatant extruded after PRP coagulation, and it may be considered as a PRP serum; the activation method to achieve granule secretion may introduce variability between products [59,69,70]. Alternatively, the platelet lysate is obtained after several freeze/thaw cycles of either PRP or Leukocyte-PRP (L-PRP) [71-73].

Importantly, studies demonstrate that MSCs expanded in PRP derived formulations maintain pluripotency along the passages [71].

3.1.3. Chondrogenic differentiation

Differentiation is of paramount importance to cartilage regeneration. Differentiated cells synthesize specific molecules unique to hyaline cartilage ECM, such as type 2 collagen and aggrecans, in adequate proportion conferring exceptional biomechanical properties to the ECM. Noteworthy, an inflammatory synovial fluid hinders the differentiation of human subchondral progenitor cells, decreasing the expression of aggrecan, type 2 collagen and cartilage oligomeric matrix protein [74]. However, PRP stimulates migration and differentiation of human subchondral cells into chondrocytes highlighting the consequences of manipulating the biological milieu.

Whether PRP drives the cell to chondrogenic differentiation *in vitro* depends on the precursor cell characteristics along with the culture system (i.e. monolayer culture, micromass, 3-D scaffolds).

Proteomic studies demonstrated that chondrocytes cultured with PRP in either mono- or 3D conditions maintained the chondrocyte phenotype or at least de-differentiation was inhibited after several days in culture [75].

3.2. Clinical trials

Conservative management of musculoskeletal conditions with PRP is becoming increasingly popular; however, clinical evidence is preliminary and limited. At present, PRP is an investigational product. However, to advance PRP the International Cellular Medical Society (ICMS) has developed guidelines for the handling and delivery of PRP and safety recommendations. The final goal is to assist physicians in performing safe therapies. Absolute contraindications for PRP administration include platelet dysfunction syndrome, critical thrombocytopenia, hemodynamic instability, septicemia, local infection at the site of the procedure and patient unwilling to accept risks.

OA is one of the most common indications for PRP injections. Most studies focus on knee OA [76-78], but there are two case series on hip OA and a prospective cohort on osteochondral lesions in the ankle [59]. These studies, merely aiming to demonstrate a clinically meaningful result (e.g., pain relief and functional improvement), have used patient-reported outcomes as end points (WOMAC, KOOS, IKDC and VAS). Importantly, clinical studies performed thus far have strongly supported the safety of PRP (no infections, worsened outcomes, or serious complication have been reported). The fact that PRP is not a potentially harmful experimental treatment is corroborated by clinical studies in other conditions and medical fields [60].

Two systematic reviews with quantitative synthesis [79] and meta-analysis [80] have evaluated the efficacy of PRP in the treatment of symptomatic knee OA [79] and the effectiveness of PRP injections for treating knee joint cartilage degenerative pathology [80]. The former study included six controlled studies (level I and II) including a total of 577 patients, 264 patients in the experimental PRP treatment. Pooled data using the WOMAC showed that PRP was better than HA injections. Similarly, pooled IKDC scores favored PRP treatment. The authors concluded that as compared with HA, multiple sequential PRP injections are beneficial for patients with mild to moderate OA at six months follow-up.

The latter study [80] was less restrictive in the inclusion criteria and included eight single-arm studies, three controlled cohorts and five randomized controlled trials with a total of 1543 patients. They compared the PRP group pooled values with the pre-treatment values and the control groups treated with HA or placebo. PRP injections showed continual efficacy up to 12 months. The benefits of PRP lasted more than HA. Injection doses equal or less than 2 lead to uncertainty in the therapeutic effects. Regarding knee severity, stratified analysis showed better results at six months in the degenerative chondropathy group (effect size: 3.90, 95%; CI: 2.54-5.26) compared with advanced OA (effect size: 1.59, 95%; CI: 0.85-2.32).

Similar findings were reported in young active patients with osteochondral lesions in the talus [59], while a comparative study in hip OA failed to show any difference between PRP and HA, after 12 months follow-up [81]. Unfortunately, a comparison between these studies is difficult due to different affected joints, differences between products, protocols and outcome measures. Indeed, as pointed out in a recent excellent review [76], several variables can interfere, such as the preparation method, the needle gauge for blood harvest and injection, the platelet concentration, storage, pre-activation and granule secretion, the leukocyte concentration, the anticoagulant and local anesthetic use, the blind or ultrasound-controlled injection, the injection volume and frequency, the disease type and severity, and patient-specific factors. For example, pure PRP and L-PRP formulations are not comparable with each other in terms of leukocyte content, platelet count and plasma volume. Moreover, the platelet and leukocyte concentration of the final L-PRP product can vary by as much as 100% [59]. Whether the differences in the clinical results are secondary to the differences in the formulation requires clarification. Similar improvements in pain and function have been observed in patients treated both with PRP and L-PRP, albeit L-PRP caused more swelling and post-injection pain [60]. It is worth mentioning that in these studies, storage of L-PRP introduces additional variability of the final product [59,60]. Regarding administration procedures, the volume and number of injections is empirically determined for each study. Although most studies involve three injections, the period between the injections is variable, ranging from 1 to 4 weeks. In knee OA, PRP is generally injected into the femoro-tibial compartment, although Sampson [82] injected PRP into the suprapatellar bursa and reported increased cartilage thickness in 6 out of 13 patients (46%). Theoretically, PRP application would be much more efficacious in patients with early post-traumatic OA before the radiographic signs become severe, but this needs further confirmation. In patients with significant irreversible bone and cartilage damage, the effect of PRPs would most likely be less impressive, even so, PRP therapy probably would still improve the patients' quality of life. Whether frequent PRP administration can delay OA progression and replacement surgery in patients with advanced OA may be a plausible hypothesis, but long-term studies using surrogate end points such as WOMAC reduction and refined imaging and biochemical markers potentially predictive of the delay of OA progression are required.

4. Hyaluronic acid and platelet rich plasma association

4.1. PRP+HA: A pericellular bioactive scaffold

It is conceivable that HA facilitates the molecular pool released from PRP to reach the target cells by creating a pericellular bioactive scaffold around the cells. This pericellular matrix may facilitate molecular diffusion and also adequate presentation of cytokines to their transmembrane receptors located in the cytoplasmic membrane of the target competent cell. Moreover, because the synovium is more cellular than the cartilage or the meniscus, and the ECM is looser, the signaling molecules will diffuse and reach the synovial cells easier. In doing so the molecular signaling pool released from PRP will reach mainly synovial cells before being degraded. Therefore molecules released from PRP will reach primarily the synovial cells and change their secretory pattern. The latter are responsible for creating the biological conditions within the joint.

Instead, cartilage has a tightly packed ECM. Although signaling molecules such as cytokines and GFs have low molecular weight, are water-soluble and diffuse easily, the number of cell targeted may be much lower than in the synovium.

Another advantage of HA+PRP is facilitation of cells division and migration as this is a common hallmark of matrices that are rich in HA. This is relevant since MSCs have been identified in the synovium and in the synovial fluid.

Assuming that we target synovial cells and MSCs from the synovial niche, whether HMW or LMW is optimal to be mixed with PRP should be investigated in the laboratory.

4.2. How PRP+HA injections may work?

Recent basic research supports the idea that HA and PRP treatments can be advantageously associated without altering the original relevant characteristics of both products. Recently, in a co-culture model, involving synovial cells and chondrocytes, Sundman et al. [83] compared the effects of PRP or HA on inflammation, as measured by TNF-α, IL-6 and IL-8 proteins; they found that, although both treatments decreased TNF-α production, IL-6 was decreased only in HA cultures, but not in PRP treated cells, suggesting that both treatments influence inflammation through different mechanisms. The expression of catabolic enzymes such as metalloproteinases was reduced in synoviocytes and chondrocytes treated with PRP but not in cells treated with HA. Moreover, the synoviocytes treated with PRP but not those treated with HA expressed HAS-2. Thus, separately, HA and PRP are beneficial for joint cells although they function through different mechanisms. Therefore, we may infer that their advantages might be additive when both products are injected. Anitua et al. [66] evaluated the potential of pure PRP to induce tendon cells and synovial fibroblasts migration and examined whether the combination of PRP with HA improves their motility *in vitro*. Human fibroblast cells were isolated from synovium and tendon biopsies and cultured by standard procedures. Therefore, PRP was obtained from a young healthy donor and added to the culture medium at different doses. Finally, the migratory capacity induced by PRP, HA, and both in association were tested. PRP stimulated the migration of fibroblasts, as well as HA, but this effect was more prominent when HA was combined with PRP. Indeed, an increase of 335% in motility was observed in the case of HA+PRP treatment compared with HA. Therefore, this *in vitro* study definitely proves that PRP improves the biological properties of HA. CD44 has been implicated in the migratory signal transduction, as well as receptor for HA-mediated motility in several cell lineages. Plasma derived GFs increase the CD44 expression, and this favors cell migration though the interaction of this receptor with extracellular HA. In another study [84], the outgrowth of rabbit chondrocytes from cartilage fragments, loaded onto a composite scaffold made of a HMW HA and autologous PRP, was evaluated. Defects were created by means of a medial arthrotomy, in rabbit knees, and cartilage fragments were collected. Therefore, membrane scaffolds with HA were prepared and cartilage fragments were loaded into the membrane. Finally, the *in vivo* defects were filled with cartilage fragment load HA scaffolds alone, or adding PRP. A histological evaluation at 6 months showed that this latter group had better results, being filled by a repair tissue with some features of hyaline cartilage. This repair tissue was better quality than that of the lesions treated with scaffold only and untreated lesions.

The idea of positive interactions between HA and PRP is supported by an elegant experiment where HA was added to GFs present in platelets. Bone morphogenetic protein (BMP) 2 plays a critical role in the embryologic development of normal cartilage, thus it may enhance reparative processes by setting in motion morphogenetic processes, including the formation of ECM. Unfortunately, the high chondrogenic potency of BMP2 is hampered by its short half life and rapid degradation in vivo. Perlecan/HSPG2, a heparan sulfate proteoglycan, represents an essential component of cartilage ECM. Due to specific receptors Perlecan can act as a depot for BMP2 storage and controlled kinetics, protecting BMP2 from proteolytic cleavage. To avoid its own diffusion and susceptibility to degradation, PlnD1 was immobilized through conjugation to a larger biocompatible carrier forming HA-based microgels (PlnD1-HA) in order to preserve BMP2 activities [85]. The efficiency of this system was tested using an experimental OA model in mice. It was observed that knees treated with PlnD1-HA/BMP2 had lesser damage compared to control knees [86]. Moreover, they had, in comparison to controls treated with Perlecan+HA, higher mRNA levels of type II collagen, proteoglycans, and xylosyltransferase 1, a rate-limiting anabolic enzyme involved in the biosynthesis of glycosaminoglycans. In conclusion, this study shows that HA can favor the stabilization of some GFs, enabling their therapeutic potential.

A synergistic anabolic actions of HA and PRP has been also demonstrated in a 3D arthritic neo-cartilage and ACLT-OA model. Indeed, the combination of HA+PRP can synergistically promote cartilage regeneration and inhibit OA inflammation [87].

Currently, no clinical studies support this basic research. There are reports, which claim excellent results of the HA+PRP association in Morton neuroma surgery [88] and in the healing of pressure ulcers and surgical wounds [89,90]. However, these findings need confirmation by controlled trials, because only one study [90] has assessed the superiority of the composite PRP/HA in the treatment of pressure ulcers, in comparison with HA or PRP, used alone.

The ability to understand and control the factors that play a role in the therapeutic effect of HA+PRP shall guide the optimization and design of the combination i.e. optimal ratio, molecular weight of HA, optimal PRP formulation.

5. Conclusions

OA is characterized by an impaired regeneration ability mainly attributed to an aberrant cycle of cartilage degradation inducing synovial inflammation and protease activities that in turn induce further joint catabolism. PRP+HA IA injections may break this vicious cycle skewing the milieu towards anti-inflammatory and chondroprotective functions.

It is definitely proved that both HA or PRP alleviate symptoms in patients with mild-moderate OA. Both treatment schedules most often involve repetitive injections, and are comparable in terms of the route of administration and safety.

The concept behind HA application is to mimic the properties of synovial fluid, that is to lubricate the hinge joint. Nevertheless, more recently, the idea that in homeostasis the synovial fluid not only lubricates the joint but provides a positive biological micro-environment has prompted research on HA signaling through hyaladherins located in the cell membrane. Unfortunately, in OA, a deleterious fluidic micro-environment is already established, with the presence of HA fragments, catabolic enzymes, and inflammatory molecules. In this context, the central concept underlying IA injection is to modify this vicious circle. Alternatively, the joint micro-environment can be modified with PRP injections that deliver multiple factors that modulate angiogenesis and inflammation as well as cell anabolism. In fact, the relationships between joint tissues (meniscus, synovium, ligaments, articular surface) and the synovial fluid are bidirectional meaning that they both (the tissues and the synovial fluid) modify and are modified. So, by injecting PRP and HA we aim to replace the ill-fluid with an "engineered fluid" providing lubrication and able to control the delivery and presentation of signaling molecules.

HA and PRP may improve OA symptoms through dissimilar biological mechanisms. Since HA and PRP are not mechanical but biological approaches, the ability of PRP+HA to change the biological status of the joint and promote tissue healing will be particularly critical during the initial stages of OA, before the onset of structural changes. Although mixing HA and PRP involves minimal manipulation, studies to verify critical aspects of the character and performance of the composite are mandatory. Several key aspects such as the molecular weight of HA and the concentration to be mixed with PRP should be analyzed. Ideally, HA tertiary structure should let spaces through which molecules can diffuse, and approach the cell membrane to interact closely with their specific receptors. Whether or not HA may help to retain PRP in the joint cavity by exerting osmotic pressure on the joint surface calls for exploration. Considering that the HA chains are constantly moving in solution, and that effective pores in this meshwork will depend on HA concentration and MW, molecules may reach the articular surfaces with different kinetics, depending on their size and hydrodynamic volumes. The future impact of HA+PRP would depend on the capacity of delivering molecules that meet the requirements of the injured joint. An efficient IA therapy would be achieved if modulatory proteins released from PRP+HA are capable of interfering with the catabolic micro-environment while modulating the inflammatory response, enhancing cell migration and proliferation, and controlling the angiogenic status as well as cell differentiation. A new device capable to mix PRP with HA in prefixed amounts is on the market. Un-published preliminary data suggest that this combination is useful in the treatment of different forms of OA but only prospective randomized double blind studies, preferably using both HA and PRP as comparators (three armed), and a selected stage of OA severity, preferable early OA, will provide sound information about the impact of this novel approach.

Author details

Michele Abate[1], Isabel Andia[2] and Vincenzo Salini[1]

*Address all correspondence to: m.abate@unich.it

1 Department of Medicine and Science of Aging, University G. d'Annunzio, Chieti, Italy

2 BioCruces/Cruces University Hospital, Barakaldo, Spain

References

[1] Felson DT. Developments in the clinical understanding of osteoarthritis. Arthritis Res Ther. 2009;11(1) 203-214.

[2] Cross M, Smith E, Hoy D, Nolte S, Ackerman I, Fransen M, Bridgett L, Williams S, Guillemin F, Hill CL, Laslett LL, Jones G, Cicuttini F, Osborne R, Vos T, Buchbinder R, Woolf A, March L. The global burden of hip and knee osteoarthritis: estimates from the global burden of disease 2010 study. Ann Rheum Dis. 2014;73(7) 1323-1330.

[3] Lawrence, RC, Helmick CG, Arnett FC, Deyo RA, Felson DT, Giannini EH, Heyse SP, Hirsch R, Hochberg MC, Hunder GG, Liang MH, Pillemer SR, Steen VD, Wolfe F. Estimates of the prevalence of arthritis and selected musculoskeletal disorders in the United States. Arthritis Reum. 1998;41(5) 778-799.

[4] Hochberg MC, Altman RD, Brandt KD, Clark BM, Dieppe PA, Griffin MR,Moskowitz RW, Schnitzer TJ. Guidelines for the medical management of osteoarthritis. Part II. Osteoarthritis of the knee. American College of Rheumatology. Arthritis Rheum. 1995;38(11) 1541-1546.

[5] Smalley WE, Griffin MR. The risks and costs of upper gastrointestinal disease attributable to NSAIDs. Gastroenterol Clin North Am. 1996; 25(2) 373-396.

[6] Roughead EE, Ramsay E, Pratt N, Gilbert, AL. NSAID use in individuals at risk of renal adverse events: an observational study to investigate trends in Australian veterans. Drug Saf. 2008;31(11) 997-1003.

[7] Mader R, Lavi I, Luboshitzky R. Evaluation of the pituitary-adrenal axis function following single intraarticular injection of methylprednisolone. Arthritis Rheum. 2005;52(3) 924-928.

[8] Meyer K, Plamer JW. The polysaccharide from the vitreous humour. J Biol Chem 1934;107 629-634.

[9] Abate M, Salini V. Hyaluronic acid in the treatment of osteoarthritis: what is new. In: Chen Q. (ed) Osteoarthritis, Diagnosis, Treatment and Surgery. Rijeka: Intech; 2012. p101-122.

[10] Reitinger S, Lepperdinger G. Hyaluronan, a ready choice to fuel regeneration: a mini review. Gerontology 2013;59 71-76.

[11] Fraser JR, Laurent TC, Laurent UB. Hyaluronan: its nature, distribution, functions and turnover. J Intern Med. 1997; 242(1) 27-33.

[12] Juranek I, Stern R, Soltes L. Hyaluronan peroxidation is required for normal synovial function: an hypothesis. Med Hypotheses. 2014;82(6) 662-666.

[13] Muto J, Yamasaki K, Taylor KR, Gallo RL. Engagement of CD44 by hyaluronan suppresses TLR4 signaling and the septic response to LPS. Mol Immunol. 2009; 47(2) 449-456.

[14] Bollyky PL, Falk BA, Wu RP, Buckner JH, Wight TN, Nepom GT. Intact extracellular matrix and the maintenance of immune tolerance: high molecular weight hyaluronan promotes persistence of induced CD4+CD25+ regulatory T cells. J Leukoc Biol. 2009; 86(3) 567-572.

[15] Abate M, Pulcini D, Di Iorio A, Schiavone C. Viscosupplementation with intra-articular hyaluronic acid for treatment of osteoarthritis in the elderly. Curr Pharm Des. 2010;16(6) 631-640.

[16] Zhang FJ, Luo W, Gao SG, Su DZ, Li YS, Zeng C, Lei GH. Expression of CD44 in articular cartilage is associated with disease severity in knee osteoarthritis. Mod Rheumatol 2013;23(6) 1186-1191.

[17] Musumeci G, Loreto C, Carnazza ML, Cardile V, Leonardi R. Acute injury affects lubricin expression in knee menisci: an immunohistochemical study. Ann Anat. 2013;195(2) 151-158.

[18] Wang LS, Du C, Toh WS, Wan AC, Gao SJ, Kurisawa M. Modulation of chondrocyte functions and stiffness dependent cartilage repair using an injectable enzymatically crosslinked hydrogel with tunable mechanical properties. Biomaterials. 2014;35(7) 2207-2217.

[19] Lurati A, Laria A, Mazzocchi D, Angela RK, Marrazza M, Scarpellini M. Effects of Hyaluronic Acid (HA) viscosupplementation on peripheral Th cells in knee and hip osteoarthritis. Osteoarthritis Cartilage. 2014 Sep 19.

[20] Zavan B, Ferroni L, Giorgi C, Calò G, Brun P, Cortivo R, Abatangelo G, Pinton P. Hyaluronic acid induces activation of the κ-opioid receptor.PLoS One. 2013;8(1) e55510.

[21] Bagga H, Burkhardt D, Sambrook P, March L. Longterm effects of intraarticular hyaluronan on synovial fluid in osteoarthritis of the knee. J Rheumatol. 2006;33(5) 946-950.

[22] Migliore A, Giovannangeli F, Granata M, Lagana B. Hylan G-F 20: review of its safety and efficacy in the management of joint pain in osteoarthritis. Clin Med Insights Arthritis Musculoskelet Disord. 2010;3 55-68.

[23] Morgen M, Tung D, Boras B, Miller W, Malfait AM, Tortorella M. Nanoparticles for improved local retention after intra- articular injection into the knee joint. Pharm Res. 2013;30(1) 257-268.

[24] Henrotin Y, Hauzeur JP, Bruel P, Appelboom T. Intra-articular use of a medical device composed of hyaluronic acid and chondroitin sulfate (Structovial CS): effects on clinical, ultrasonographic and biological parameters. BMC Res Notes. 2012;5 407.

[25] Dong J, Jiang D, Wang Z, Wu G, Miao L, Huang L. Intra-articular delivery of liposomal celecoxib-hyaluronate combination for the treatment of osteoarthritis in rabbit model. Int J Pharm. 2013;441(1-2) 285-290.

[26] Lu HT, Sheu MT, Lin YF, Lan J, Chin YP, Hsieh MS, Cheng CW, Chen CH. Injectable hyaluronic-acid-doxycycline hydrogel therapy in experimental rabbit osteoarthritis. BMC Vet Res. 2013;9 68.

[27] Migliore A, Massafra U, Bizzi E, Tormenta S, Cassol M, Granata M. Duration of symptom relief after intra-articular injection of hyaluronic acid combined with sorbitol (anti-ox-vs) in symptomatic hip osteoarthritis. Int J Immunopathol Pharmacol. 2014;27(2) 245-252.

[28] Miller LE, Block JE. US-Approved Intra-Articular Hyaluronic Acid Injections are Safe and Effective in Patients with Knee Osteoarthritis: Systematic Review and Meta-Analysis of Randomized, Saline-Controlled Trials. Clin Med Insights Arthritis Musculoskelet Disord. 2013;6 57-63.

[29] Bannuru RR, Natov NS, Dasi UR, Schmid CH, McAlindon TE. Therapeutic trajectory following intra-articular hyaluronic acid injection in knee osteoarthritis-meta-analysis. Osteoarthritis Cartilage. 2011;19(6) 611-619.

[30] Henrotin Y, Chevalier X, Deberg M, Balblanc JC, Richette P, Mulleman D, Maillet B, Rannou F, Piroth C, Mathieu P, Conrozier T; Osteoarthritis Group of French Society of Rheumatology.. Early decrease of serum biomarkers of type II collagen degradation (Coll2-1) and joint inflammation by hyaluronic acid intra-articular injections in

patients with knee osteoarthritis: a research study part of the Biovisco study. J Orthop Res. 2013;31(6) 901-917.

[31] Migliore A, Tormenta S, Laganà B, Piscitelli P, Granata M, Bizzi E, Massafra U, Giovannangeli F, Maggi C, De Chiara R, Iannessi F, Sanfilippo A, Camminiti M, Pagano MG, Bagnato G, Iolascon G. Safety of intra-articular hip injection of hyaluronic acid products by ultrasound guidance: an open study from ANTIAGE register. Eur Rev Med Pharmacol Sci. 2013 Jul;17(13) 1752-1759.

[32] Paoloni M, Di Sante L, Dimaggio M, Bernetti A, Mangone M, Di Renzo S, Santilli V. Kinematic and kinetic modifications in walking pattern of hip osteoarthritis patients induced by intra-articular injections of hyaluronic acid. Clin Biomech (Bristol, Avon). 2012;27(7) 661-665.

[33] Migliore A, Bella A, Bisignani M, Calderaro M, De Amicis D, Logroscino G, Mariottini F, Moreschini O, Massafra U, Bizzi E, Laganà B, Piscitelli P, Tormenta S. Total hip replacement rate in a cohort of patients affected by symptomatic hip osteoarthritis following intra-articular sodium hyaluronate (MW 1,500-2,000 kDa) ORTOBRIX study. Clin Rheumatol. 2012;31(8) 1187-1196.

[34] Migliore A, Bizzi E, Massafra U, Bella A, Piscitelli P, Laganà B, Tormenta S. The impact of treatment with hylan G-F 20 on progression to total hip arthroplasty in patients with symptomatic hip OA: a retrospective study. Curr Med Res Opin. 2012;28(5) 755-760.

[35] Migliore A, Granata M, Tormenta S, Laganà B, Piscitelli P, Bizzi E, Massafra U, Alimonti A, Maggi C, De Chiara R, Iannessi F, Sanfilippo A, Sotera R, Scapato P, Carducci S, Persod P, Denaro S, Camminiti M, Pagano MG, Bagnato G, Iolascon G. Hip viscosupplementation under ultra-sound guidance riduces NSAID consumption in symptomatic hip osteoarthritis patients in a long follow-up. Data from Italian registry. Eur Rev Med Pharmacol Sci. 2011;15(1) 25-34.

[36] Abate M, Schiavone C, Salini V. Hyaluronic acid in ankle osteoarthritis: why evidence of efficacy is still lacking? Clin Exp Rheumatol. 2012;30(2) 277-281.

[37] DeGroot H 3rd, Uzunishvili S, Weir R, Al-omari A, Gomes B. Intra-articular injection of hyaluronic acid is not superior to saline solution injection for ankle arthritis: a randomized, double-blind, placebo-controlled study. J Bone Joint Surg Am. 2012;94(1) 2-8.

[38] Salk RS, Chang TJ, D'Costa WF, Soomekh DJ, Grogan KA. Sodium hyaluronate in the treatment of osteoarthritis of the ankle: a controlled, randomized, double-blind pilot study. J Bone Joint Surg Am. 2006;88(2) 295-302.

[39] Cohen MM, Altman RD, Hollstrom R, Hollstrom C, Sun C, Gipson B. Safety and efficacy of intra – articular sodium hyaluronate (Hyalgan) in a randomized, double-blind study for osteoarthritis of the ankle. Foot and Ankle International. 2008;29(7) 657-663.

[40] Karatosun V, Unver B, Ozden A, Ozay Z, Gunal I. Intra-articular hyaluronic acid compared to exercise therapy in osteoarthritis of the ankle. A prospective randomized trial with long-term follow-up. Clinical and experimental rheumatology. 2008;26(2) 288-294.

[41] Carpenter B, Motley T. The role of viscosupplementation in the ankle using hylan G-F 20. Journal of Foot & Ankle Surgery. 2008; 47(5) 377-384.

[42] Han SH, Park do Y, Kim TH. Prognostic factors after intra-articular hyaluronic acid injection in ankle osteoarthritis. Yonsei Med J. 2014;55(4) 1080-1086.

[43] Lucas Y Hernandez J, Darcel V, Chauveaux D, Laffenêtre O. Viscosupplementation of the ankle: a prospective study with an average follow-up of 45.5 months. Orthop Traumatol Surg Res. 2013;99(5) 593-599.

[44] Cunnington J, Marshall N, Hide G, Bracewell C, Isaacs J, Platt P, Kane D. A randomized, double-blind, controlled study of ultrasound-guided corticosteroid injection into the joint of patients with inflammatory arthritis. Arthritis Rheum. 2010; 62(7) 1862-1869.

[45] Merolla G, Bianchi P, Porcellini G. Ultrasound-guided subacromial injections of sodium hyaluronate for the management of rotator cuff tendinopathy: a prospective comparative study with rehabilitation therapy. Musculoskelet Surg. 2013;97 49-56.

[46] Merolla G, Sperling JW, Paladini P, Porcellini G. Efficacy of Hylan G-F 20 versus 6-methylprednisolone acetate in painful shoulder osteoarthritis: a retrospective controlled trial. Musculoskelet Surg. 2011;95(3) 215-224.

[47] Kwon YW, Eisenberg G, Zuckerman JD. Sodium hyaluronate for the treatment of chronic shoulder pain associated with glenohumeral osteoarthritis: a multicenter, randomized, double-blind, placebo-controlled trial. J Shoulder Elbow Surg. 2013;22(5) 584-594.

[48] Salini V, De Amicis D, Abate M, Natale MA, Di Iorio A. Ultrasound-guided hyaluronic acid injection in carpometacarpal osteoarthritis: short-term results. Int J Immunopathol Pharmacol. 2009;22(2) 455-460.

[49] Ingegnoli F, Soldi A, Meroni PL. Power Doppler sonography and clinical monitoring for hyaluronic Acid treatment of rhizarthrosis: a pilot study. J Hand Microsurg. 2013;3(2) 51-54.

[50] Guarda-Nardini L, Rossi A, Ramonda R, Punzi L, Ferronato G, Manfredini D. Effectiveness of treatment with viscosupplementation in temporomandibular joints with or without effusion. Int J Oral Maxillofac Surg. 2014;43(10) 1218-1223.

[51] Su N, Yang X, Liu Y, Huang Y, Shi Z. Evaluation of arthrocentesis with hyaluronic acid injection plus oral glucosamine hydrochloride for temporomandibular joint osteoarthritis in oral-health-related quality of life. J Craniomaxillofac Surg. 2014;42(6) 846-851.

[52] Triantaffilidou K, Venetis G, Bika O. Efficacy of hyaluronic acid injections in patients with osteoarthritis of the temporomandibular joint. A comparative study. J Craniofac Surg. 2013;24(6) 2006-2009.

[53] Manfredini D, Guarda-Nardini L, Ferronato G. Single-needle temporomandibular joint arthrocentesis with hyaluronic acid injections. Preliminary data after a five-injection protocol Minerva Stomatol. 2009;58(10) 471-478.

[54] El-Hakim IE, Elyamani AO. Preliminary evaluation of histological changes found in a mechanical arthropatic temporomandibular joint (TMJ) exposed to an intra-articular Hyaluronic acid (HA) injection, in a rat model. J Craniomaxillofac Surg. 2011;39(8) 610-614.

[55] Guarda-Nardini L, Ferronato G, Favero L, Manfredini D. Predictive factors of hyaluronic acid injections short-term effectiveness for TMJ degenerative joint disease. J Oral Rehabil. 2011;38(5) 315-320.

[56] Fuchs S, Erbe T, Fischer HL, Tibesku CO. Intraarticular hyaluronic acid versus glucocorticoid injections for nonradicular pain in the lumbar spine. J Vasc Interv Radiol. 2005;16(11) 1493-1498.

[57] Cleary M, Keating C Poynton AR. Viscosupplementation in lumbar facet joint arthropathy: a pilot study. J Spinal Disord Tech. 2008;21(1) 29-32.

[58] Chazerain P, Rolland D, Cordonnier C, Ziza JM. Septic hip arthritis after multiple injections into the joint of hyaluronate and glucocorticoid. Rev Rhum Engl Ed. 1999;66(7-9) 436.

[59] Andia I, Abate M. Platelet-rich plasma: underlying biology and clinical correlates. Regen Med. 2013;8(5) 645-658.

[60] Andia I, Abate M. Knee osteoarthritis: hyaluronic acid, platelet-rich plasma or both in association? Expert Opin Biol Ther. 2014;14(5) 635-649.

[61] Andia I, Maffulli N. Platelet-rich plasma for managing pain and inflammation in osteoarthritis. Nat Rev Rheumatol. 2013;9(12) 721-730.

[62] Manferdini C, Maumus M, Gabusi E, Piacentini A, Filardo G, Peyrafitte JA, Jorgensen C, Bourin P, Fleury-Cappellesso S, Facchini A, Noël D, Lisignoli G.. Adipose-derived mesenchymal stem cells exert anti-inflammatory effects on chondrocytes and synoviocytes from osteoarthritis patients through prostaglandin E2. Arthritis Rheum. 2013;65(5) 1271-1281.

[63] Murphy MB, Blashki D, Buchanan RM, Yazdi IK, Ferrari M, Simmons PJ, Tasciotti E. Adult and umbilical cord blood-derived platelet-rich plasma for mesenchymal stem cell proliferation, chemotaxis, and cryo preservation. Biomaterials. 2012;33(21) 8-16.

[64] Xie X, Zhang C, Tuan RS. Biology of platelet-rich plasma and its clinical application in cartilage repair. Arthritis Res Ther. 2014 Feb 25;16(1) 204.

[65] Kulawig R, Kruger JP, Klein O, et al. Identification of fibronectin as a major factor in human serum to recruit subchondral mesenchymal progenitor cells. Proc Nat. Acad Sci USA. 2013;110(12) 4563-4568.

[66] Anitua E, Sanchez M, De la Fuente M, Zalduendo MM, Orive G. Plasma rich in growth factors (PRGF-Endoret) stimulates tendon and synovial fibroblasts migration and improves the biological properties of hyaluronic acid. Knee Surg Sports Traumatol Arthrosc. 2012;20(9) 1657-1665.

[67] Anitua E, Sánchez M, Nurden AT, Zalduendo MM, de la Fuente M, Azofra J, Andía I. Platelet-released growth factors enhance the secretion of hyaluronic acid and induce hepatocyte growth factor production by synovial fibroblasts from arthritic patients. Rheumatology (Oxford). 2007;46(12) 1769-1772.

[68] Drengk A, Zapf A, Sturmer EK, Sturmer KM, Frosch KH. Influence of platelet-rich plasma on chondrogenic differentiation and proliferation of chondrocytes and mesenchymal stem cells. Cells Tissues Organs. 2009;189(5) 317-326.

[69] Harrison S, Vavken P, Kevy S, Jacobson M, Zurakowski D, Murray MM. Platelet activation by collagen provides sustained release of anabolic cytokines. Am J Sports Med. 2011;39(4),729-34.

[70] Cavallo C, Filardo G, Mariani E, Kon E, Marcacci M, Pereira Ruiz MT, Facchini A, Grigolo B. Comparison of platelet-rich plasma formulations for cartilage healing: an in vitro study. J Bone Joint Surg Am. 2014;96(5) 423-429.

[71] Griffiths S, Baraniak PR, Copland IB, Nerem RM, McDevitt TC. Human platelet lysate stimulates high-passage and senescent human multipotent mesenchymal stromal cell growth and rejuvenation in vitro. Cytotherapy. 2013;15(12) 1469-1483.

[72] Assirelli E, Filardo G, Mariani E, Kon E, Roffi A, Vaccaro F, Marcacci M, Facchini A, Pulsatelli L. Effect of two different preparations of platelet-rich plasma on synoviocytes. Knee Surg Sports Traumatol Arthrosc. 2014 Jun 19.

[73] Braun HJ, Kim HJ, Chu CR, Dragoo JL. The effect of platelet-rich plasma formulations and blood products on human synoviocytes: implications for intra-articular injury and therapy. Am J Sports Med. 2014; 42(5) 1204-1210.

[74] Krüger JP, Endres M, Neumann K, Stuhlmüller B, Morawietz L, Häupl T, Kaps C. Chondrogenic differentiation of human subchondral progenitor cells is affected by synovial fluid from donors with osteoarthritis or rheumatoid arthritis. J Orthop Surg Res. 2012;7 10.

[75] Spreafico A, Chellini F, Frediani B, Bernardini G, Niccolini S, Serchi T, Collodel G, Paffetti A, Fossombroni V, Galeazzi M, Marcolongo R, Santucci A. Biochemical investigation of the effects of human platelet releasates on human articular chondrocytes. J Cell Biochem. 2009;108(5) 1153-1165.

[76] Pourcho AM, Smith J, Wisniewski SJ, Sellon JL. Intraarticular Platelet-Rich Plasma Injection in the Treatment of Knee Osteoarthritis: Review and Recommendations. Am J Phys Med Rehabil. 2014 May 29.

[77] Rodriguez-Merchan EC. Intraarticular Injections of Platelet-rich Plasma (PRP) in the Management of Knee Osteoarthritis. Arch Bone Jt Surg. 2013;1(1) 5-8.

[78] Guler O, Mutlu S, Isyar M, Seker A, Kayaalp ME, Mahirogullari M. Comparison of short-term results of intraarticular platelet-rich plasma (PRP) and hyaluronic acid treatments in early-stage gonarthrosis patients. Eur J Orthop Surg Traumatol. 2014 Aug 2.

[79] Khoshbin A, Leroux T, Wasserstein D, Marks P, Theodoropoulos J, Ogilvie-Harris D, Gandhi R, Takhar K, Lum G, Chahal J. The efficacy of platelet-rich plasma in the treatment of symptomatic knee osteoarthritis: a systematic review with quantitative synthesis. Arthroscopy. 2013;29(12) 2037-2048.

[80] Chang KV, Hung CY, Aliwarga F, Wang TG, Han DS, Chen WS. Comparative effectiveness of platelet-rich plasma injections for treating knee joint cartilage degenerative pathology: a systematic review and meta-analysis. Arch Phys Med Rehabil. 2014;95(3) 562-575.

[81] Battaglia M, Guaraldi F, Vannini F, Rossi G, Timoncini A, Buda R, Giannini S. Efficacy of ultrasound-guided intra-articular injections of platelet-rich plasma versus hyaluronic acid for hip osteoarthritis. Orthopedics. 2013;36(12):e1501-8.

[82] Sampson S, Reed M, Silvers H, Meng M, Mandelbaum B. Injection of platelet-rich plasma in patients with primary and secondary knee osteoarthritis: a pilot study. Am J Phys Med Rehabil. 2010;89(12) 961-969.

[83] Sundman EA, Cole BJ, Karas V, Della Valle C, Tetreault MW, Mohammed HO, Fortier LA. The Anti-inflammatory and Matrix Restorative Mechanisms of Platelet-Rich Plasma in Osteoarthritis. Am J Sports Med. 2014;42(1) 35-41.

[84] Marmotti A, Bruzzone M, Bonasia DE, Castoldi F, Rossi R, Piras L, Maiello A, Realmuto C, Peretti GM. One-step osteochondral repair with cartilage fragments in a composite scaffold. Knee Surg Sports Traumatol Arthrosc. 2012;20(12) 2590-2601.

[85] Srinivasan PP, McCoy SY, Jha AK, Yang W, Jia X, Farach-Carson MC, Kirn-Safran CB. Injectable perlecan domain 1-hyaluronan microgels potentiate the cartilage repair effect of BMP2 in a murine model of early osteoarthritis. Biomed Mater. 2012;7(2) o24109.

[86] Sánchez M, Azofra J, Anitua E, Andía I, Padilla S, Santisteban J, Mujika I. Plasma rich in growth factors to treat an articular cartilage avulsion: a case report. Med Sci Sports Exerc 2003;35(10) 1648-1652.

[87] Chen WH, Lo WC, Hsu WC, Wei HJ, Liu HY, Lee CH, Tina Chen SY, Shieh YH, Williams DF, Deng WP. Synergistic anabolic actions of hyaluronic acid and platelet-rich

plasma on cartilage regeneration in osteoarthritis therapy. Biomaterials. 2014;35(36) 9599-9607.

[88] De Angelis B, Lucarini L, Orlandi F, Agovino A, Migner A, Cervelli V, Izzo V, Curcio C. Regenerative surgery of the complications with Morton's neuroma surgery: use of platelet rich plasma and hyaluronic acid. Int Wound J 2013;10(4) 372-376.

[89] Cervelli V, Lucarini L, Spallone D, Palla L, Colicchia GM, Gentile P, De Angelis B. Use of platelet-rich plasma and hyaluronic acid in the loss of substance with bone exposure. Adv Skin Wound Care. 2011;24(4) 176-181.

[90] Ramos-Torrecillas J, García-Martínez O, Luna-Bertos ED, Ocaña-Peinado FM, Ruiz C. Effectiveness of Platelet-Rich Plasma and Hyaluronic Acid for the Treatment and Care of Pressure Ulcers. Biol Res Nurs. 2014 May 20.

6

Structural and Functional features of Major Synovial Joints and Their Relevance to Osteoarthritis

Xiaoming Zhang, Brian Egan and Jinxi Wang

1. Introduction

Osteoarthritis (OA) is considered to be an organ disease that may affect all of the articular and peri-articular tissues such as articular cartilage, synovium, ligament, capsule, subchondral bone, and peri-articular muscles [1-3]. Understanding the structural and functional features of the joint is of great significance for the diagnosis and treatment of OA. Although OA can occur in any synovial joint in the body, it mainly attacks the joints responsible for weight/load bearing such as the knee, hip, hand, and ankle joints. In this chapter, we will focus only on the structural and functional features of the major synovial joints and their relevance to osteoarthritis.

2. Shoulder (glenohumeral) joint

The glenohumeral joint is a ball-and-socket joint formed by the shallow glenoid cavity of the scapula and the head of the humerus. The joint cavity is slightly deepened by a ring-shaped fibrocartilage structure called the "glenoidal labrum", which attaches to the edge of the glenoid cavity. Because of its structure, the joint has a wide range of movement in all directions. However, its wide range of mobility is accompanied by instability. Only about 1/3 of the humeral head surface area attaches to the glenoid cavity. The humeral head is held onto the glenoid cavity by the rotator cuff muscles, namely, the supraspinatus, infraspinatus, teres minor, and subscapularis. These four muscles are located superior, posterior, and anterior on three sides around the joint cavity.

The fibrous joint capsule originates from the margin of the glenoid cavity and attaches to the anatomical neck of the humerus. The arrangement of the joint capsule is remarkably loose, particularly inferiorly when the arm is fully adducted (in anatomical position), allowing great separation between the bones of the joint and freedom of motion [4]. There are two apertures: one opens toward the intertubercular groove (sulcus) of the humerus to allow the long head of the biceps tendon to travel into the joint cavity, the other opens to the subscapularis bursa located anterior and inferior to the coracoid process of the scapula. The synovial membrane is lined up the inner surface of the joint capsule. In addition, it forms a tubular sheath wrapping the long head of the biceps tendon and extends into the intertubercular groove.

There are two intrinsic ligaments that are part of the joint capsule, the glenohumeral ligament that strengthens the anterior portion of the capsule and the coracohumeral ligament that is located superiorly. In addition, the transverse humeral ligament holds the long head of the biceps brachii muscle tendon inside the intertuberbular groove, and the coraco-acromial ligament stabilizes the glenohumeral joint from above.

The supraspinatus muscle tendon travels laterally in between the acromion of the scapula and the superior aspect of the joint capsule and attaches to the greater tubercle of the humerus. A synovial bursa called the "subacromial/subdeltoid bursa" is located in between the acromion and the muscle tendon to prevent friction of the latter against the bone. A second bursa associated with the glenohumeral joint is located anterior-inferiorly to the coracoid process at the neck of the scapula. It protects the tendon of the subscapularis muscle from friction against the neck of scapula. This bursa communicates with the joint cavity.

The movement of the glenohumeral joint is in three axes plus circumduction. The extensive range of movement of the joint is due to its structural feature, a large humeral head articulating with a small glenoid cavity and a loose joint capsule. Many muscles move the glenohumeral joint including the thoracoappendicular muscles (muscles that originate from the thoracic wall and attach to the humerus) and scapulohumeral muscles (muscles that originate from the scapula and attach to the humerus).

The glenohumeral joint is supplied by the anterior and posterior circumflex humeral arteries and the suprascapular artery. The joint is innervated by the axillary and lateral pectoral nerves[5].

Commonly seen injuries to the glenohumeral joint and its associated bursae are the following:

a. Subacromial/subdeltoid bursitis due to wear-and-tear.

b. Supraspinatus tendonitis, usually as a further development of subacromial bursitis.

c. Bicipital tendonitis, an inflammatory process of the long head of the biceps tendon inside the intertubercular groove. This process can be accompanied by tendon rupture, and/or transverse humeral ligament tear.

d. Subscapular bursa inflammation (bursitis).

e. Dislocation of the glenohumeral joint, which often happens with the humeral head dislocating inferiorly. If the dislocated humeral head is positioned anterior to the long head of the triceps brachii muscle tendon, it is called an "anterior dislocation". Risk factors for shoulder injury include athletic participation, male gender, and young or old age [6,7].

Young, active individuals can experience dislocation or partial-dislocation of the shoulder during exercise, practice, or competitive events. In prospective cohort studies of young military populations, 3% to 6% sustained shoulder dislocations or partial-dislocations were observed [8,9].

f. Fracture at the surgical neck of the humerus. This fracture often causes axillary nerve injury.

g. Joint instability. Shoulder instability is a significant problem due to the structural features of the shoulder joint. Studies of young and adult patients revealed the chance of recurrent shoulder instability after standard non-operative treatment at 55% to 67%, with the young male population presenting recurring injuries at an 87% rate during a five year follow-up[8,10]. Randomized clinical trials demonstrated that surgical stabilization of the shoulder is more effective to prevent the recurrence of injury than immobilization and rehabilitation alone [11-13]. Identifying specific structural risks associated with shoulder instability is another way to combat recurrent shoulder dislocations.

OA in the glenohumeral joint. Primary OA in the glenohumeral joint is relatively uncommon, and occurs more often in women and patients over the age of 60 [14,15]. In younger patients, it is usually caused by injuries to the joint that occurred several years earlier such as joint dislocation, fracture, rotator cuff tear, and glenoid labrum injury.

3. Elbow joint

The elbow joint is a complex structure involving three bones, the humerus, ulna, and radius, articulating together. There are three joints wrapped within one joint capsule: the humeroulnar joint, the humeroradial joint, and the proximal radioulnar joint.

The humeroulnar joint is formed between the trochlear of the humerus and the trochlear notch of the ulna. It is a typical hinge joint capable of flexion and extension. The humeroradial joint is formed between the capitulum of the humerus and the head of the radius. The capitulum is a ball shaped structure that allows the head of the radius, which is a disc-shaped structure articulating with the capitulum on its flat surface, to move in two directions: flexion and extension, plus axial rotation against the capitulum. The proximal radioulnar joint is formed between the head of the radius (round surface) and the radial notch of the ulna. The radial structure rotates against the ulnar structure when the forearm carries out pronation and supination actions.

The fibrous joint capsule surrounds the elbow joint on four sides with the anterior and posterior sides weaker than those on the medial and lateral sides. Therefore, elbow joint dislocation often happens anteriorly or posteriorly. Synovial membrane lines the inner surface of the fibrous joint capsule.

The fibrous joint capsule thickens on the medial and lateral sides to become medial (ulnar) or lateral (radial) collateral ligaments. The ulnar collateral ligament is a triangular shaped ligament containing three components: the anterior cord-like band (strongest), the posterior fan-like band, and the oblique band. The radial collateral ligament is fan-shaped and connects the lateral epicondyle of the humerus with the annular ligament of the radial head. The annular ligament is a ring-shaped ligament that surrounds the circumference of the disc-shaped radial head and fixes it to the radial notch of the ulna.

The movement of the elbow joint includes flexion/extension and pronation/supination. There are more than a dozen muscles across the elbow joint that participate in moving the joint. Blood is supplied to the elbow joint by anastomosing branches from the humeral artery, radial artery, and ulna artery. Musculocutaneous, radial, and ulnar nerves innervate this joint.

OA in the elbow joint: The elbow is one of the least affected joints by osteoarthritis because of its well matched joint surfaces and strong stabilizing ligaments. As a result, the elbow joint can tolerate large forces across it without becoming unstable. Development of osteoarthritis in elbow joint is usually due to previous injuries to the joint.

4. Wrist (radiocarpal) joint

The wrist joint is a condyloid joint. The proximal joint surface is the distal end of the radius and the articular disc. The distal joint surface is formed by three of the proximal row of carpal bones (scaphoid, lunate, and triquetrum). The ulna and pisiform are not involved in wrist joint formation. The articular disc is a triangular-shaped fibrocartilage structure that connects the styloid process of the ulna to the distal end of the radius. The distal end of the ulna is located proximal to the articular disc and thus does not contact the carpal bones.

The fibrous joint capsule is strengthened by several ligaments which are all part of the fibrous joint capsule. Anteriorly, there is the palmar radiocarpal ligament. Posteriorly, there is the dorsal radiocarpal ligament. On the medial side, there is the ulnar collateral ligament which attaches to the ulnar styloid process. On the lateral side, there is the radial collateral ligament which attaches to the radial styloid process. The synovial membrane lines the internal surface of the fibrous joint capsule and forms numerous synovial folds.

The movement of the wrist joint involves flexion/extension, abduction/adduction, and circumduction. Many muscles from the forearm to the hand move this joint. The wrist joint is supplied by the palmar and dorsal carpal arches which are branches of the radial and ulnar arteries. The innervation of this joint is by median, radial, and ulnar nerves.

OA in the wrist joint: There are different causes, both idiopathic and traumatic, of wrist osteoarthritis. Traumatic causes of wrist OA include injuries to ligament, articular carti- lage, and bone. Although injuries to many wrist ligaments can lead to progressive wrist arthrosis, a chronic scapholunate ligament tear in particular is known to produce intercar- pal instability, altered wrist kinematics and joint loading, and degeneration of the radiocar- pal joint. Fracture and subsequent nonunion of the scaphoid also leads to a series of predictable degenerative changes. Wrist OA can also occur secondary to an intra-articular fracture of the distal radius or ulna or from an extra-articular fracture resulting in malunion and abnormal joint loading [16].

5. Hand joints

There are several groups of joints in the hand. From proximal to distal, the groups are:

a.   Intercarpal joints: These are the joints between the carpal bones within each row and between the proximal and distal rows. They are plane types joints with little movement, and most of them share a common joint cavity.

b.   Carpometacarpal and intermetacarpal joints: These are the joints between the distal row of the carpal bones and the metacarpal bones and also between each metacarpal bone. They are grouped together because they share a common joint cavity. They are all plane types joints except for the carpometacarpal joint of the thumb (1st digit), which is a saddle type joint.

c.   Metacarpophalangeal joints: These are joints between the metacarpal bones and the proximal phalanges. They are condyloid joints allowing bi-directional movements (flexion/extension and adduction/abduction).

d.   Interphalangeal joints: These are the joints between each phalange. They are hinge types joints.

OA in hand: Hand OA is a prevalent disorder. It is not one single disease, but a heterogeneous group of disorders. It may appear as osteophyte or joint space narrowing, interphalangeal nodal, or thumb base erosion [17-19].

6. Hip joint

The hip joint is a ball-and-socket joint formed by the head of the femur (ball) and the acetabulum of the pelvis (socket). It is a very stable joint that bears all the weight of the upper body yet maintains a wide range of movement.

The head of the femur is covered by articular cartilage except for the center where a depression called the "fovea" allows for the attachment of the ligament to the femoral head.

The acetabulum is formed by the fusion of three pelvic bones: pubis, ischium, and ilium. It is a hemispherical hollow socket facing anteriolaterally. The edge of the acetabulum is called the "acetabular rim", which is covered by semilunar-shaped articular cartilage called the "lunate surface of the acetabulum". It is an incomplete circle with the inferior part missing. The missing inferior segment is called the "acetabular notch". This notch is bridged by the "transverse acetabular ligament", which is part of a fibrocartilaginous ring that attaches to the margin of the acetabulum. This lip-shaped ring structure is called the "acetabular labrum". It increases the articular surface of the acetabulum by 10%. The central region of the acetabulum is not covered by any articular cartilage; rather, it is filled with a fat pad. This region is called the "acetabular fossa", which has a thin wall from the ischium and communicates with the acetabular notch (Figure 1).

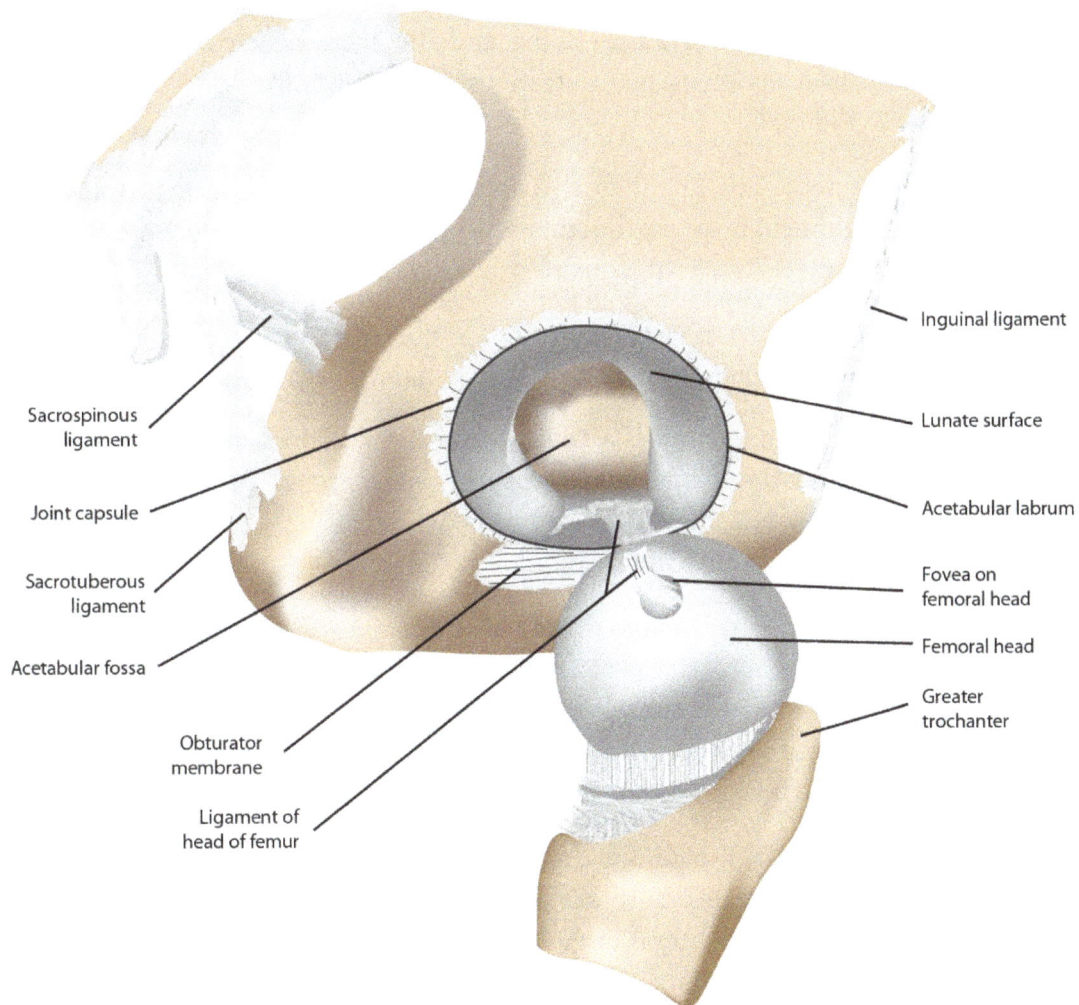

Figure 1. An illustration showing the lateral view of the hip joint. The ligament of the head of the femur has been transected and the femoral head has been dislocated to show the internal structure of the acetabulum.

More than half of the femoral head fits into the acetabulum making the joint the most stable for weight bearing.

The capsule of the hip joint is strong in its fibrous layer. It attaches just outside the acetabular rim proximally and the femoral neck, intertrochanteric line, and greater trochanter distally. Most of the fibers of this joint capsule run in a spiral direction between its two ends. This is particularly true when the hip joint is extended at a standing position (anatomical position). At this position, the joint capsule is tightened, pushing the head of the femur against the acetabulum firmly. When the hip joint is flexed, such as when one is in a sitting position, the spiral joint capsule fibers are "unwound" becoming straight. The straightened joint capsule fibers are longer than their spiral state making the joint capsule loosen for more mobility. The synovial membrane lines up the inner surface of the fibrous joint capsule and forms synovial folds at the femoral neck.

There are three intrinsic joint ligaments that are part of the joint capsule.

a.   Iliofemoral ligament: A Y-shaped ligament located anterior-superiorly to the joint. It attaches to the anterior inferior iliac spine and the acetabular rim proximally and the intertrochanteric line distally. It is the strongest ligament of the body preventing overextension of the hip joint.

b.   Pubofemoral ligament: A ligament located anterior-inferiorly bridging the pubic bone and the iliofemoral ligament. It works together with the latter to prevent overextension of the hip joint. It also protects the joint from over-abduction.

c.   Ischiofemoral ligament: A ligament located posteriorly between the ischium and the femoral neck/greater trochanter.

The ligament of the head of the femur is actually a synovial fold located inside the joint cavity. It attaches to the fovea of the head of the femur at one end and the transverse acetabular ligament at the other. There is a small artery running inside this ligament. It is a weak ligament of little importance for the stability of the joint.

The movement of the hip joint is extensive in all three axes (flexion/extension, abduction/adduction, and medial/lateral rotation) plus circumduction. Its movement is also affected by the positions of the knee and the vertebral column. Muscles in the gluteal region, lumbar region, anterior thigh, medial thigh, and posterior thigh are involved when moving the hip joint. Some muscles move the joint in more than one direction.

The major blood supply to the hip joint is the retinacular arteries arising from the medial and lateral circumflex femoral arteries. Both are branches of the profunda femoris artery or the femoral artery. The medial and lateral circumflex arteries travel along the intertrochanteric ridge and the intertrochanteric line of the femur and anastomose with each other. The retinacular arteries branch off from the circumflex arteries and travel along the neck of the femur to reach the femoral head and the hip joint. When fracture happens to the neck of the femur, retinacular arteries are injured resulting in reduced blood supply to the femoral head and the hip joint.

"Hilton's Law" states that the nerve that innervates the muscles moving the joint also innervates the joint. The following nerves innervate the muscles that move the hip joint: femoral nerve, obturator nerve, and superior and inferior gluteal nerves.

OA in the hip joint: In addition to idiopathic OA, acetabular fracture is a known cause of post-traumatic OA of the hip joint [20]. Acetabular dysplasia is predictive of hip OA and subsequent hip arthroplasty [21]. An increased prevalence of radiographic hip OA and osteophytosis is observed in high bone mass (HBM) cases compared with controls [22]. In addition, the development of knee OA is related to variations in hip and pelvic anatomy [23].

7. Knee joint

The knee joint is formed by three bones: femur, tibia, and patella. It is basically a hinge joint for flexion and extension with additional motions such as gliding (between the femur and patella), rolling (between the femur and tibia), and rotation (between the femur and tibia). There are three articulations in this joint: medial femorotibial (between the medial condyles of the femur and the tibia), lateral femorotibial (between the lateral condyles of the femur and the tibia), and femoropatellar (between the femur and the patella). The articulating surfaces of the femur are ball-shaped, whereas the articulating surfaces of the tibia are flat. When they articulate with each other, it is like two balls placed on a warped table top, making the articulation very unstable. Ligaments, menisci, and muscles strengthen the knee joint (Figure 2).

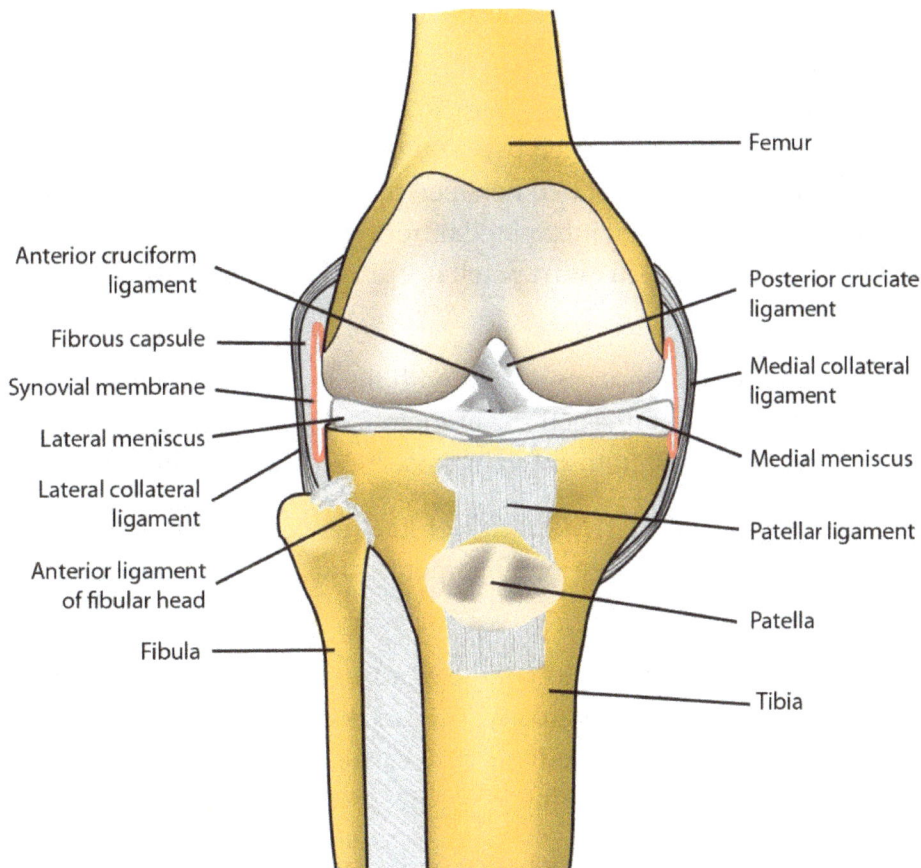

Figure 2. An illustration showing the anterior view of the knee joint with major intra-articular and peri-articular tissues. The patellar ligament has been reflected downward with the attached patella.

The fibrous capsule of the knee joint thickens in some areas to become the intrinsic joint ligaments. Anteriorly, the fibrous capsule merges with the quadriceps tendon, the patella, and the patellar ligament so that these structures become part of the anterior fibrous joint capsule. Posteriorly, the fibrous joint capsule has an opening at the medial condyle of the tibia. This opening allows the tendon of the popliteus muscle to exit the joint capsule and attach to the tibia.

The synovial membrane lines the inside surface of the fibrous joint capsule. In the center of the joint where the intercondylar fossa houses the anterior and posterior cruciate ligaments, the synovial membrane leaves the posterior fibrous capsule and reflects anteriorly into the intercodyle fossa area forming the "infrapatella synovial fold". This synovial fold excludes the cruciate ligaments and the infrapatella fat pad from the joint cavity and almost sub-divides the knee joint cavity into medial and lateral halves. This unique anatomical feature allows surgeons to approach the cruciate ligaments through the posterior fibrous capsule without entering the joint cavity. However, the synovial membrane does not cover the following joint structures: articular cartilages on femur and tibia, the posterior surface of the patella, and the menisci.

There are about 12 bursae around the knee joint; some of them communicate with the joint cavity.

Anteriorly, there are 5 bursae. The suprapatellar bursa is a large, deep bursa located above the patella and under the quadriceps tendon. It communicates with the joint cavity. The synovial membrane of the knee joint becomes the lining of this bursa. There are 2 prepatella bursae: the subtendinous prepatellar bursa is located between the patellar tendon and the patella and the subcutaneous prepatellar bursa is located between the skin and the patellar tendon. There are also 2 infrapatellar bursae: the deep infrapatellar bursa is located between the patellar tendon and the tibia and the subcutaneous infrapatellar bursa is located between the skin and the patellar tendon.

Posteriorly, there are several bursae associated with the muscle attachments around the knee joint such as the gastrocnemius bursae, the semimembranosus bursa, and the popliteus bursa. These bursae are less clinically significant than those located in the anterior aspect of the knee.

The knee joint is strengthened by two groups of ligaments, external ligaments and internal ligaments. There are five external knee joint ligaments, and most of them are part of the fibrous joint capsule (intrinsic ligaments).

The patellar ligament is the distal portion of the quadriceps tendon when it wraps the patella and goes on to insert into the tibial tuberosity. On each side of the patellar ligament extending from the aponeurosis of the vastus medialis and vastus lateralis, are the medial and lateral "patellar retinacula", which help to maintain the position of the patella.

There are two collateral ligaments on each side of the knee joint. The medial (tibial) collateral ligament (MCL or TCL) is a flat, broad band of the fibrous joint capsule. Its fibers continue into the medial meniscus connecting the two. When the MCL is injured, the medial meniscus is mostly involved. The lateral (fibular) collateral ligament (LCL or FCL) is a cord-like strong extracapsular ligament. It attaches to the fibular head splitting the tendon of the biceps femoris muscle. It is separated from the joint capsule by the tendon of the popliteus muscle, and therefore is not connected to the lateral meniscus.

The oblique and arcuate popliteal ligaments are located posteriorly to the knee joint and strengthen the joint capsule posteriorly.

The internal or intra-articular ligaments include the cruciate ligaments and the meniscal ligaments. The cruciate ligaments are located inside the fibrous joint capsule in the intercondylar fossa but outside the synovial membrane, and therefore outside the joint cavity. They cross each other and play the most important role in maintaining the contact between the femur and the tibia when the knee is flexed. Whatever position the knee joint is at, one of the cruciate ligaments is maintained in tension.

The anterior cruciate ligament (ACL) arises from the anterior intercondylar area of the tibia posterior to the attachment of the medial meniscus, travels posterior-laterally, and attaches to the medial surface of the lateral condyle of the femur. When the ACL travels across the posterior cruciate ligament (PCL), it is on the lateral side of the PCL. The ACL prevents the posterior movement of the femur from the tibial plateau when the knee is extended. When the knee joint is flexed, the ACL prevents the anterior movement of the tibia from the femur [24,25].

The posterior cruciate ligament (PCL) arises from the posterior intercondylar area of the tibia, travels anteriorly on the medial side of the ACL, and attaches to the lateral surface of the medial condyle of the femur. It is stronger than the ACL. When the knee joint is extended, the PCL prevents the anterior movement of the femur from the tibial plateau. When the knee is flexed, the PCL prevents the posterior movement of the tibia from the femur.

Because of the anatomical relationship between the two cruciate ligaments, the medial rotation of the tibia is limited to about $10°$ when the knee is flexed. This is because the ACL is pushed against the PCL and the latter blocks the ACL from moving medially during the rotation. Under the same situation but reversing direction, the lateral rotation of the tibia is about $60°$ because the two cruciate ligaments are moving away from each other.

The menisci are crescent-shaped fibrocartilage structures located on the articular surface of the tibia. They are thicker at the external margins and thin in the central edges, thereby deepening the surface of the tibial articular surface. They attach to the intercondylar area of the tibia with their ends and to the fibrous joint capsule on each side. Other than these attachments, the menisci are free of attachment to other joint structures. Therefore, they are mobile along with the knee joint movement. The medial meniscus is C-shaped, attaches to the medial collateral ligament and is less mobile. The lateral meniscus is almost O-shaped and is more movable.

The movement of the knee joint is essentially flexion and extension. During these actions, the patella glides against the femur and the femur rolls against the tibial plateau. When the knee joint is in the fully extended position with the foot on the ground, the femur may rotate $5°$medially along its longitudinal axis on the tibial plateau. This is the locking of the knee. When the knee is "locked", the knee joint is stable for weight bearing and the thigh and leg muscles can briefly relax. To "unlock" the knee, the popliteus muscle rotates the femur laterally about $5°$ [26-28].

When the knee joint is extended, the contacting area between the femur and the tibia moves anteriorly; when the knee is flexed, this contacting area moves posteriorly. As a result, the menisci, particularly the lateral meniscus, moves anteriorly during extension, and posteriorly during flexion.

The blood supply to the knee joint is from the genicular arteries branched from the popliteal artery. Extensive anastomoses form around the knee joint. The nerve innervation of the knee joint follows Hilton's law by femoral, obturator, and sciatic nerves.

The knee joint is the most vulnerable joint for injury. Structures that are most frequently injured are the ACL, MCL, and the medial meniscus. Because of its weight bearing feature, the knee joint is also the most affected joint for OA [29-31].

8. Ankle joint

The ankle joint is a hinge joint involving three bones: distal tibia, distal fibula, and superior surface of talus. The distal end of the tibia forms an L-shaped joint surface with its horizontal aspect articulating with the talus from above and its vertical aspect articulating with the talus on the medial side. The distal end of the tibia forms the medial malleolus. The fibula articulates with the talus on the lateral side and forms the lateral malleolus. The distal tibia and distal fibula are connected together by ligaments forming an open rectangular recess like a mortise facing inferiorly. The superior surface of the talus sits inside the mortise like a trochlea to form the ankle joint with three articular surfaces, superior and medially by tibia and laterally by fibula.

The superior articular surface of the talus is not rectangular in shape, but rather trapezoidal with a wider anterior measure and a narrower posterior measure. When the ankle joint is dorsiflexed, the wider anterior portion of the talus sits in the mortise formed by the tibia and fibula. In this situation, there is little room for the talus to move inside the joint cavity. Therefore, the ankle joint is most stable when the foot is dorsiflexed. On the contrary, when the ankle joint is plantarflexed, the narrower posterior portion of the talus sits inside the mortise and there is more room laterally for the talus to move. In this situation, the ankle joint is unstable and is vulnerable to injuries.

The joint capsule of the ankle joint is loose anteriorly and posteriorly but strengthened on each side by collateral ligaments. Synovial membrane lines the internal surface of the fibrous capsule.

The ligaments of the ankle joint can be grouped into those that stabilize the tibia and the fibula and those that are located on each side of the joint.

There is an interosseous ligament located deep between the tibia and the fibula. In addition, there are the anterior superior tibiofibular ligament, anterior inferior tibiofibular ligament in the front, and posterior tibiofibular ligament at the back. All of these ligaments strengthen the bond between tibia and fibula and stabilize the ankle joint.

On the lateral side of the ankle, the fibrous joint capsule is reinforced by the lateral ligaments of the ankle. They are intrinsic joint ligaments (being part of the fibrous joint capsule) and are actually three separate structures (Figure 3A).

a.   Anterior talofibular ligament – from the lateral malleolus to talus.

b. Posterior talofibular ligament – from the lateral malleolus to talus at the back.

c. Calcaneofibular ligament – from lateral malleolus to the lateral surface of the calcaneus.

The medial ligament of the ankle is also referred to as the deltoid ligament of the ankle. It is a fan-shaped ligament that originates from the medial malleolus and attaches to several bones distally. From anterior to posterior in sequence, the portions of the medial ligament of the ankle are the anterior tibiotalar part, the tibionavicular part, the tibiocalcaneal part, and the posterior tibiotalar part (Figure 3C).

The major movements of the ankle joint are dorsiflexion and plantarflexion. The ankle joint can slightly abduct and adduct. When the foot is in plantarflexion in combination with adduction, the movement is inversion (Figure 3B). When the foot is in dorsiflexion in combination with abduction, the ankle joint is carrying out eversion (Figure 3D).

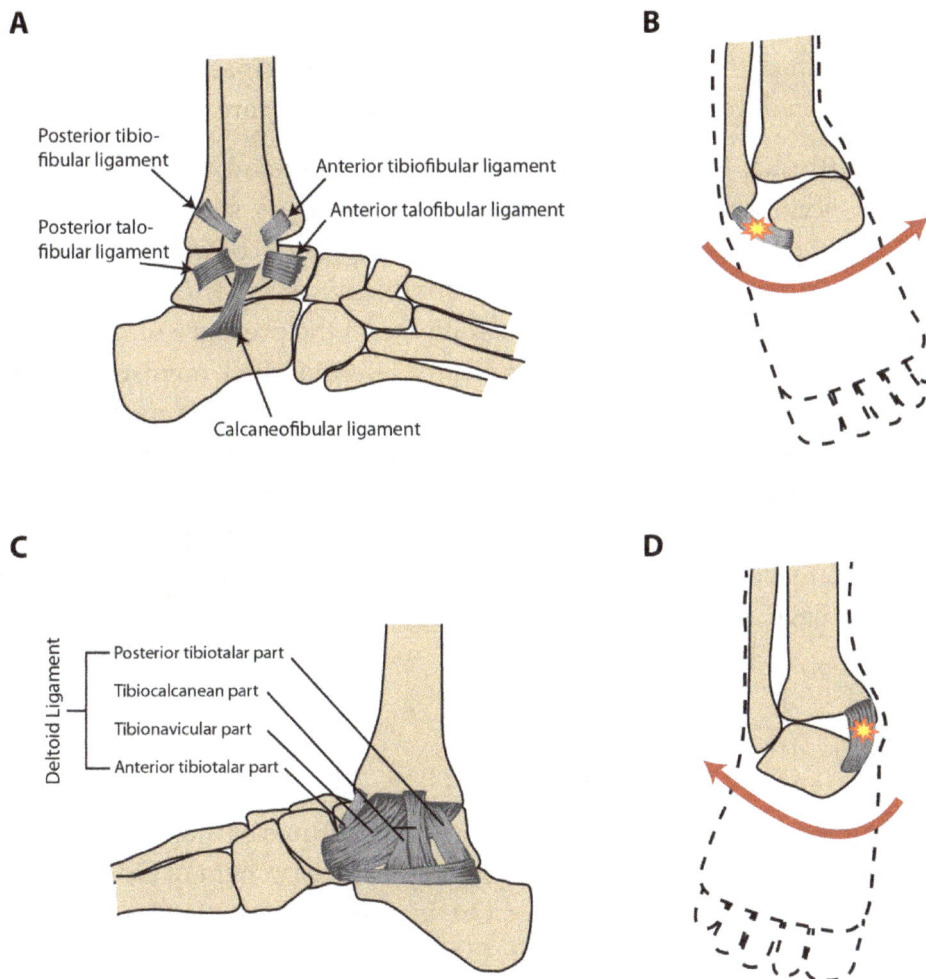

Figure 3. (A) A representation of major lateral ligaments of the ankle and the tibiofibular ligaments. (B) A typical inversion injury of the ankle that leads to damage of the lateral ankle ligaments. (C) The deltoid ligament which is the primary medial ankle ligament complex. (D) A typical eversion injury of the ankle that results in damage to the medial ligaments of the ankle.

The blood supply to the ankle joint is via the anterior tibial artery, the posterior tibial artery, and the fibular artery which is a branch of the posterior tibial artery. The nerve innervation is by the tibial nerve and the deep fibular nerve.

Ankle joint injury: The ankle is a second joint that demonstrates a high susceptibility to injury. A severe injury of major ligaments of the ankle may cause instability of the joint.

Like knee injuries, ankle injuries often occur during participation in sports or exercise; consequently, populations of athletes are often used in incidence studies. For example, ankle injuries are estimated to account for 14% of all athletic injuries, with sprains to ankle ligaments accounting for over 75% of ankle injuries [32-34]. The anterior talofibular ligament is the most commonly injured ankle ligament, involved in an estimated 85% of sprains sustained during United States high school sports [35]. A major problem accompanying ankle injury is the high rate of recurrence associated with chronic ankle instability. Approximately 15% of all ankle sprains occur in ankles with previous ligament injury[35]. Current models of chronic ankle instability (CAI) identify sufferers as experiencing—individually or in combination—mechanical instability, perceived instability, and recurrent sprains. Further characterizing patients with CAI by specific impairment, activity limitations, and participation restrictions, could help in the design of targeted treatments and injury reduction programs[36].

Ankle joint osteoarthritis: Idiopathic OA is common in the hand, foot, knee, spine, and hip joints, but rarely occurs in the ankle joint mainly due to its stable anatomical structure. However, the risk of post-traumatic OA in the ankle appears to be at least as great as the risk in the other joints. Differences among joints in congruity, articular cartilage thickness, force transmission across the joint surfaces, joint stability, and the presence of menisci could make some joints more vulnerable to OA. For example, the knee has thick menisci but the ankle does not. In addition, the ankle joint has a smaller bearing surface and is more constrained. The distal tibial articular surface has much thinner cartilage than the proximal tibial articular surface. Mechanical loading on the articular surface of the distal tibia after chondral damage causes higher subchondral bone strains than the loading on the proximal tibial articular surface. These differences may make the distal tibial articular surface more vulnerable to degradation of cartilage and development of OA [37-42].

9. Conclusion

This chapter summarizes the structural and functional features of major synovial joints of the human body and their relevance to joint injury and the development of OA. Although OA can affect any synovial joint, the prevalence of OA in specific joints is closely related to their structural and functional features. Idiopathic OA rarely occurs in the ankle, wrist, elbow, and shoulder, but it is common in the hand, foot, knee, spine, and hip joints. The risk of post-traumatic OA in the ankle, wrist, elbow, and shoulder appears to be as great as the risk in the hand, foot, knee, and hip. Differences among joints in articular surface congruity, articular cartilage thickness, mechanical force transmission, ligament structure-related joint stability, and the presence of menisci could make some joints more vulnerable to the development of

OA. A better understanding of the structural and functional features of major synovial joints of the human body may help us develop more effective strategies for the prevention and treatment of OA.

Acknowledgements

This work was supported in part by the U.S. National Institutes of Health (NIH)/NIAMS grant R01 AR059088, the U.S. Department of Defense medical research grant W81XWH-12-1-0304, and the Harrington Distinguished Professorship Endowment. The authors thank Mr. Zhaoyang Liu for editorial assistance.

Author details

Xiaoming Zhang[1], Brian Egan[2] and Jinxi Wang[2*]

*Address all correspondence to: jwang@kumc.edu

1 Department of Anatomy and Cell Biology, University of Kansas School of Medicine, Kansas City, USA

2 Department of Orthopedic Surgery, University of Kansas School of Medicine, Kansas City, USA

References

[1] Brandt KD, Dieppe P, Radin E. Etiopathogenesis of osteoarthritis. Med Clin North Am. 2009;93(1):1-24, xv.

[2] Brandt KD, Radin EL, Dieppe PA, van de Putte L. Yet more evidence that osteoarthritis is not a cartilage disease. Ann Rheum Dis. 2006;65(10):1261-1264.

[3] Loeser RF, Goldring SR, Scanzello CR, Goldring MB. Osteoarthritis: a disease of the joint as an organ. Arthritis Rheum. 2012;64(6):1697-1707.

[4] Gray H. Gray's Anatomy. Edinburgh: C. Livingstone; 1989.

[5] Moore KL, Dalley AF, Agur AMR. Upper Limb. In: Moore KL, Dalley AF, Agur AMR (eds.) Clinically Oriented Anatomy 7th ed. 2014; Wolters Kluwer I Lippincott Williams & Wilkins, Philadelphia, pp793-819.

[6] Zacchilli MA, Owens BD. Epidemiology of shoulder dislocations presenting to emergency departments in the United States. J Bone Joint Surg Am. 2010;92(3):542-549.

[7] Owens BD, Agel J, Mountcastle SB, Cameron KL, Nelson BJ. Incidence of glenohumeral instability in collegiate athletics. Am J Sports Med. 2009;37(9):1750-1754.

[8] Owens BD, Duffey ML, Nelson BJ, DeBerardino TM, Taylor DC, Mountcastle SB. The incidence and characteristics of shoulder instability at the United States Military Academy. Am J Sports Med. 2007;35(7):1168-1173.

[9] Owens BD, Campbell SE, Cameron KL. Risk factors for posterior shoulder instability in young athletes. Am J Sports Med. 2013;41(11):2645-2649.

[10] Robinson CM, Howes J, Murdoch H, Will E, Graham C. Functional outcome and risk of recurrent instability after primary traumatic anterior shoulder dislocation in young patients. J Bone Joint Surg Am. 2006;88(11):2326-2336.

[11] Kirkley A, Griffin S, Richards C, Miniaci A, Mohtadi N. Prospective randomized clinical trial comparing the effectiveness of immediate arthroscopic stabilization versus immobilization and rehabilitation in first traumatic anterior dislocations of the shoulder. Arthroscopy. 1999;15(5):507-514.

[12] Kirkley A, Werstine R, Ratjek A, Griffin S. Prospective randomized clinical trial comparing the effectiveness of immediate arthroscopic stabilization versus immobilization and rehabilitation in first traumatic anterior dislocations of the shoulder: long-term evaluation. Arthroscopy. 2005;21(1):55-63.

[13] Jakobsen BW, Johannsen HV, Suder P, Sojbjerg JO. Primary repair versus conservative treatment of first-time traumatic anterior dislocation of the shoulder: a randomized study with 10-year follow-up. Arthroscopy. 2007;23(2):118-123.

[14] Nakagawa Y, Hyakuna K, Otani S, Hashitani M, Nakamura T. Epidemiologic study of glenohumeral osteoarthritis with plain radiography. J Shoulder Elbow Surg. 1999;8(6):580-584.

[15] Raymond AC, McCann PA, Sarangi PP. Magnetic resonance scanning vs axillary radiography in the assessment of glenoid version for osteoarthritis. J Shoulder Elbow Surg. 2013;22(8):1078-1083.

[16] Weiss KE, Rodner CM. Osteoarthritis of the wrist. J Hand Surg Am. 2007;32(5): 725-746.

[17] Kloppenburg M, Kwok WY. Hand osteoarthritis--a heterogeneous disorder. Nat Rev Rheumatol. 2012;8(1):22-31.

[18] Kwok WY, Kloppenburg M, Marshall M, Nicholls E, Rosendaal FR, Peat G. The prevalence of erosive osteoarthritis in carpometacarpal joints and its clinical burden in symptomatic community-dwelling adults. Osteoarthritis Cartilage. 2014;22(6): 756-763.

[19] Kwok WY, Kloppenburg M, Marshall M, Nicholls E, Rosendaal FR, van der Windt DA, Peat G. Comparison of clinical burden between patients with erosive hand os-

teoarthritis and inflammatory arthritis in symptomatic community-dwelling adults: the Keele clinical assessment studies. Rheumatology (Oxford). 2013;52(12):2260-2267.

[20] Lawyer TJ, Jankowski J, Russell GV, Stronach BM. Prevalence of post-traumatic osteoarthritis in morbidly obese patients after acetabular fracture fixation. J Long Term Eff Med Implants. 2014;24(2-3):225-231.

[21] Thomas GE, Palmer AJ, Batra RN, Kiran A, Hart D, Spector T, Javaid MK, Judge A, Murray DW, Carr AJ, Arden NK, Glyn-Jones S. Subclinical deformities of the hip are significant predictors of radiographic osteoarthritis and joint replacement in women. A 20 year longitudinal cohort study. Osteoarthritis Cartilage. 2014;22(10):1504-1510.

[22] Hardcastle SA, Dieppe P, Gregson CL, Hunter D, Thomas GE, Arden NK, Spector TD, Hart DJ, Laugharne MJ, Clague GA, Edwards MH, Dennison EM, Cooper C, Williams M, Davey Smith G, Tobias JH. Prevalence of radiographic hip osteoarthritis is increased in high bone mass. Osteoarthritis Cartilage. 2014;22(8):1120-1128.

[23] Weidow J, Mars I, Karrholm J. Medial and lateral osteoarthritis of the knee is related to variations of hip and pelvic anatomy. Osteoarthritis Cartilage. 2005;13(6):471-477.

[24] Takeda K, Hasegawa T, Kiriyama Y, Matsumoto H, Otani T, Toyama Y, Nagura T. Kinematic motion of the anterior cruciate ligament deficient knee during functionally high and low demanding tasks. J Biomech. 2014;47(10):2526-2530.

[25] Oberlander KD, Bruggemann GP, Hoher J, Karamanidis K. Knee mechanics during landing in anterior cruciate ligament patients: A longitudinal study from pre- to 12 months post-reconstruction. Clin Biomech (Bristol, Avon). 2014;29(5):512-517.

[26] Liu H, Wu W, Yao W, Spang JT, Creighton RA, Garrett WE, Yu B. Effects of knee extension constraint training on knee flexion angle and peak impact ground-reaction force. Am J Sports Med. 2014;42(4):979-986.

[27] Markolf KL, Jackson SR, Foster B, McAllister DR. ACL forces and knee kinematics produced by axial tibial compression during a passive flexion-extension cycle. J Orthop Res. 2014;32(1):89-95.

[28] McClelland JA, Feller JA, Menz HB, Webster KE. Patterns in the knee flexion-extension moment profile during stair ascent and descent in patients with total knee arthroplasty. J Biomech. 2014;47(8):1816-1821.

[29] Hayashi D, Felson DT, Niu J, Hunter DJ, Roemer FW, Aliabadi P, Guermazi A. Preradiographic osteoarthritic changes are highly prevalent in the medial patella and medial posterior femur in older persons: Framingham OA study. Osteoarthritis Cartilage. 2014;22(1):76-83.

[30] Valdes AM, Suokas AK, Doherty SA, Jenkins W, Doherty M. History of knee surgery is associated with higher prevalence of neuropathic pain-like symptoms in patients with severe osteoarthritis of the knee. Semin Arthritis Rheum. 2014;43(5):588-592.

[31] van der Esch M, Knol DL, Schaffers IC, Reiding DJ, van Schaardenburg D, Knoop J, Roorda LD, Lems WF, Dekker J. Osteoarthritis of the knee: multicompartmental or compartmental disease? Rheumatology (Oxford). 2014;53(3):540-546.

[32] Fong DT, Hong Y, Chan LK, Yung PS, Chan KM. A systematic review on ankle injury and ankle sprain in sports. Sports Med. 2007;37(1):73-94.

[33] Nelson AJ, Collins CL, Yard EE, Fields SK, Comstock RD. Ankle injuries among United States high school sports athletes, 2005-2006. J Athl Train. 2007;42(3):381-387.

[34] Fong DT, Man CY, Yung PS, Cheung SY, Chan KM. Sport-related ankle injuries attending an accident and emergency department. Injury. 2008;39(10):1222-1227.

[35] Swenson DM, Collins CL, Fields SK, Comstock RD. Epidemiology of U.S. high school sports-related ligamentous ankle injuries, 2005/06-2010/11. Clin J Sport Med. 2013;23(3):190-196.

[36] Hiller CE, Kilbreath SL, Refshauge KM. Chronic ankle instability: evolution of the model. J Athl Train. 2011;46(2):133-141.

[37] Buckwalter JA, Martin JA. Osteoarthritis. Adv Drug Deliv Rev. 2006;58(2):150-167.

[38] Coester LM, Saltzman CL, Leupold J, Pontarelli W. Long-term results following ankle arthrodesis for post-traumatic arthritis. J Bone Joint Surg Am. 2001;83-a(2): 219-228.

[39] Lubbeke A, Salvo D, Stern R, Hoffmeyer P, Holzer N, Assal M. Risk factors for post-traumatic osteoarthritis of the ankle: an eighteen year follow-up study. Int Orthop. 2012;36(7):1403-1410.

[40] McKinley TO, Bay BK. Trabecular bone strain changes associated with cartilage defects in the proximal and distal tibia. J Orthop Res. 2001;19(5):906-913.

[41] Stufkens SA, Knupp M, Horisberger M, Lampert C, Hintermann B. Cartilage lesions and the development of osteoarthritis after internal fixation of ankle fractures: a prospective study. J Bone Joint Surg Am. 2010;92(2):279-286.

[42] Tochigi Y, Buckwalter JA, Martin JA, Hillis SL, Zhang P, Vaseenon T, Lehman AD, Brown TD. Distribution and progression of chondrocyte damage in a whole-organ model of human ankle intra-articular fracture. J Bone Joint Surg Am. 2011;93(6): 533-539.

7

Specific Proteases for Osteoarthritis Diagnosis and Therapy

Xiao-Yu Yuan, Liping Zhang and Yuqing Wu

1. 1. Introduction

1.1. Osteoarthritis (OA)

1.1.1. Causes and Symptoms of Osteoarthritis

Osteoarthritis is the most common style of arthritis, and this complicated and chronic degenerative joint disease is extremely found in adults and especially in old people. It mostly affects the whole joint structures associated with progressive changes in cartilage, menisci, ligaments and subchondral bone.[1-3] The cartilage covers the end of joint bones and provides slippery touch during movement, so it is obvious that the degradation of the cartilage extracellular matrix is a central feature of this disease. Normal articular cartilage makes bones frictionless with each other, and additionally it can also reduce the damage caused by shock of movement. [4] However, in osteoarthritis the top layer of articular cartilage wears out and even breaks down, which initiates the bone rubbing against each other, and therefore causes pain, sclerosis, swelling and loss of organ function in joint. As time going on, the symptoms are increasing in frequency and severity, finally the shape of joint changes with deformity, bone spurs may also occur at the edges of joints, bits of bones even fractures and floats among the joint space.

According to the pre-existing investigations, osteoarthritis has affected the health of a growing number of people world-widely.[5] Though osteoarthritis will not endanger the life safety of sufferers, its occurrence and development may not only seriously threaten people's physical fitness, but also directly reduce their quality of life.

It is well known that the loss of cartilage is concerned with the etiology of osteoarthritis. [1] The articular cartilage failure is triggered by several correlate factors, such as genetic, metabolic, and biomechanical factors with secondary components inflammation which react mutually. Until now the pathogenesis has not been wholly revealed due to the multi-factorial pathological mechanism of osteoarthritis, though many groups have researched for a long time.[6-10] Moreover, other risk factors including obesity, older age, joint injury, family history, over using, bone density, defect in joint cartilage contribute to osteoarthritis progression.[11-14]

Based on the above description, it is not hard to see that there must be osteoarthritis syndrome with a series of heterogeneous presentations,[15] such as **a)** joint pain, also the major clinical manifestation; **b)** joint stiffness, especially morning stiffness; **c)** functional disorder, like joint instability and activity limitation. These symptoms of osteoarthritis develop slowly and get serious increasingly with time.

Osteoarthritis is short of the physical and biochemical integrity of a joint, and also presents as a mono-arthritis, oligo-arthritis or a poly-arthritis, with several distinct patterns which exist in most ethnic and racial groups.[16] The common feature of osteoarthritis is characterized by the early inflammation followed by degeneration of chondrocytes including irreversible biodegradation. Then osteoarthritis appears as transformation of whole joint structures including degradation of the articular cartilage, menisci and ligaments, and these are also accompanied by other performance, such as joint space narrowing (JSN), bone marrow lesions, synovial inflammation, changes of subchondral bone and generation of osteophytes at the joint edge (See Figure 1).[2, 10, 13, 17] The degradative process of cartilage is widely considered to be regulated by the protease involved in osteoarthritis.[4, 6, 10, 18]

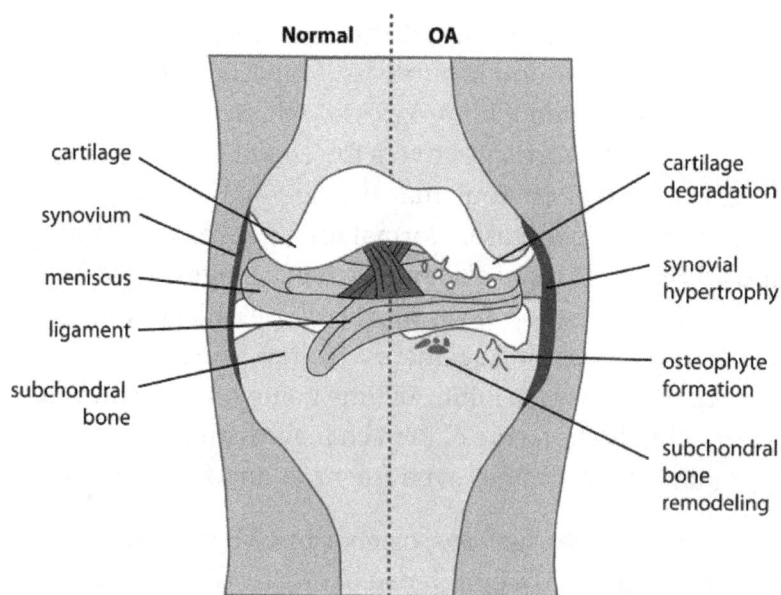

Figure 1. Diagrammatic presentation of normal and osteoarthritic joint.[10]

As the major mediators of collagen and proteoglycan cleavage, two classes of proteases are thought to be responsible for the degradation of cartilage components in osteoarthritis. It was thought that the collagen degradation is majorly due to the action of matrix metalloproteinase (MMP) collagenases. Mort *et al.* have indicated that members of both MMP and ADAMTS (a disintegrin and metalloproteinase with thrombospondin motifs) families are important mediators of the degradation of proteoglycans.[19] At the same time there is evidence for the role of the cysteine protease cathepsin K in collagen degradation in articular cartilage as revealed by Konttinen *et al.*.[20] The cleavage of cartilage proteins often occurs at specific sites on these molecules, resulting in the generation of characteristic N- and C-terminal epitopes which can be used for the production of antibodies specific for these cleavage products (anti-neoepitope antibodies).[21] Recent years, Chan *et al.* have also reported that the increased chondrocyte sclerostin may protect against cartilage degradation in osteoarthritis.[22]

1.2. Importance of osteoarthritis diagnosis and therapy

Currently the total number of osteoarthritis patients in world-wide is more than 600 million. There are about 1/6 of people in Asia suffering from osteoarthritis at some stage of their life, among which patients account for 10% of the total population in China, and are increasing in recent years. It is even estimated that the number may reach to 150 million by 2015. In addition, it has been reported that a lifetime risk of OA-specific morbidity of about 45% for the knee and 25% for the hip.[23] The National Healthy and Nutrition Examination Survey of USA points out that the symptoms and signs of clinical osteoarthritis are only in 12% of 6913 people, aged among from 25 to 74 years, and X-ray results of osteoarthritis appeared in at least one site occupy 33%.[24] It will be worse that 53% of osteoarthritis patients may lead to disability, loss of joint function and the ability to work.

Unfortunately, the disease-modifying drugs for osteoarthritis are not available currently, the drugs have the role of analgesic effect and symptom improvement, but they do not involve the OA pathology and change the abnormal structure. Even though some styles of drugs can slow down and reverse the degradation of cartilage, they produce the desired result tardily, and the curative effect only can maintain for a short period. Osteoarthritis has become the largest disease causing disability and is known as "no-lethal cancer", it is so harmful to human health, and the related research about it has been carried out.[25-27]

While there is no complete cure for OA until now, the early detection followed by efficient therapy may slow down its detrimental effects. Apparently, a diagnostic system that enables early and reliable diagnosis of this degenerative joint disease is necessary,[28] such as bio-chemical test and imageological diagnosis (X-ray or/and NMR examination). **a)** biochemical test: recent years, the special biochemical marker have been drawn attention, hydroxylysyl-pyridinoline, heoxylysylpyridinoline, C-reactive protein, Serum amyloid A and so on are all used to calculate the OA; **b)** imageological diagnosis: the diagnosis base on radiology mani-festation of OA through X-ray or/and NMR examination. However, the imaging technique can not accurately, selectively evaluate quantitative property of articular cartilage. In addition, once it is diagnosed as osteoarthritis, the disease has proceeded into the mid- or late- period, and the opportune moment and prompt treatment to patients are all missed, so the new technology and strategy need to be further developed. Treatments are also limited to relieve the symptoms and surgically replace the affected joints. Therefore, to minimize the damage, understanding the early symptoms of bone disease will help to detect and treat the disease. The development of bone-related diagnostic and therapeutic programs will be essential,[29] and a wide range of work in the past years has proved that several proteases might related directly to osteoarthritis.

2. Diagnosis of osteoarthritis in targeting specific proteases

2.1. Cathepsin B (Cath B)

As a cysteine proteinase, cathepsin B is a lysosomal cysteine protease, which belongs to the papain surper-family and has been implicated in the pathology of a number of important human disease, including cancer and arthritis.[30] It has been shown to be up-regulated in patients with rheumatoid arthritis,[31] and components of the estracellular matrix are shown to be substrates for this protease.[32] Cathepsin B is active in aggrecan and cartilage,[33-34] cleaves the aggrecan G1-G2 domain fragment, and engenders two fragments from the cleavage at Gly-Val bond to the metalloproteinase cleavage site. For example, Fosang *et al.* have revealed that cathepsin B degraded the proteoglycan extensively producing several bands of faster migration and therefore it can be used as a biomarker of diagnosis of OA.[35]

Then Lai's group took twelve male nude mice to investigate early diagnosis of osteoarthritis on a molecular basis, by using the developed cathepsin B sensitive near-infrared (NIR) fluorescent probe.[36] Firstly, they injected collagenase (1.0%, w/v) into the right knee joint to induce osteoarthritis and the left knee joint served as a comparison. Secondly, the cathepsin B sensitive near-infrared fluorescence probe was activated, which could radiate an intensive NIR fluorescence signal. Finally, the NIR fluorescence signals were caught by an optical imaging system which could receive an emission wavelength of 680–720 nm. Using this mechanism, they discovered that 3-fold difference in signal intensity between osteoarthritic and normal joints can be detected after 24h intravenous injection (see Figure 2). Therefore, it is believed that cathepsin B activatable NIR fluorescence probe can offer a potential new imaging technology for early osteoarthritis diagnosis.

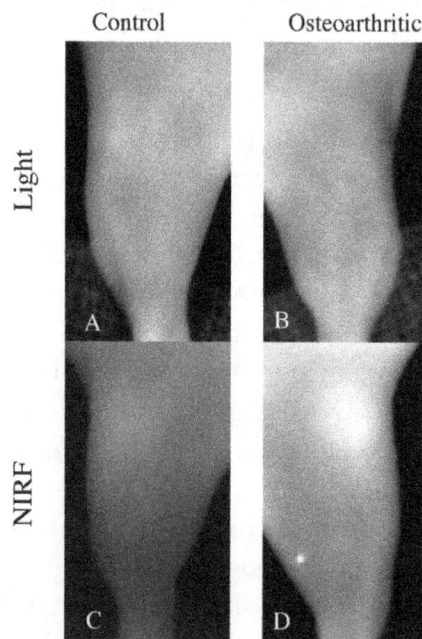

Figure 2. Near infrared fluorescence reflectance imaging, which were taken 24 h after intravenous injection of the cathepsin B sensitive auto-quenched probe in a representative animal; (A and B) white light images, (C and D) NIRF images.[36]

2.2. Lactate Dehydrogenase (LDH)

LDH-4 and LDH-5 play an important role in anaerobic metabolism of articular cartilage. In early 1975, Weseloh and Fiegelmann began to realize the importance of LDH-isoenzym patterns in human cartilage, and attempted to evaluate it. The result of experience was that LDH-5 dominates with an average of 75.3%, whereas the LDH-4 (21.7%) and the LDH-3 (3.2%) were considerably lower, which was significant for the later study. [37]

As we know from previous literatures, degenerative joint diseases were deemed to associate with increased LDH activity in the synovial fluid. In order to verify the distribution of LDH, Eveline *et al.* have made a study to examine healthy and degenerative stifle joints for the goal of clarifying the origin of LDA in synovial fluid through many technical means, such as transmission electron microscopy (TEM), immunolabeling and enzyme cytochemistry. And then all techniques corroborated that the presence of LDH in chondrocytes and in the inter-territorial matrix of degenerative stifle joints. Whereas LDH is retained in healthy cartilage due to permeability limitations, it is released into synovial fluid through abrasion as well as through unrestricted diffusion as a result of degradation of collagen and increased water content in degenerative joints.[38]

In addition, the spectrophotometric technique using the pyruvate to lactate conversion was taken to measure the total LDH activity, while agar gel electrophoresis followed by a tetrazolium enzymatic staining reaction was used to establish the LDH isoenzyme patterns. Veys *et al.* have found long before that the cases of arthritis had high LDH activity both in cellular material and in cell-free fluid. Moreover, these cases also had an increased percentage of LDH-5 in the cellular extract. It was concluded that the LDH could be a symbol reflecting the degree of arthritis and used to the diagnosis of early OA.[39]

3. Therapeutics of osteoarthritis in targeting specific proteases

3.1. Sclerostin (SOST)

Sclerostin is a kind of extracellular protease (see Figure 3). As it is well known, the SOST gene encodes for the secreted protein sclerostin.[40] The expression of SOST in the adult body exclusively is produced by osteocytes located in bones. Therefore, sclerostin is considered as negatively modulating osteoblast development and bone formation.[41-42]

At first it was thought that sclerostin might implement its regulatory function *via* acting as a modulator of bone morphogenetic proteins (BMPs).[43] Afterwards the accumulating evidence showed that sclerostin interferes with the Wnt signaling pathway due to binding to the Wnt co-receptor LRP5 and consequently regulating bone growth.[44-45] SOST restrained the express of Wnt signaling, which was important in the skeletal development[41, 46] and could regulate the activity of β-catenin. It was also reported that excess SOST could lead to chondrocyte apoptosis and cartilage damage, namely arthritis, through suppressing the normal function of β-catenin.[47] At the same time, the study performed by Blom *et al.* have shown that superabundant β-catenin would produce a procatabolic effect in the cartilage and promote

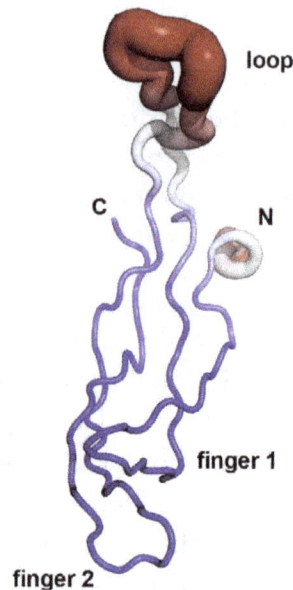

Figure 3. "Sausage" plot of the averaged minimized structure of murine sclerostin showing the highly flexible regions of mSOST. Regions colored in blue structurally marked the highly defined areas, regions marked in red are highly disordered.[51]

chondrocyte hypertrophy directly related with osteoarthritic pathology. Therefore, moderate sclerostin would be necessary to keep β-catenin at an appropriate level, and it would be a crucial indicator in the treatment or diagnosis of osteoarthritis.[48-50] Of note is that, the importance of Wnt/β-catenin signaling in the pathogenesis of osteoarthritis in humans has not been well understood. For example, the findings in preclinical studies using anti-sclerostin therapy in animal models of osteoarthritis have been disappointing, with no reported benefit on cartilage remodeling during aging or mechanical injury.[50] In addition, the role of sclerostin in the pathogenesis of osteoarthritis in humans has not yet been well defined, and the potential utility of treating osteoarthritis with interventions that alter sclerostin is not known. Still, we are surely pleased to see that summary of SOST in therapeutics of OA will be performed.

3.2. Matrix Metalloproteinases (MMPs) and Adamalysin with Thrombospondin Motifs (ADAMTS)

A significant characteristic of osteoarthritis is the degradation of the extracellular cartilage tissue. According to the previous reports it is widely known that the structural component of the matrix is mainly composed of collagen and aggrecan, which are regulated by the proteolytic enzymes, MMPs and ADAMTs.

3.2.1. MMPs

The collagen found primarily in the cartilage ECM is type II collagen, which appears as the fibrillar network (see Figure 4) and offers strong elasticity to the cartilage matrix. It will be difficult to be repaired for cartilage once the collagen was lost (see Figure 5).[52-53] Matrix metalloproteinases (MMP) comprises a family of zinc-dependent enzymes, they are called collagenases which possess the collagenolytic abilities that degrade extracellular matrix components.[54] These proteases regulate the initial cleavage of the collagen triple helix, occurring at 3/4 of the distance from the amino-terminal end of each chain, forming collagen fragments of 3/4 and 1/4 length.[55] To be directly related to these processes there are three kinds of collagenases: collagenase-1 or interstitial collagenase (MMP-1); collagenase-2 or neutrophil collagenase (MMP-8); and collagenase-3 (MMP-13). In addition, MMP-13 is considered as the primary collagenase in collagen degradation.[6-57] Neuhold *et al.* showed that MMP-13 transgenic animals exhibited joint pathology which strongly resembled osteo-arthritis. Such a result provided direct evidence in support of a role for this proteinase in the pathology of this disease.[18]

3.2.2. ADAMTS

Aggrecan is a large proteoglycan including chondroitin sulphate and keratan sulphate glycosaminoglycan moieties, and is crucial for bringing water to the cartilage matrix which gives joints the ability to bear the heavy load. Aggrecan plays such a good role, short of it can lead to the articular cartilage softening and loss of fixed charges, then the joint function will be reduced and even forfeited.[58] Aggrecan molecules possess two major cleavage sites in the interglobular domain (IGD) region of the core protein. Without the G1 domain, aggrecan molecules can be free in and out of the cartilage matrix, leading to the lack of cartilage function. [59] The first cleavage site at the Asn341-Phe342 bond, creating the neoepitope VDIPEN, is found to be generated by MMPs.[60] The second site at the Glu373-Ala374 bond, creating the NITEGE neoepitope, is found to be very important and results from aggrecan cleavage, which is associated with lots of pathologies.

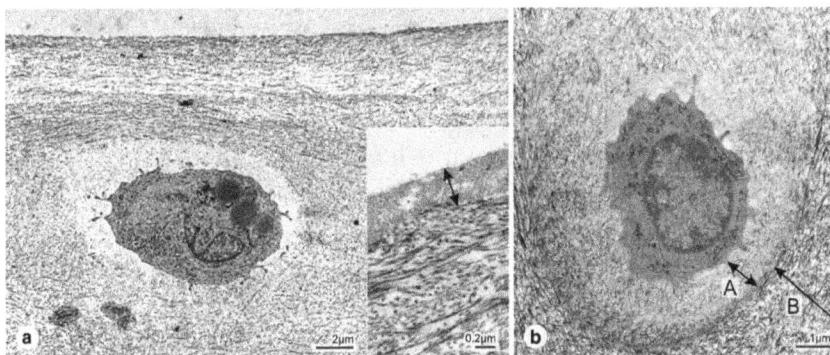

Figure 4. Electron micrographs of healthy cartilage. **a)** A dense superficial network of collagen fibers running in paral-lel with the articular surface is present. Chondrocytes contain numerous organelles and vesicles. *Inset* An amorphous layer (*double arrow*) extends at the surface. Underneath, densely packed collagen fibers run in parallel with the articular surface. **b)** Territorial (A) and interterritorial (B) zones of extracellular matrix are clearly demarcated. Note the large nucleus and abundance of organelles in the chondrocyte.[38]

Related studies have shown that ADAMTS-5 is a pivotal enzyme for cutting the Glu373~Ala374 bond, and the inhibitors of ADAMTS-5 can debase the aggrecan decomposition effectively. So ADAMTS-5 is important in osteoarthritis of individuals and responsible for aggrecan degra-

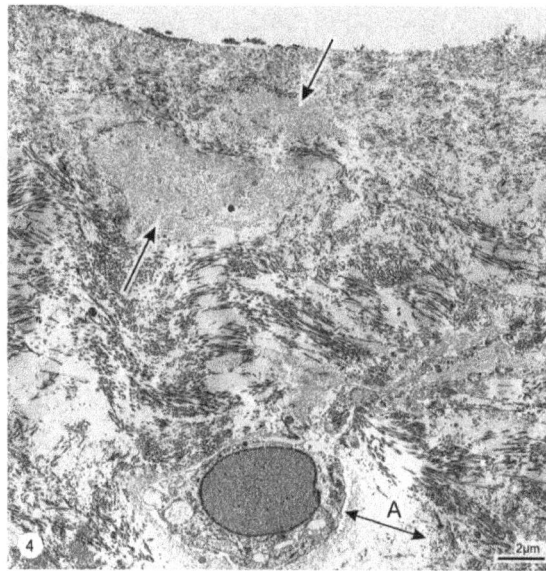

Figure 5. Electron micrograph of degenerative cartilage. The amorphous layer is missing, and the articular surface is uneven. Collagen Wbers are loosely packed and arranged at random. Note amorphous foci in the extracellular matrix (arrows). (A) Territorial extracellular matrix.[38]

dation in normal and diseased cartilage.[61] A new drug, AGG523, in targeting ADAMTS-5 and ADAMTS-4 for therapeutics has entered clinical trials phase I. Studies by Glasson *et al.* and Majumdar *et al.* carried out with ADAMTS-5 knockout and ADAMTS-4/-5 double knockout mice showed that these animals were more resistant to cartilage degradation after destabilizing knee surgery.[62-63] However, in human, assumed damaging polymorphisms in the ADAMTS-5 gene does not show any modification in selectivity to osteoarthritis.[64] The search for the most important aggrecanase in human osteoarthritis is still going.[65]

3.3. Cathepsin K

Cathepsin K (Cath K) is a cysteine proteinase of papain family. It has been implicated in the resorption of the bone matrix. Like most of the proteinases, cathepsin K is synthesized and secreted from the cell as an inactive proenzyme, it should be noted that cathepsin K is secreted from macrophage and synovial fibroblasts. Cathepsin K cleaves the triple-helical type II collagen[66], and the special distribution of cathepsin K in osteoarthritic cartilage suggests an important role of this protease in the etiopathogenesis of osteoarthritis.

Early in 2004, Morko *et al.* took transgenic mice which were predisposed to early osteoarthritis because of harboring a short deletion mutation and their non-transgenic litter mates as controls for study.[53] They used the immunohistochemistry and morphometry to investigate the distribution of cathepsin K in the knee joints. In the knee joints of transgenic mice, Cathepsin K was found near sites of matrix destruction in articular chondrocytes, particularly in calcified cartilaginous matrix and proliferating cells. It indicted that cathepsin K played an important role in the pathogenesis of osteoarthritis. They also gave an explain that cathepsin K could digest cartilage matrix components, therefore, it was considered to contribute to the progression of osteoarthritic damage. Such studies have provided new clew for the development of treatments aimed at holding back cartilage degeneration.[53]

4. Inhibition of proteases related to OA

There is currently no disease-modifying OA drug available, and treatment is limited to symptomatic relief or surgical replacement of affected joints. There is thus considerable interest in developing effective treatments that can halt or reverse the progression of the disease.

4.1. Inhibition of sclerostin

Till date, it is well documented that SOST inhibition is effective for treatment of osteoporosis. Tanners group have performed the DNA aptamer selectively against sclerostin, and characterized DNA aptamer-sclerostin binding affinity.[67] Aptamers can be used for therapeutic purposes and have been investigated in major disease such as osteoarthritis and osteoporosis.[68]

There are several potential advantages of using aptamers for osteoarthritis and osteoporosis. Nucleic acids show good pharmacokinetic parameters in cartilage and joints, and many therapeutic targets tend to be extracellular so that the challenge of cross-membrane delivery of the nucleic acid can be avoided. Furthermore, aptamers also hold particular promise in conjunction with other technologies such as fluorescent nanoclusters which open up new possibilities for diagnostic imaging. At last the stable aptamers display effective and specific dose-dependent inhibition of sclerostin's antagonistic effect on Wnt activity. Their studies have provided an alternative approach to inhibit sclerostin function with therapeutic potential.

However, there is no pre-clinical or clinical evidence to show its efficacy for the treatment of osteoarthritis. Its role in OA treatment is still under premature. É. Abed *et al.* explored the role played by Sirtuin 1 and SOST on the abnormal mineralization and cWnt signaling in human osteoarthritic subchondral osteoblast (OA Ob). The results indicated that high level of SOST was responsible, in part for the reduced cWnt and mineralization of human OA Ob, which in turn is linked with abnormal SIRT1 levels in these pathological cells.[69] A recent study found that absence of sclerostin in mice with genetic knockout of sclerostin did not alter development of age-dependent osteoarthritis, and that anti-sclerostin therapy with a monoclonal antibody in rats with post-traumatic osteoarthritis had no effect on articular cartilage remodeling.[50] Anyway, antisclerostin therapy has appeared be a promising approach to the treatment of osteoporosis, while Wnt/β-catenin signaling has also been implicated in the pathogenesis of osteoarthritis, with the potential for therapeutic intervention yet to be determined.[70]

4.2. Inhibition of MMPs and ADAMTs

According to the reports, it is known that the MMPs can be effectively inhibited by TIMP-1, -2, -3, -4.[71] Similar to MMPs, ADAMTS family members can also be inhibited effectively by TIMPs.[72-73] It is illustrated that TIMPs is a significant candidate of blocking cartilage degradation. And of particular note is that TIMP-3 can inhibit several ADAM/ADAMTS proteinases, as reported in lots of existed literatures, while TIMP-1 shows ability to inhibit ADAMTS-10.[72-77] In addition, it is also reported that TIMP-3 can be endocytosed and degraded by chondrocytes,[78] suggesting that its activity in cartilage may be regulated post-translationally rather than transcriptionally.[10]

Wayne *et al.* have demonstrated that inhibition of full-length ADAMTS-4 by TIMP-3 was enhanced in the presence of aggrecan, and this interaction was mediated largely through the binding of aggrecan and the spacer domains of ADAMTS-4 to form a complex with an improved binding affinity for TIMP-3 over free ADAMTS-4. Therefore, the results also indicated that the cartilage environment could modulate the function of protease-inhibitor systems and have relevance for therapeutic approaches to aggrecanase modulation.[79]

ADAMTS-2 is an activity necessary for the formation of extracellular matrix and responsible for cleaving the N-propeptides of procollagens I–III. Wang *et al.* have shown that TIMP-3 inhibited ADAMTS-2 *in vitro* with apparent K_i values of 160 and 602 nM, in the presence of heparin or without respectively. In a word, TIMP-3 was shown to inhibit procollagen processing by cells.[80]

4.3. Inhibition of cathepsin K

Cathepsin K contains a highly conserved catalytic triad Cys25, His159, and Asn175 within its active site. And in design of the cathepsin K inhibitors, there are several key elements that need to be considered, its inhibitors must be reversible so as to prevent antigenicity arising from covalent modification of proteins *via* irreversible, such as aldehydes, ketones and nitriles. These reversible inhibitors have become more crucial in recent years because they combine strongly to the cathepsin K with low reactivity towards cellular nucleophiles.[81] In addition, the selectivity of inhibitors towards cathepsin K and other cysteine are also desirable to avoid side effects.[82]

4.3.1. Aldehydes and ketones

Aldehydes and ketones modulate cathepsin K activity *via* hemiacetal/thiohemiacetal and bond formation. Some representatives of aldehyde- and ketone-based reversible covalent cathepsin K inhibitors have reached stages of clinical trials.[83-84]

Since selectivity is important when designing potential drugs to avoid undesired toxicities, Boros *et al.* have obtained several of selective aldehyde-based inhibitors[85] and some of them presented at least 500-fold more potent for cathepsin K than cathepsin B or L. These results gave the encouragement that the aldehyde-based inhibitors could be developed as an anti-OA drug in targeting Cath K. In addition, cyclic ketone was also indicated as the inhibitors of the cysteine protease cathepsin K.

Crystallographic and structure-activity (SA) studies on acyclic ketone-based inhibitors of cathepsin K have guided the design and identification of two series of cyclic ketone inhibitors. Marquis *et al.* have found that the 3-amidopyrrolidin-4-one inhibitors were bound into the active site of the cathepsin K with two alternate directions. Epimerization issues associated with the labile alpha-amino ketone diastereomeric center contained within these inhibitor classes has proven to limit their utility.[86] The results showed that the heterogeneous ketone inhibitors have different influence on the practical application.

4.3.2. Nitriles

Inhibitors for papain-like cysteine are derived from peptides, they contains electrophilic group and have been shown to covalently interact with the thiol group at the active site of cathepsin K under formation a thioimidate adduct. Among many types of inhibitors, nitriles have received much attention in recent study.[87-88]

Three chemical classes of nitrile-containing inhibitors of cysteine proteases are known as: **a)** cyanamides,[89] **b)** aromatic nitriles,[90] and **c)** aza-nitrile derivatives, which includes a P1 aza-amino nitrile.[91-93] Among these inhibitors the aza-nitrile derivatives are the optimal ones due to the unique properties such as proteolytical stabilization, reversible binding and excellent inhibitory activity.[94]

In 2013, Ren and Yuan *et al.* in our research group has synthesized two new series of cathepsin K inhibitors. The first series with P2-P3 amide linker have both high selectivity and potency, especially the *meta*-triaryl compound **13** is significantly more potent to cathepsin K (K_i = 0.0031 nM). The second series without the P2-P3 amide linkage have showed a remarkable improvements, the triaryl *meta*-product **13'** possessed a favorable balance between potency (K_i = 0.29 nM) and selectivity of cathepsin K over L, S, B (320-, 1784-, 8566-fold). Such a selective improvement would be useful to avoid harmful side effects in practical applications of the inhibitors.[94-95]

5. Conclusion and perspective

A significant improvement about scientific cognition of osteoarthritis have been achieved in the past decades, both the aggrecan and collagen play a supporting role in cartilage. It is indisputable that there is a close relationship between the component lost and cartilage degradation, and people are becoming increasingly aware that osteoarthritis is a serious joint disease which is adjusted by proteases and is performed as the degradation of the cartilage extracellular matrix. In addition, we also summarized the profoundly reorganizations that risk factors for OA contain obesity, sports injury, joint instability, particular muscle weakness, genetic, occupational factors and so on. These are related with mechanical, genetic, metabolic factors launch and hold the biochemical changes result the joint dysfunction.

As stated above, a wide range of work in the past years has proved that several proteases are intertwined with osteoarthritis and focused upon in clinical trails. Sclerostin, MMPs, ADAMTS, cathepsins and LDH have become key targets in the development of the diagnosis and treatment of osteoarthritis, and significant progress has been made over the decades. It is no doubt that international co-work in this area will made great progress in the near future and lead to some effective treatment methods in order to alleviate the symptoms and hamper the progression of osteoarthritis.

Acknowledgements

This work was supported by the National Natural Science Foundation of China (21373101, 20973073, and 91027027) and the Innovation Program of the State Key Laboratory of Supra-molecular Structure and Materials, Jilin University.

Author details

Xiao-Yu Yuan[1], Liping Zhang[2] and Yuqing Wu[1*]

*Address all correspondence to: yqwu@jlu.edu.cn

1 State Key Laboratory of Supramolecular Structure and Materials, Jilin University, Changchun, China

2 Grain and Oil Food Processing Key Laboratory of Jilin Province, Jilin Business and Technology College, Changchun, China

References

[1] Lotz M., Martel-Pelletier J., Christiansen C., Brandi M.-L., Bruyère O., Chapurlat R., Collette J., Cooper C., Giacovelli G., Kanis J. A., Karsdal M. A., Kraus V., Lems W. F., Meulenbelt I., Pelletier J.-P., Raynauld J.-P., Reiter-Niesert S., Rizzoli R., Sandell L. J., Van Spil W. E., Reginster J.-Y., Value of biomarkers in osteoarthritis: current status and perspectives. *Ann. Rheum. Dis.*, 2013, 72, 1756.

[2] Goldring M. B., Goldring S. R., Articular cartilage and subchondral bone in the pathogenesis of osteoarthritis. *Ann. N. Y. Acad. Sci.*, 2010, 1192, 230.

[3] Felson D. T., Developments in the clinical understanding of osteoarthritis. *Arthritis Res. Ther.*, 2009, 11, 203.

[4] Farley J., Dejica V. M., Mort J. S., Proteases and cartilage degradation in osteoarthri-tis. 2012. p399-418. In book: Principles of Osteoarthritis - Its Definition, Character, Derivation and Modality-Related Recognition; Chaptor 16.

[5] Wieland H. A., Michaelis M., Kirschbaum B. J., Rudolphi K. A., Osteoarthritis - an untreatable disease? *Nat. Rev. Drug Discov.*, 2005, 4, 331.

[6] van den Berg W. B., Osteoarthritis year 2010 in review: pathomechanisms. *Osteoarthr. Cartilage*, 2011, 19, 338.

[7] Punzi L., Oliviero F., Laboratory investigations in osteoarthritis. *Aging Clin. Exp. Res.*, 2005, 42, 279.

[8] Krasnokutsky S., Attur M., Palmer G., Samuels J., Abramson S. B., Current concepts in the pathogenesis of osteoarthritis. *Osteoarthr. Cartilage*, 2008, 16, S1.

[9] Heijink A., Gomoll A. H., Madry H., Drobnič M., Filardo G., Espregueira-Mendes J., Van Dijk C. N., Biomechanical considerations in the pathogenesis of osteoarthritis of the knee. *Knee Surg. Sport. Tr. A.*, 2012, 20, 423.

[10] Troeberg L., Nagase H., Proteases involved in cartilage matrix degradation in osteoarthritis. *BBA-Proteins Proteom.*, 2012, 1824, 133.

[11] NHS choices. Causes of osteoarthritis. http://www.nhs.uk/Conditions/Osteoarthritis/Pages/Causes.aspx (accessed 27 Aug. 2014)

[12] WebMD. pain management: osteoarthritis. http://www.webmd.com/pain-management/guide/pain-management-osteoarthritis?page=2 (accessed 10 Dec. 2013)

[13] Felson D. T., Developments in the clinical understanding of osteoarthritis. *Arthritis Res. Ther.*, 2009, 11, 203.

[14] Heinegård D., Saxne T., The role of the cartilage matrix in osteoarthritis. *Nat. Rev. Rheumatol.*, 2011, 7, 50.

[15] Chan K. K. W., Wu R. W. K., Symptoms, signs and quality of life (Qol) in osteoarthritis (OA). 2012, p25-40. In book: Principles of osteoarthritis - its definition, character, Derivation and modality – related recognition; Chaptor 2.

[16] van Saase J. L., van Romunde L. K., Cats A., Vandenbroucke J. P., Valkenburg H. A., Epidemiology of osteoarthritis: zoetermeer survey. comparison of radiological osteoarthritis in a Dutch population with that in 10 other populations. *Ann. Rheum. Dis.*, 1989, 48, 271.

[17] Attur M., Krasnokutsky-Samuels S., Samuels J., Abramson S. B., Prognostic biomarkers in osteoarthritis. *Curr. Opin. Rheumatol.*, 2013, 25, 136.

[18] Neuhold L. A., Killar L., Zhao W., Sung M.-L. A., Warner L., Kulik J., Turner J., Wu W., Billinghurst C., Meijers T., Poole A. R., Babij P., DeGennaro L. J., Postnatal expression in hyaline cartilage of constitutively active human collagenase-3 (MMP-13) induces osteoarthritis in mice. *J. Clin. Invest.*, 2001, 107, 35.

[19] Mort J. S., Billington C. J., Articular cartilage and changes in arthritis: matrix degradation. *Arthritis Res.*, 2001, 3, 337.

[20] Konttinen Y.T., Mandelin J., Li T.F., Salo J., Lassus J., Liljestrom M., Hukkanen M., Takagi M., Virtanen I., Santavirta S., Acidic cysteine endoproteinase cathepsin K in the degeneration of the superficial articular hyaline cartilage in osteoarthritis. *Arthritis Rheum.*, 2002, 46, 953.

[21] Mort J. S., Flannery C. R., Makkerh J., Krupa J. C., Lee E. R., The use of anti-neoepi-tope antibodies for the analysis of degradative events in cartilage and the molecular basis for neoepitope specificity. *Biochem. Soc. Symp.*, 2003, 70, 107.

[22] Chan B. Y., Fuller E. S., Russell A. K., Smith S. M., Smith M. M., Jackson M. T., Cake M. A., Read R. A., Bateman J. F., Sambrook P. N., Little C. B., Increased chondrocyte sclerostin may protect against cartilage degradation in osteoarthritis. *Osteoarthr. Cartilage*, 2011, 19, 874.

[23] Cooper C., Arden N. K., Excess mortality in osteoarthritis. *Brit. Med. J.*, 2011, 8, 342

[24] Lawrence R. C., Helmick C. G., Arnett F. C., Deyo R. A., Felson D. T., Giannini E. H., Heyse S. P., Hirsch R., Hochberg M. C., Hunder G. G., Liang M. H., Pillemer S. R., Steen V. D., Wolfe F., Estimates of the prevalence of arthritis and selected musculos-keletal disorders in the United States. *Arthritis Rheum.*, 1998, 41, 778.

[25] Sandy J. D., A contentious issue finds some clarity: on the independent and comple-mentary roles of aggrecanase activity and MMP activity in human joint aggrecanoly-sis. *Osteoarthr. Cartilage*, 2006, 14, 95.

[26] Xu L., Peng H., Glasson S., Lee P. L., Hu K., Ijiri K., Olsen B. R., Goldring M. B., Li Y., Increased expression of the collagen receptor discoidin domain receptor 2 in articular cartilage as a key event in the pathogenesis of osteoarthritis. *Arthritis Rheum.*, 2007, 56, 2663.

[27] Ferrell W. R., Kelso E. B., Lockhart J. C., Plevin R., McInnes I. B., Protease-activated receptor 2: a novel pathogenic pathway in a murine model of osteoarthritis. *Ann. Rheum. Dis.*, 2010, 69, 2051.

[28] Pearle A. D., Warren R. F., Rodeo S. A., Basic science of articular cartilage and osteo-arthritis. *Clin. Sport Med.*, 2005, 24, 1.

[29] Little C. B., Fosang A. J., Is cartilage matrix breakdown an appropriate therapeutic target in osteoarthritis - insights from studies of aggrecan and collagen proteolysis? *Curr. Drug Targets*, 2010, 11, 561.

[30] Tuek B., Turk D., Turk V., Lysosomal cysteine proteases: more than scavengers. *Biochim. Biophys. Acta.*, 2000, 1477, 98.

[31] Keyszer G., Redlich A., Haupl T., Zacher J., Sparmann M., Entgethum U., Gay S., Burmester G. R., Differential expression of cathepsins B and L compared with matrix metalloproteinases and their respective inhibitors in rheumatoid arthritis and osteo-arthritis: a parallel investigation by semiquantitative reverse transcriptase-polymer-ase chain reaction and immunohistochemistry. *Arthritis Rheum.*, 1998, 41, 1378.

[32] Buttle D. J., Handley C. J., Ilic M. Z., Saklatvala J., Murata M., Barrett A. J., Inhibition of cartilage proteoglycan release by a specific inactivator of cathepsin B and an inhib-itor of matrix metalloproteinases. Evidence for two converging pathways of chondro-cyte-mediated proteoglycan degradation. *Arthritis Rheum.*, 1993, 36, 1709.

[33] Bayliss M. T., Ali S. Y., Studies on cathepsin B in human articular cartilage. *Biochem. J.*, 1978, 171, 149.

[34] Hernandez-Vidala G., Jeffcott L. B., Davies M. E., Immunolocalization of cathepsin B in equinedyschondroplastic articular cartilage. *Vet. J.*, 1998, 156, 193.

[35] Fosang A. J.,. Neamell P. J, Last K., Hardingham T. E., Murphy G., Hamilton J. A., The interglobular domain of cartilage aggrecan is cleaved by PUMP, gelatinases, and Cathepsin B. *J. Biol. Chem.*, 1992, 267, 19470.

[36] Lai W.-F., T., Chang C.-H., Tang Y., Bronson R. and Tung C.-H., Early diagnosis of osteoarthritis using cathepsin B sensitive near-infrared fluorescent probes. *Osteo-Arthr. Cartilage*, 2004, 12, 239.

[37] Weseloh G., Fiegelmann A., Distribution of the isoenzym lactatdehydrogenase in human cartilage. *Arch. orthop. UnfaltChir.*, 1975, 83, 345.

[38] Walter E. L. C., Spreng D., Schmöckel H., Schawalder P., Tschudi P., Friess A. E., Stoffel M. H., Distribution of lactate dehydrogenase in healthy and degenerative canine stifle joint cartilage. *Histochem. Cell Biol.*, 2007, 128, 7.

[39] Veys E. M., Wieme R. J., Lactate dehydrogenase in synovial fluid diagnostic evaluation of total activity and isoenzyme patterns. *Ann. rheum. Dis.*, 1968, 27, 569.

[40] Balemans W., Ebeling M., Patel N., van Hul E., Olson P., Dioszegi M., Lacza C., Wuyts W., van Den Ende J., Willems P., Paes-Alves A. F., Hill S., Bueno M., Ramos F. J., Tacconi P., Dikkers F. G., Stratakis C., Lindpaintner K., Vickery B., Foernzler D., van Hul W., Increased bone density in sclerosteosis is due to the deficiency of a novel secreted protein (SOST). *Hum. Mol. Genet.*, 2001, 10, 537.

[41] Poole K. E., van Bezooijen R. L., Loveridge N., Hamersma H., Papapoulos S. E., Lowik C. W., Reeve J., Sclerostin is a delayed secreted product of osteocytes that inhibits bone formation. *FASEB J.*, 2005, 19, 1842.

[42] van Bezooijen R. L., Roelen B. A., Visser A., van der Wee-Pals L., Wilt E., Karperien M., Hamersma H., Papapoulos S. E., ten Dijke P., Lowik C.W., Sclerostin is an osteocyte-expressed negative regulator of bone formation, but not a classical BMP antagonist. *J. Exp. Med.*, 2004, 199, 805.

[43] Winkler D. G., Sutherland M. K., Geoghegan J. C., Yu C., Hayes T., Skonier J. E., Shpektor D., Jonas M., Kovacevich B. R., Staehling-Hampton K., Appleby M., Brunkow M. E., Latham J. A., Osteocyte control of bone formation via sclerostin, a novel BMP antagonist. *EMBO J.*, 2003, 22, 6267.

[44] Li X., Zhang Y., Kang H., Liu W., Liu P., Zhang J., Harris S. E., Wu D., Sclerostin binds to LRP5/6 and antagonizes canonical Wnt signaling. *J. Biol. Chem.*, 2005, 280, 19883.

[45] Semenov M., Tamai K., He X., SOST is a ligand for LRP5/LRP6 and a Wnt signaling inhibitor. *J. Biol. Chem.*, 2005, 280, 26770.

[46] van Bezooijen R. L., Svensson J. P., Eefting D., Visser A., van der Horst G., Karperien M. Quax P. H A, Vrieling H., Papapoulos S. E, ten Dijke P. Löwik C. W G M, Wnt but not BMP signaling is involved in the inhibitory action of sclerostin on BMP-stimulated bone formation. *J. Bone Miner Res.*, 2007, 22, 19.

[47] Weng L. H., Wang C. J., Ko J. Y., Sun Y. C., Su Y. S., Wang F. S., Inflammation induction of Dickkopf-1 mediates chondrocyte apoptosis in osteoarthritic joint. *Osteoarthr. Cartilage*, 2009, 17, 919.

[48] Blom A. B., Brockbank S. M., van Lent P. L., van Beuningen H. M., Geurts J., Takahashi N., van der Kraan P. M., van de Loo F. A., Schreurs B. W., Clements K., Newham P., van den Berg W. B., Involvement of the Wnt signaling pathway in experimental and human osteoarthritis: prominent role of Wnt-induced signaling protein 1. *Arthritis Rheum.*, 2009, 60, 501.

[49] Deal C., Potential new drug targets for osteoporosis. *Nat. Rev. Pract. Rheumatol.*, 2009, 5, 20.

[50] Li, X. Ominsky M. S., Niu Q. T., Sun N., Daugherty B., D'Agostin D., Kurahara C., Gao Y., Cao J., Gong J., Asuncion F., Barrero M., Warmington K., Dwyer D., Stolina M., Morony S., Sarosi I., Kostenuik P. J., Lacey D. L., Simonet W. S., Ke H. Z., Paszty C., Targeted deletion of the sclerostin gene in mice results in increased bone formation and bone strength. *J. Bone Miner. Res.*, 2008, 23, 860.

[51] Weidauer S. E., Schmieder P., Beerbaum M., Schmitz W., Oschkinat H., Mueller T. D., NMR structure of the Wnt modulator protein Sclerostin. *Biochem. Bioph. Res. Co.*, 2009, 380, 160.

[52] Karsdal M. A., Madsen S. H., Christiansen C., Henriksen K., Fosang A. J., Sondergaard B. C., Cartilage degradation is fully reversible in the presence of aggrecanase but not matrix metalloproteinase activity. *Arthritis Res. Ther.*, 2008, 10, R63.

[53] Morko J. P., SÖderstrÖm M., Sä ämänen A-M K., Salminen H. J., Vuorio E. I., Up regulation of cathepsin K expression in articular chondrocytes in a transgenic mouse model for osteoarthritis. *Ann. Rheum. Dis.*, 2004, 63, 649.

[54] Poole A.R., Alini M., Hollander A. P., Cellular biology of cartilage degradation. 1995, p163-204. In book: Mechanism and models in rheumatoid arthritis.

[55] Harris E. D., Krane S. M., Collagenases. *New Engl. J. Med.*, 1974, 291, 605.

[56] Johnson A. R., Pavlovsky A. G., Ortwine D. F., Prior F., Man C. F., Bornemeier D. A., Banotai C. A., Mueller W. T., McConnell P., Yan C., Baragi V., Lesch C., Roark W. H., Wilson M., Datta K., Guzman R., Han H. K., Dyer R. D., Discovery and characterization of a novel inhibitor of matri x metalloprotease-13 that reduces cartilage damage in vivo without joint fibroplasia side effects. *J. Biol. Chem.*, 2007, 282, 27781.

[57]   Piecha D., Weik J., Kheil H., Becher G., Timmermann A., Jaworski A., Burger M., Hofmann M. W., Novel selective MMP-13 inhibitors reduce collagen degradation in bovine articular and human osteoarthritis cartilage explants. *Inflamm. Res.*, 2010, 59, 379.

[58]   Maroudas A. I., Balance between swelling pressure and collagen tension in normal and degenerate cartilage. *Nature*, 1976, 260, 808.

[59]   Sandy J. D., Neame P. J., Boynton R. E., Flannery C. R., Catabolism of aggrecan in cartilage explants. Identification of a major cleavage site within the interglobular domain. *J. Biol. Chem.*, 1991, 266, 8683.

[60]   Sandy J. D.; Flannery C. R., Neame P. J., Lohmander L. S., The structure of aggrecan fragments in human synovial fluid. Evidence for the involvement in osteoarthritis of a novel proteinase which cleaves the Glu 373-Ala 374 bond of the interglobular domain. *J. Clin. Invest.*, 1992, 89, 1512.

[61]   Plaas A., Osborn B., Yoshihara Y., Bai Y., Bloom T., Nelson F., Mikecz K., Sandy J. D., Aggrecanolysis in human osteoarthritis: confocal localization and biochemical characterization of ADAMTS5-hyaluronan complexes in articular cartilages. *Osteoarthr. Cartilage*, 2007, 15, 719.

[62]   Glasson S. S., Askew R., Sheppard B., Carito B., Blanchet T., Ma H. L., Flannery C. R., Peluso D., Kanki K., Yang Z., Majumdar M. K., Morris E. A., Deletion of active ADAMTS5 prevents cartilage degradation in a murine model of osteoarthritis. *Nature*, 2005, 434, 644.

[63]   Majumdar M. K., Askew R., Schelling S., Stedman N., Blanchet T., Hopkins B., Morris E. A., Glasson S. S., Double-knockout of ADAMTS-4 and ADAMTS-5 in mice results in physiologically normal animals and prevents the progression of osteoarthritis. *Arthritis Rheum.*, 2007, 56, 3670.

[64]   Rodriguez-Lopez J., Mustafa Z., Pombo-Suarez M., Malizos K. N., Rego I., Blanco F. J., Tsezou A., Loughlin J., Gomez-Reino J. J., Gonzalez A., Genetic variation including nonsynonymous polymorphisms of a major aggrecanase, ADAMTS-5, in susceptibility to osteoarthritis. *Arthritis Rheum.*, 2008, 58, 435.

[65]   Fosang A. J., Rogerson F. M., Identifying the human aggrecanase. *Osteoarthr. Cartilage*, 2010, 18, 1109.

[66]   Dejica V. M., Mort J. S., Laverty S., Percival M. D., Antoniou J., Zukor D. J., Poole A. R., Cleavage of Type II Collagen by Cathepsin K in Human Osteoarthritic Cartilage. *Am. J. Pathol.*, 2008, 173, 161.

[67]   Shum K. T., Chan C., Leung C. M., Tanner J. A., Identification of a DNA aptamer that inhibits sclerostin's antagonistic effect on Wnt signaling. *Biochem. J.*, 2011, 434, 493.

[68]   Dassie J. P., Giangrande P. H., Current progress on aptamer-targeted oligonucleotide therapeutics. *Ther. Deli.*, 2013, 4, 1527.

[69] Abed É., Couchourel D., Delalandre A., Duval N., Pelletier J.-P., Martel-Pelletier J., Lajeunesse D, Lowsirtuin 1 levels in human osteoarthritis subchondral osteoblasts lead to abnormal sclerostin expression which decreases Wnt/β-catenin activity, *Bone,* 2014, 59, 28.

[70] Michael Lewiecki E., Role of sclerostin in bone and cartilage and its potential as a therapeutic target in bone diseases. *Ther Adv Musculoskel Dis.,* 2014, 6 (2) 48.

[71] Brew K., Nagase H., The tissue inhibitors of metalloproteinases (TIMPs): an ancient family with structural and functional diversity. *Biochim. Biophys. Acta,* 2010, 1803, 55.

[72] Amour A., Knight C. G., Webster A., Slocombe P. M., Stephens P. E., Knauper V., Docherty A. J., Murphy G. The in vitro activity of ADAM-10 is inhibited by TIMP-1 and TIMP-3. *FEBS Lett.,* 2000, 473, 275.

[73] Kashiwagi M., Tortorella M., Nagase H., Brew K., TIMP-3 is a potent inhibitor of aggrecanase 1 (ADAM-TS4) and aggrecanase 2 (ADAM-TS5). *J. Biol. Chem.,* 2001, 276, 12501.

[74] Loechel F., Fox J. W., Murphy G., Albrechtsen R., Wewer U. M., ADAM 12-S cleaves IGFBP-3 and IGFBP-5 and is inhibited by TIMP-3. *Biochem. Biophys. Res. Co.,* 2000, 278, 511.

[75] Amour A., Slocombe P. M., Webster A., Butler M., Knight C. G., Smith B. J., Stephens P. E., Shelley C., Hutton M., Knauper V., Docherty A. J., Murphy G., TNF-α converting enzyme (TACE) is inhibited by TIMP-3. *FEBS Lett.,* 1998, 435, 39.

[76] Visse, R., Nagase H., Matrix metalloproteinases and tissue inhibitors of metalloproteinases: structure, function, and biochemistry. *Circ. Res.,* 2003, 92, 827.

[77] Baker A. H., Edwards D. R., Murphy G., Metalloproteinase inhibitors: biological actions and therapeutic opportunities. *J. Cell Sci.,* 2002, 115, 3719.

[78] Troeberg L., Fushimi K., Khokha R., Emonard H., Ghosh P., Nagase H., Calcium pentosan polysulfate is a multifaceted exosite inhibitor of aggrecanases. *FASEB J.,* 2008, 22, 3515.

[79] Wayne G. J., Deng S.-J., Amour A., Borman S., Matico R., Carter H. L., Murphy G., TIMP-3 inhibition of ADAMTS-4 (Aggrecanase-1) is modulated by interactions between aggrecan and the C-terminal domain of ADAMTS-4. *J. Bio. Chem.,* 2007; 282, 20991.

[80] Wang W.-M., Ge G., Lim N. H., Nagase H., Greenspan D. S., TIMP-3 inhibits the procollagen N-proteinase ADAMTS-2. *Biochem. J.,* 2006, 398, 515.

[81] Frizler M., Stirnberg M., Sisay M. T., Gütschow M., Development of Nitrile-Based Peptidic Inhibitors of Cysteine Cathepsins. *Curr. Top. Med. Chem.,* 2010, 10, 294.

[82] Deaton D. N., Tavares F. X., Design of Cathepsin K inhibitors for Osteoporosis. *Curr. Top. Med. Chem.,* 2005, 5, 1639.

[83] Stoch S. A., Wagner J. A., Cathepsin K inhibitors: a novel target for osteoporosis therapy. *Clin. Pharmacol. Ther.*, 2008, 83, 172.

[84] Reesink H. W., Zeuzem S., Weegink C. J., Forestier N., van Vliet A., van de Wetering de Rooij J., McNair L., Purdy S., Kauffman R., Alam J., Jansen P. L., Rapid decline of viral RNA in hepatitis C patients treated with VX-950: a phase Ib, placebocontrolled, randomized study. *Gastroenterology*, 2006, 131, 997.

[85] Boros E. E., Deaton D. N., Hassell A. M., McFadyen R. B., Miller A. B., Miller L. R., Paulick M. G., Shewchuk L. M., Thompson J. B., Willard D. H., Wright L. L., Exploration of the P2-P3 SAR of aldehyde cathepsin K inhibitors. *Bioorg. Med. Chem. Lett.*, 2004, 14, 3425.

[86] Marquis R. W., Ru Y., Zeng J., Trout R. E., LoCastro S. M., Gribble A. D., Witherington J., Fenwick A. E., Garnier B., Tomaszek T., Tew D., Hemling M. E., Quinn C. J., Smith W. W., Zhao B., McQueney M. S., Janson C. A., D'Alessio K., Veber D. F., Cyclic ketone inhibitors of the cysteine protease cathepsin K. *J. Med. Chem.*, 2001, 44, 725.

[87] Bondebjerg J., Fuglsang H., Valeur K. R., Pedersen J., Naerum L., Dipeptidyl nitriles as human dipeptidyl peptidase I inhibitors. *Bioorg. Med. Chem. Lett.*, 2006, 16, 3614.

[88] Frizler M., Lohr F., Lülsdorff M., Gütschow M., Facing the *gem*-Dialkyl effect in enzyme inhibitor design: preparation of homocycloleucine-based azadipeptide nitriles. *Chem. Eur. J.*, 2011, 17, 5256.

[89] Deaton D. N., Hassell A. M., McFadyen R. B., Miller A. B., Miller L. R., Shewchuk L. M., 9Tavares F. X., Willard D. H., Wright L. L., Novel and potent cyclic cyanamide-based cathepsin K inhibitors. *Bioorg. Med. Chem. Lett.*, 2005, 15, 1815.

[90] Altmann E., Cowan-Jacob S. W., Missbach M., Novel purine nitrile derived inhibitors of the cysteine protease cathepsin K. *J. Med. Chem.*, 2004, 47, 5833.

[91] Leung-Toung R., Zhao Y., Li W., Tam T. F., Karimian K., Spino M., Thiol proteases: inhibitors and potential therapeutic targets. *Curr. Med. Chem.*, 2006, 13, 547.

[92] Löser R., Gut J., Rosenthal P. J., Frizler M., Gütschow M., Andrews K. T., Antimalarial activity od azadipeptide nitriles. *Bioorg. Med. Chem. Lett.*, 2010, 20, 252.

[93] Loh Y., Shi H., Hu M., Yao S. Q., "Click" synthesis of small molecule–peptide conjugates for organelle-specific delivery and inhibition of lysosomal cysteine proteases. *Chem. Commun.*, 2010, 46, 8407.

[94] Ren X.-F., Li H.-W., Fang X., Wu Y., Wang L., Zou S., Highly selective azadipeptide nitrile inhibitors for cathepsin K: design, synthesis and activity assays. *Org. Biomol. Chem.*, 2013, 11, 1143.

[95] Yuan X.-Y., Fu D.-Y., Ren X.-F., Fang X., Wang L., Zou S., Wu Y., Highly selective aza-nitriles inhibitors for cathepsin K, structural optimization and molecular modeling. Org. Biomol. Chem., 2013, 11, 5847.

8

Classifications and Definitions of Normal Joints

Xiaoming Zhang, Darryl Blalock and Jinxi Wang

1. Introduction

The anatomical definition of a joint (articulation) is the location where two or more bones, or any rigid parts of the skeleton, connect with each other. It forms a mechanical support to the skeleton and allows a variety of movements in different ranges between the rigid skeletal elements. Some joints, such as the sutures between cranial bones, allow very little or no movement. Other joints, such as the shoulder and hip joints, allow free movement in a large range [1].

2. Joint classification

Joints differ from each other by their tissue formation, function, structure, and movement.

2.1. Types of joints by tissue formation

When the articulating bones are connected, the connection may mainly involve three types of tissues – fibers, cartilages, or synovial membrane. Therefore, joints are generally classified according to these three tissues.

The fibrous joints are united by dense connective fibers such as the sutures between cranial bones, the interosseous membrane in the forearm, and the socket articulation between the root of the tooth and the alveolar processes of the maxilla and the mandible. The interosseous membrane allows movement between the two articulating bones. This type of fibrous joint is classified as "syndesmoses" (discussed below). The root of the tooth and its alveolar process associate in a manner similar to how a cone-shaped peg fits into a socket. There is very little room to move in this type of joint, which is defined as "gomphosis".

The cartilaginous joints have cartilage in between articulating bones to form a cartilaginous plate or disc. An example of a primary cartilaginous joint is the epiphyseal plate of a long bone, which disappears after puberty. An example of a secondary cartilaginous joint is the intervertebral disc between each vertebra.

The synovial joint is also called the "diarthrodial joint" and is formed by three basic components – the joint cavity, the joint (articular) cartilage which covers the surfaces of articulating bones, and the joint capsule which is composed of a synovial membrane layer lining up the joint cavity and a fibrous layer outside the synovial membrane. In addition, a synovial joint may have ligaments that form a portion of the fibrous joint capsule or ligaments that exist inside the joint capsule (Figure 1). Cartilaginous discs, such as the menisci in the knee joint, may also be found inside the joint cavity.

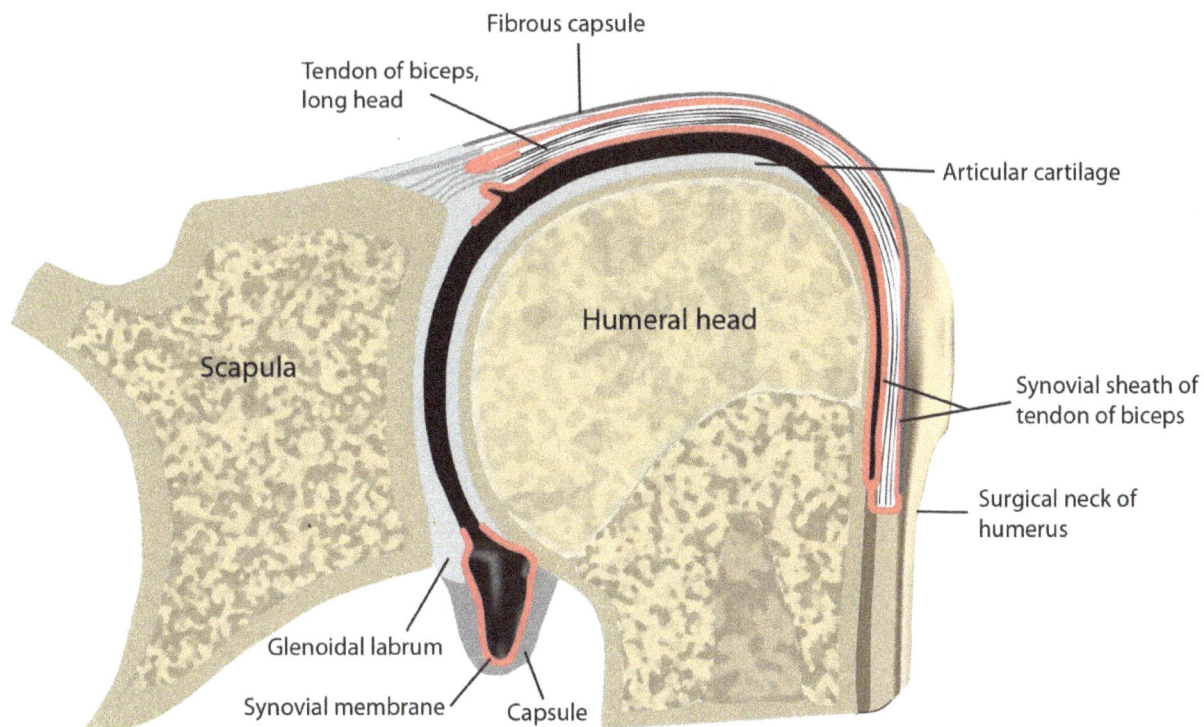

Figure 1. An illustration of the shoulder joint shows that the synovial membrane (red) lines the inner surface of the fibrous capsule. The joint/synovial cavity is marked in black. The tendon of the long head of the biceps passes through the joint and is enclosed in a tubular sheath of synovial membrane, which is continued around the tendon into the intertubercular sulcus as far as the surgical neck of the humerus.

2.2. Types of joints by tissue formation and mobility

Synarthroses joint: A fibrous type of joint that allows very little or no movement under normal conditions. If a joint is formed with an intervening tissue (fibrous connective tissue, cartilage, or bone) in between the two joint forming elements, it is a "synarthroses" joint. This type of joint usually has limited mobility. The above mentioned suture joints between cranial bones and the gomphosis are synarthroses joints.

Diarthroses joint: If a joint has a space in between the two joint forming elements, it is a "diarthroses" joint. Synovial joints are diathroses joints and their mobility varies in a large range.

Synostoses joint: This term is used to define when two bones fuse with each other under either normal or abnormal conditions. Normally, cranial bones fuse together when a child reaches adulthood, or when the diaphysis and epiphysis fuses in puberty. Abnormal fusion of bones may occur too early in development such as the early fusion of cranial bones (craniostenosis) or when bones are abnormally joined together such as the synostosis of the cervical vertebrae.

Syndesmoses joint: It refers to fibrous joints containing either an interosseous membrane or a ligament that allows movement. The distal tibiofibular joint is a typical syndesmosis joint.

Synchondroses joint: A cartilaginous joint containing a hyaline cartilage in between the two joined bones. The primary cartilaginous joint with an epiphyseal plate between the epiphysis and the diaphysis of a long bone is a typical synchondrosis joint. The joint between the first rib and the sternum (not including any other ribs) is also a synchondroses joint. However, the intervertebral discs are not considered synchondroses joints because they are composed of fibrous cartilage. They, along with the joint between the pubic bones, are instead referred to as "symphysis" joints.

2.3. Types of joints categorized by structure and movement.

Joints develop into different physical forms. As a result, the structural formation of a joint determines its movement. There are six types of joints in this category and they are all synovial joints (Figure 2).

Pivot type: A round bony process fits into a bony groove permitting rotation. For example, the atlanto-axial joint (between C1 and the Dens of C2 vertebrae).

Ball and socket type: A ball shaped bony head fits into a concavity allowing movement in several axes. The glenohumeral (shoulder) and hip joints are ball and socket type joints.

Plane type: The joint surfaces of both bones are flat against each other. Gliding action in one direction (uniaxial) can happen in this type of joint, for example, the acromioclavicular joint.

Hinge type: A joint forms like a door hinge allowing only one direction (uniaxial) movement, for example, the elbow joint.

Saddle type: The opposing articular surfaces are both saddle shaped. As a result, this type of joint can move in two directions (biaxial), for example, the carpometacarpal joint of the thumb.

Condyloid type: A rounded bony prominence of one bone articulates with a shallow indentation of another bone. This type joint allows two direction (biaxial) movement as well as circumduction, for example, the metacarpophalangeal joints.

Atlanto-axial joint
(Pivot-type joint)

Dens

Axis (C1)

Axis (C2)

Hip joint
(Ball-and-socket-type joint)

Acetabelum

Head of femur

Acromioclavicular joint
(Plane-type joint)

Clavicle

Acronium of scapula

Elbow joint
(Hinge-type joint)

Humerus

Radius

Ulna

Carpometacarpal joint
(Saddle-type joint)

Trapezium

First metacarpal

Metacarpophalangeal joint
(Condyloid-type joint)

Metacarpal

Proximal phalanx

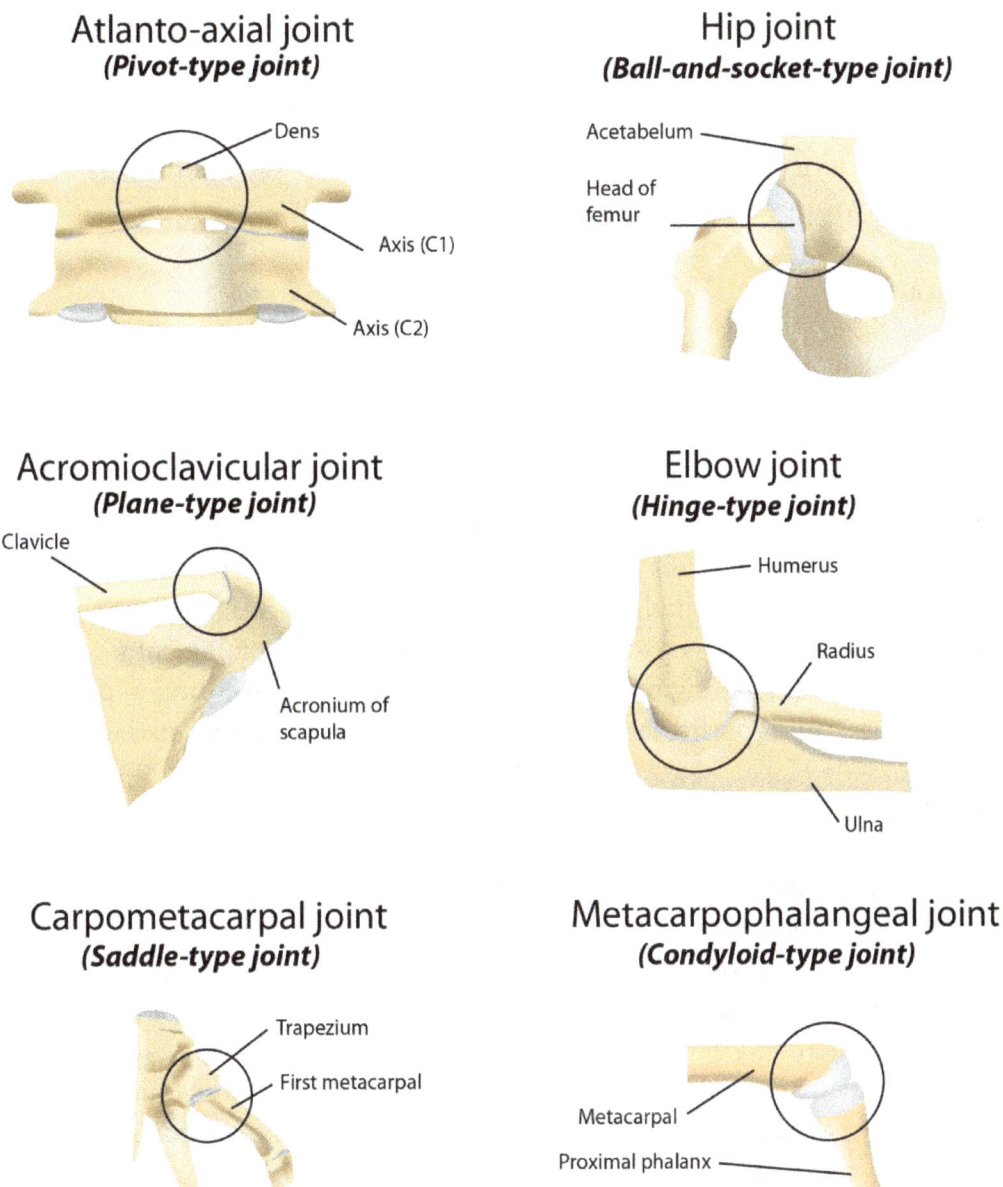

Figure 2. Diagrammatic illustrations show the structural features of six different types of human joints.

3. Cartilage associated with joints

Cartilage is a semi-rigid type of connective tissue composed of cells called chondrocytes and a large amount (>95%) of specialized extracellular matrix. Chondrocytes are scattered among the matrix and located in spaces called "lacunae".

A primary cartilaginous joint (synchondroses) such as the epiphyseal plate contains hyaline cartilage. The secondary cartilaginous joints (symphyses) such as the intervertebral discs contain fibrous cartilage. In synovial joints, a layer of hyaline cartilage "caps" the articulating surfaces of each joint-forming bone. This particular cartilage is called "articular cartilage". Articular cartilage provides smooth, low-friction, gliding surfaces for free movement. It also absorbs mechanical impacts placed on the articulating bones [1].

Cartilage is usually covered on its external surface by a thin layer of connective tissue named "perichondrium". However, perichondrium does not cover articular cartilage, the epiphyseal plate, and cartilage immediately under the skin such as the cartilage at the ear and nose.

Based on the characteristics of its matrix, cartilage is classified as the following and each type has its own different appearance and mechanical property [2].

3.1. Hyaline cartilage

Hyaline cartilage is named such because of the glassy (transparent) appearance of its matrix in living state. The matrix contains predominantly water (60-80%), with type II collagen fibers (~15%), chondroitin sulfate proteoglycan aggregates (~9%), and adhesive non-collagen glycoproteins (~5%) [2]. The highly hydrated matrix is due to the high content of proteoglycans, which allows water molecules to bind and stay. The hydrated matrix permits diffusion of small metabolites and nutrients as well as providing resilience to mechanical pressures during weight bearing. The matrix is made by the chondrocytes, which continuously remodel the matrix throughout life in response to mechanical, chemical, and biological signals. However, as the body ages, this remodeling process slows down or stops, resulting in degradation that surpasses synthesis. This is particularly the case in articular cartilage located in synovial joints.

3.2. Fibrocartilage

Fibrocartilage is a combination of hyaline cartilage and dense regular connective tissue [2]. The chondrocytes in fibrous cartilage appear similar to those in the hyaline cartilage. These cells make various amounts of type I and type II collagen fibers resulting in different proportions of type I and type II collagen in fibrocartilages at different regions of the body. Fibrocartilage can be found in intervertebral discs, pubic symphysis, articular discs inside several joint cavities, and the menisci in the knee joint. There is no perichondrium surrounding the fibrocartilages in these regions. Fibrocartilage functions much like a shock absorber for joints.

3.3. Elastic cartilage

Elastic cartilage is characterized by hyaline cartilage containing elastic fibers with the presence of elastin in its matrix. This type of cartilage is found mainly in the external ear, the wall of external acoustic meatus, the auditory (Eustachian) tube, and the epiglottis of the larynx [2].

4. Definition, structure, and function of joint tissues

4.1. Articular cartilage

Articular cartilage is a highly specialized viscoelastic hyaline cartilage that is found overlying the bone ends in synovial joints and forming the joint surface [3,4]. Articular cartilage has all the characteristics of hyaline cartilage with some additional features of its own.

Human articular cartilage is normally 2-4 mm thick and does not have a perichondrium on either the surface side that faces the joint cavity or the deep side that connects to the bone [3]. It has a limited intrinsic capacity to heal and repair, and is closely related to joint health.

From the joint surface to subchondral bone, a cross section of articular cartilage can be divided into four zones under the microscope (Figure 3).

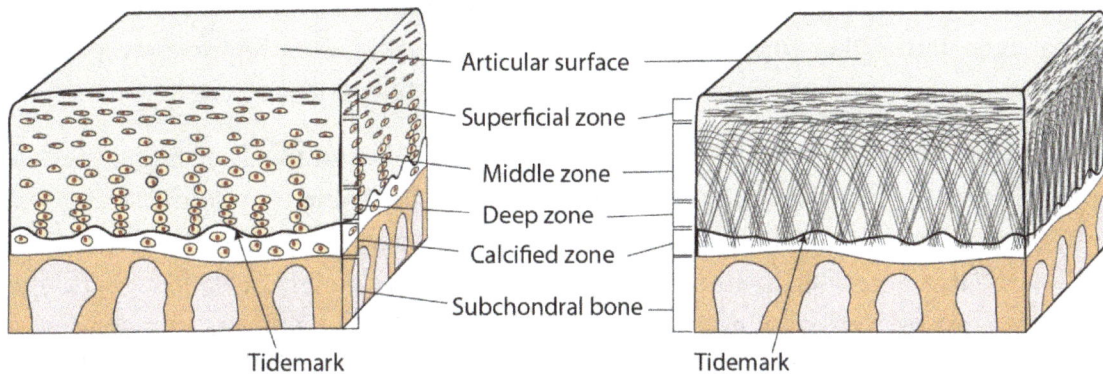

Figure 3. Illustrations showing the zonal features of human articular cartilage and subchondral bone. **Left panel** (chondrocyte organization): The superficial zone chondrocytes are small and flattened, which are orientated parallel to the joint surface. The middle zone chondrocytes are rounded and oriented randomly. The deep zone chondrocytes are grouped in columns or clusters. **Right panel:** Collagen orientation in articular cartilage. In the superficial (tangential) zone, small and medium-sized collagen fibrils aggregate into bundles that are aligned parallel to the joint surface. In the middle and deep zones, collagen fibrils aggregate into larger bundles and are aligned more perpendicular to the joint surface.

The superficial (tangential) zone contains numerous elongated and flattened chondrocytes. These cells are surrounded by dense type II collagen fibril fascicles arranged parallel to the surface [2]. This zone occupies 10-20% of the articular cartilage's thickness and is in contact with synovial fluid. It bears sheer, tensile, and compressive forces imposed on the articular surface [3].

The intermediate (middle or transitional) zone is deep to the superficial zone and contains randomly distributed round chondrocytes. Collagen fibers are generally organized in an oblique orientation to the surface. It occupies 40-60% of the thickness of articular cartilage and mainly resists compressive forces.

The deep (radial) zone has round chondrocytes arranged in short columns perpendicular to the joint surface. Collagen fibers located between cell columns are thick and are generally perpendicular to the joint surface. The proteoglycan content is the highest among all the zones while water concentration is low. It occupies about 30% of the thickness of articular cartilage and provides additional resistance to compressive forces [5,6].

The calcified zone contains a small amount of chondrocytes and a large amount of calcified matrix. A smooth and heavily calcified line called the "tidemark" separates this zone from the deep zone. The primary role of the calcified zone is to firmly secure articular cartilage to subchondral bone. This highly organized structure is responsible for the unique mechanical properties of articular cartilage.

In addition to the histologically defined zones, the matrix distribution of articular cartilage is distinguished in three regions [3].

The pericellular matrix is a thin layer adjacent to the cell membrane completely surrounding the chondrocyte. It contains mainly proteoglycans, glycoproteins, and other noncollagenous proteins. This matrix region may function to initiate signal transduction within cartilage.

The territorial matrix is thicker and surrounds the pericellular matrix. It is composed mostly of fine collagen fibrils that form a network around the cells. This region may protect the cartilage cells against mechanical stresses when there are substantial forces loaded.

The interterritorial region is the largest and refers to the collagen fibrils arranged parallel to the surface in the superficial zone, obliquely in the middle zone, and perpendicular in the deep zone. It contributes the most to the biomechanical properties of articular cartilage. The extracellular matrix accounts for approximately 95% of the dry weight of articular cartilage [4]. The primary macromolecule found in articular cartilage is type II collagen, which represents 90-95% of the total collagen content. The remaining are collagen types I, IV, V, VI, IX, and XI. The second largest group of macromolecules is proteoglycans which consist of a protein core with covalently linked glycosaminoglycan chains (GAGs). The main proteoglycans found in articular cartilage include aggrecan, decorin, biglycan and fibromodulin with aggrecan being the most abundant. Negatively charged carboxyl and sulfate groups found on these GAGs, namely keratin sulfate and chondroitin sulfate, have a high affinity for water [2,3].

The renewal process of mature articular cartilage is very slow due to the stable type II collagen structure and the long half-life of GAGs. The matrix degrading enzyme metalloproteinase activity is also low [2,3].

4.2. Synovial membrane (synovium)

Synovial membrane is the inner layer of the joint capsule facing the joint cavity and synovial fluid. The synovium lines the joint cavity producing synovial fluid that lubricates the joint surfaces and provides nutrition to the articular cartilage [7]. The synovial membrane is composed of two layers; the surface layer consisting of one or two layers of synovial cells and the underlying connective tissue layer.

There are two types of synovial cells. Type A synovial cells are macrophage-like cells whereas type B cells are fibroblast-like. These cells secrete hyaluronic acid and glycoprotein molecules, which are part of the synovial fluid lubricating the joint surfaces. There is no basal lamina separating the synovial cells from the underlying connective tissue. This connective tissue contains a rich network of fenestrated capillaries, which allow plasma to flow out of blood circulation and enter the joint cavity. The filtered plasma content combines with hyaluronic acid, glycoproteins, and leukocytes becoming the synovial fluid [8,9]. Normal synovial fluid appears clear to pale yellow in color, transparent, and contains less than 200 white blood cells/μl [10].

4.3. Joint capsule

The joint capsule is essential to the proper function of synovial joints. It forms the seal that contains synovial fluid within the joint, imparts passive stability by limiting joint movement, and provides active stability via its proprioceptive nerve endings [11]. It is composed of collagen fibers that are firmly adhered to bone through a fibrocartilaginous attachment. Localized thickenings of the capsule form capsular ligaments that provide strong points of fixation to bone. Tendons commonly attach to the joint capsule and occasionally replace it as is the case with the quadriceps and patellar tendons in the anterior knee. Blood vessels and nerves pass through the joint capsule supplying both the capsule and the underlying synovium. Nerve endings in the joint capsule are thought to be proprioceptive and play an important role in the active protection of the capsule and associated ligaments by reflex control of the appropriate musculature [11].

4.4. Tendon

Tendon is a tough band of fibrous connective tissue that usually connects muscle to bone. Tendons are mainly composed of type I collagen fibers arranged in fascicles and bands. Proteoglycans are primarily responsible for holding the collagen fibrils together. Specialized fibroblast cells called "tenocytes" exist in tendons and are responsible for collagen synthesis in tendon. Tendon is surrounded by a loose connective tissue layer called "peritendineum", which blends with the periosteum when the tendon attaches to the bone [12-14].

At the site of tendon insertion, parallel collagen fibers penetrate through the periosteum and insert into the mineralized fibrocartilage zone of the bone. Elastic fibers function to prevent overstretching and cartilage cells function to resist transverse shortening at the tendon insertion site [15].

Tendons contain some, but not many blood vessels. Enhanced physical activity can increase blood flow in the tendon. In regions where the tendons wrap around bony pulleys, blood supply is largely reduced. Tendons also have nerve supply in various degrees [12].

4.5. Ligament

Ligaments can be defined as dense bands of collagenous fibers that span a joint and are anchored to bone at either end [16]. Like tendon, ligament is made of dense connective tissue consisting mainly of type I collagen. Some ligaments are located outside the joint cavity; others are inside the joint cavity. Some ligaments are discrete structures that stand alone such as the cruciate ligaments in the knee; some are regional thickenings of the joint capsule as a part of the fibrous layer of the joint capsule. The primary function of ligaments is to provide passive stability to a joint through a normal range of motion under an applied load. Bundles of collagen fibrils form the majority of the ligament substance [17]. These fibrils are typically aligned in the direction of tension applied to the ligament during normal joint motion.

The ligament-bone interface is a complex structure that has been described as two distinct insertion types: direct and indirect. Direct insertion involves passage of a ligament directly into cortical bone. The superficial ligament collagen fibers merge with the fibrous layer of the periosteum while the majority of the insertion consists of deeper fibers directly penetrating the cortex [17]. These deep fibers pass through ligament substance, fibrocartilage, mineralized fibrocartilage and finally into bone. This direct insertion typically occurs at a right angle to the bone. In contrast, indirect insertions typically occur more obliquely. This type of insertion is less common and usually involves a wide surface area of insertion along the bone surface as opposed to directly into the cortex [17]. These insertions are believed to allow gradual transmission of force between ligament and bone.

4.6. Subchondral bone

The bony component lying under (deep to) the calcified zone of the articular cartilage is called subchondral bone, which can be separated into two distinct anatomic entities: subchondral bone plate and subchondral trabecular bone.

The subchondral bone plate is the thin cortical lamella, lying parallel to and immediately under the calcified cartilage. This cortical endplate is a penetrable structure and is invaded by channels that provide a direct link between articular cartilage and subchondral trabecular bone. A number of arterial and venous vessels, as well as nerves penetrate through the channels and send tiny branches into calcified cartilage, communicating between the calcified cartilage and the trabeculae bone [18-20].

Compared to the subchondral bone plate, the sunchondral trabecular bone is more porous and metabolically active, containing blood vessels, sensory nerves, and bone marrow. It exerts important shock-absorbing and supportive functions in normal joints and may also be important for cartilage nutrient supply and metabolism [18,19].

Subchondral bone changes are important features of osteoarthritis (OA), suggesting that subchondral bone plays a vital role in the pathogenesis of OA [21-23]. Bone marrow edema-like lesions (BMELs), which are strongly associated with pain among patients with OA, are frequently identified by magnetic resonance imaging (MRI) in patients with progressive OA. BMELs are also observed in the healthy, asymptomatic population and predict an increased risk of OA [24,25].

5. Conclusion

This chapter describes the classification of different types of joints based on their structural and functional features. The anatomical and functional features of six different types of human joints are demonstrated. Definitions and structures of specific joint tissues associated with the function of joints such as the joint cartilage, synovial membrane, joint capsule, tendon, ligament, ligament-bone interface, and subchondral bone are described in great detail. The clinical relevance of specific joint structures to joint injury, joint instability, and the development of OA is discussed at both macro- and micro-anatomical levels.

Acknowledgements

This work was supported in part by the U.S. National Institutes of Health (NIH)/NIAMS grant R01 AR059088, the U.S. Department of Defense medical research grant W81XWH-12-1-0304, and the Harrington Distinguished Professorship Endowment. The authors thank Mr. Brian Egan and Mr. Zhaoyang Liu for their graphic and editorial assistance.

Author details

Xiaoming Zhang[1], Darryl Blalock[2] and Jinxi Wang[2]

*Address all correspondence to: jwang@kumc.edu

1 Department of Anatomy and Cell Biology, University of Kansas School of Medicine, Kansas City, USA

2 Department of Orthopedic Surgery, University of Kansas School of Medicine, Kansas City, USA

References

[1] Moore KL, Dalley AF, Agur AMR.. Introduction to Clinically Oriented Anatomy. In: Moore KL, Dalley AF, Agur AMR (eds.), Clinically Oriented Anatomy, 7th ed. 2014; Wolters Kluwer Lippincott Williams & Wilkins, Philadelphia, p25-29.

[2] Ross MH, Pawlina W. Cartilage. In: Ross MH and Pawlina W. (eds.) Histology: A text and Atlas 6th ed. 2011; Wolters Kluwer Lippincott Williams & Wilkins, Philadelphia, pp198-217.

[3] Sophia Fox AJ, Bedi A, Rodeo SA. The basic science of articular cartilage: structure, composition, and function. Sports Health. 2009;1(6):461-468.

[4] Alford JW, Cole BJ. Cartilage restoration, part 1: basic science, historical perspective, patient evaluation, and treatment options. Am J Sports Med. 2005;33(2):295-306.

[5] Curtin WA, Reville WJ. Ultrastructural observations on fibril profiles in normal and degenerative human articular cartilage. Clin Orthop Relat Res. 1995(313):224-230.

[6] Minns RJ, Steven FS. The collagen fibril organization in human articular cartilage. J Anat. 1977;123(Pt 2):437-457.

[7] Firestein GS, Kelley WN. Kelley's textbook of rheumatology. 9th ed. Philadelphia, PA: Elsevier/Saunders; 2013.

[8]   Edwards JC. The nature and origins of synovium: experimental approaches to the study of synoviocyte differentiation. J Anat. 1994;184 (Pt 3):493-501.

[9]   Vandenabeele F, De Bari C, Moreels M, Lambrichts I, Dell'Accio F, Lippens PL, Luyten FP. Morphological and immunocytochemical characterization of cultured fibroblast-like cells derived from adult human synovial membrane. Arch Histol Cytol. 2003;66(2):145-153.

[10] Thompson JC. Basic Science. In: Thompson JC (eds.) Netter's Concise Orthopaedic Anatomy 2nd ed. 2010; Saunders/Elsevier, Philadelphia, p20.

[11] Ralphs JR, Benjamin M. The joint capsule: structure, composition, ageing and disease. J Anat. 1994;184 (Pt 3):503-509.

[12] Benjamin M, Kaiser E, Milz S. Structure-function relationships in tendons: a review. J Anat. 2008;212(3):211-228.

[13] Connizzo BK, Yannascoli SM, Soslowsky LJ. Structure-function relationships of postnatal tendon development: a parallel to healing. Matrix Biol. 2013;32(2):106-116.

[14] Thorpe CT, Birch HL, Clegg PD, Screen HR. The role of the non-collagenous matrix in tendon function. Int J Exp Pathol. 2013;94(4):248-259.

[15] Schuenke M, Schulte E, Schumacher U. The Muscles. In: Schuenke M, Schulte E, Schumacher U. (eds.) Thieme Atlas of Anatomy, general anatomy and musculoskeletal system. 2006; Thieme, Stuttgart, p42.

[16] Frank CB. Ligament structure, physiology and function. J Musculoskelet Neuronal Interact. 2004;4(2):199-201.

[17] DeLee J, Drez D, Miller MD. DeLee & Drez's orthopaedic sports medicine : principles and practice. 3rd ed. Philadelphia: Saunders/Elsevier; 2010.

[18] Li G, Yin J, Gao J, Cheng TS, Pavlos NJ, Zhang C, Zheng MH. Subchondral bone in osteoarthritis: insight into risk factors and microstructural changes. Arthritis Res Ther. 2013;15(6):223.

[19] Madry H, van Dijk CN, Mueller-Gerbl M. The basic science of the subchondral bone. Knee Surg Sports Traumatol Arthrosc. 2010;18(4):419-433.

[20] Milz S, Putz R. Quantitative morphology of the subchondral plate of the tibial plateau. J Anat. 1994;185 (Pt 1):103-110.

[21] Baker-LePain JC, Lane NE. Role of bone architecture and anatomy in osteoarthritis. Bone. 2012;51(2):197-203.

[22] Burr DB, Gallant MA. Bone remodelling in osteoarthritis. Nat Rev Rheumatol. 2012;8(11):665-673.

[23] Weinans H, Siebelt M, Agricola R, Botter SM, Piscaer TM, Waarsing JH. Pathophysiology of peri-articular bone changes in osteoarthritis. Bone. 2012;51(2):190-196.

[24] Link TM, Steinbach LS, Ghosh S, Ries M, Lu Y, Lane N, Majumdar S. Osteoarthritis: MR imaging findings in different stages of disease and correlation with clinical findings. Radiology. 2003;226(2):373-381.

[25] Wluka AE, Hanna F, Davies-Tuck M, Wang Y, Bell RJ, Davis SR, Adams J, Cicuttini FM. Bone marrow lesions predict increase in knee cartilage defects and loss of cartilage volume in middle-aged women without knee pain over 2 years. Ann Rheum Dis. 2009;68(6):850-855.

9

Biomechanics of Cartilage and Osteoarthritis

Herng-Sheng Lee and Donald M. Salter

1. Introduction

The etiology of osteoarthritis (OA) is not known with certainty. Undoubtedly, many factors contribute to articular cartilage failure but consistently abnormal biomechanics appear central to the condition. Indeed it is recognized that mechanical loading that is either below or in excess of the physiology range leads cartilage degeneration. There are currently no cures for OA and no effective pharmacological treatments that slow or halt disease progression. Physical activity is one of the most widely prescribed non-pharmacological therapies for OA management, based on its ability to limit pain and improve physical function. The detailed mechanisms underlying these beneficial effects of exercise and physical therapy are largely unknown. Structural integrity is important for joint function and can be lost as a consequence of a range of physical, biomechanical and inflammatory factors. This chapter will overview how joint loading influences cartilage structure and how mechanical loading is perceived by chondrocytes resulting in cellular responses that are either chondroprotective or promoting inflammatory and catabolic responses initiating and progressing OA.

2. Mechanical integrity of joint structure

The synovial or diarthrodial joint allows movement between bones and permits transmission of mechanical loads. The mechanical integrity of the joint elements including articular cartilage, synovium, subchondral bone, joint capsule, ligaments and periarticular connective tissues cooperates to provide optimal function. Loss of mechanical integrity results in a range of pathological changes within the joint recognized as osteoarthritis.

In a synovial joint the articulating bone ends are covered by a thin, highly hydrated specialized connective tissue, articular cartilage. A high interstitial fluid content distinguishes cartilage from most other connective tissues and contributes to the mechanical properties of the tissue

[1,2]. The major components of articular cartilage are type II collagen, proteoglycans, noncollagenous proteins and glycoproteins. Type II collagen forms the fibrillar meshwork which provides tensile strength [3-6] and entraps aggregating hydrophilic proteoglycans which help maintain the high tissue hydration [7-9]. Disruption of the fibrillar meshwork or loss of proteoglycan results in an in-ability of cartilage to distribute loads and its contribution to near frictionless joint movement leading, in time, to progressive structural damage and pathological features of OA.

3. Articular cartilage responses to mechanical loading *in vivo*

Mechanical loading within a physiological range is necessary to maintain joints in a healthy state. During normal daily activity articular cartilage is exposed to a range of mechanical forces during joint movement. Peak forces across the human hip and knee joints have been shown to reach 4 and 7 times body weight, respectively, during normal walking [10,11]. In vivo, mechanical loading is applied cyclically and the cells within cartilage, chondrocytes, are exposed to a composite of radial, tangential and shear stresses [12]. The effects of mechanical load bearing on the development and microscopic structure of the articular cartilage have been studied in some detail [13]. Elevated loading increases cartilage thickness, causes hypertrophy of the superficial zone chondrocytes, and increases the amount of intercellular matrix [14-17]. In normal human joints, load-bearing areas of the cartilage are thicker with a higher proteoglycan concentration and are mechanically stronger than non-load-bearing regions of the same joint [18-20]. Increasing weight-bearing of joints, in a variety of animal models, leads to elevation of proteoglycan content within articular cartilage [15,16,21-23]. In contrast, removal of load bearing leads to a reduction in proteoglycan content [13]. In a dog model, immobilization of a joint by placing a leg in a cast leads to cartilage atrophy, loss of Safranin O staining, and a decrease in its uronic acid content [21]. These changes are reversible on remobilization. Mechanical regulation is also an important factor for chondrogenesis and has been involved in the development of cell-based therapies for cartilage degeneration and disease [24].

3.1. Mechanical stress within articular cartilage

Articular cartilage is exposed to surprisingly large mechanical loads during joint movement. Using an instrumented hip prosthesis mechanical stresses have been measured in a 74-year-old female [25]. Rising from a chair, pressures in the hip joint cartilage can reach nearly 20 MPa and during walking, pressures cycle between atmospheric and 3-4 MPa at a frequency of around 1 Hz. With walking or running forces at the joint surface may vary from near zero to several times the whole body weight within a period of 1 second [10,11]. Loading of articular cartilage generates a combination of tensile, compressive and shear stress in the material. The tensile modulus of healthy human articular cartilage varies from 5-25 MPa, depending on the site of movement on the joint surface (i.e., high or low weight bearing regions), and the depth and orientation of the test specimen relative to the joint surface [4,26]. The compressive modulus varies from 0.4-2.0 MPa [27,28]. Articular cartilage responds to shearing forces by both stretching and deformation of the solid matrix. The dynamic shear modulus is within the range of 0.2-2.0 MPa for healthy bovine or canine cartilage [29-31]. These physiological stresses are important regulators of cartilage metabolism and integrity as mechanical loading serves to maintain fluid flow and ion phase function within the tissue and act to stimulate chondrocyte metabolism [32].

4. Articular cartilage explant and chondrocyte responses to mechanical loading *in vitro*

Rodan et al. [33] studied the effects of application of compressive forces (80 g/cm^2) to chick tibial epiphyses (16-day-old embryos) in culture and found that glucose consumption reduced to half of controls. Twenty four hours after the release of pressure, glucose utilization again increased, approaching control levels. The same pressure also stimulated thymidine incorporation into DNA. Exposing chick tibial epiphyses to continuous compressive forces (60 g/cm^2, equal to 5.865 kPa) caused a reduction of both cAMP and cGMP [34]. An equivalent hydrostatic pressure applied directly to cells isolated from chick tibial epiphyses also affects cyclic nucleotide accumulation [34]. Veldhuijzen et al. developed a model system that exposed cultured monolayer chondrocytes on the walls of tissue culture tubes to intermittent compressive forces of 12.8 kPa for 6 hours at a frequency of 0.3 Hz [35]. Contrary to the effect of continuous compressive forces, intermittent compressive forces caused a rise in levels of cAMP and a reduction in DNA synthesis. Palmoski and Brandt [36] studied the effects of both static and intermittent mechanical stress on full-thickness plugs of canine articular cartilage. When the plugs were exposed to compressive force using a regime of 60 sec on/60 sec off, glycosaminoglycan synthesis was reduced to 30-60% of controls. However, when a regime of 4 sec on/ 11 sec off was employed, the glycosaminoglycan synthesis increased by 34%, although protein synthesis and DNA, uronic acid, and water content remained unaltered indicating that different frequencies of cyclical strain produce differences in metabolic activity within chondrocytes.

Some models designed to test the effects of mechanical force on chondrocytes in vitro have focused on the effects of cell stretching. In these models there is usually deformation of a cell-laden, flexible membrane which can be regulated according to (1) the method of deformation of the membrane - by control of either the displacement or the force, and (2) the shape and mounting of the deformable membrane - either a circular membrane held at its periphery or

displacement include (a) a vacuum driven diaphragm (silicone elastomer membrane, 2.5 mm in thickness) [38,39], (b) pin shaped displacement (silicone elastomer membrane, 0.254 mm in thickness) [40], (c) glass dome displacement (polytetrafluoroethylene membrane, 0.025 mm in thickness) [41,42], (d) air or fluid displacement (polyurethane membrane, 0.094 mm in thickness) [43-45], and (e) a circular groove displacement (silicone elastomer membrane, 0.076 mm in thickness; polyurethane membrane, 0.094 mm in thickness) [46,47]. The Flexercell™ strain unit [38] consists of a computer-controlled vacuum unit and a baseplate on which are held the culture dishes. These dishes have a flexible base. A vacuum is applied to the dishes via the baseplate. When a precise vacuum level is applied to the system, the bases of the culture plates are deformed by known percentage elongation that is maximal at the edge of the culture dish, but decreases towards the center. Using the system, straining the base of a culture dish leads to strain of the attached cultured cells. When the vacuum is released, the bases of the dishes return to their original conformation.

By stretching a supportive flexible membrane on which chondrocytes were cultured, Lee et al. [48] found that a cyclic 10% mechanical stretch for 8 hours increased glycosaminoglycan synthesis and decreased protein and collagen synthesis. DeWitt et al. [49] showed increased radiosulphate and ^{14}C-glucosamine incorporation into glycosaminoglycans by chick epiphyseal chondrocytes in high density cultures subjected to a 5.5% strain at a frequency of 0.2 Hz. Protein synthesis after 24 hours mechanical strain remained unchanged. Using the Flexercell™ strain system, Fujisawa et al. [50] investigated the influence of cyclic tension force on the metabolism of cultured chondrocytes. Two levels of force (5 kPa or 15 kPa) and three frequencies 30 cycles/min (1 sec on/1 sec off), 0.5 cycles/min (1 sec on/119 sec off) and 0.25 cycles/min (1 sec on/239 sec off) were used. Both 5 and 15 kPa of high frequency cyclic mechanical stress for 48 hours significantly inhibited the syntheses of DNA, proteoglycan, collagen, and protein. The expression of interleukin-1, matrix metalloproteinase (MMP)-2 and MMP–9 mRNA were induced by 15 kPa of high frequency force. The production of pro- and active-MMP-9 which would lead to cartilage breakdown in vivo was also increased at this pressure and frequency of stimulation. Reducing the applied frequency decreased the inhibition of proteoglycan synthesis. Mechanical stretch producing 25% maximal elongation at a frequency of 0.05 Hz for 48 hours also induces the expression of high molecular weight heat shock protein (HSP) 105 kDa in the human chondrocytic cell line CS-OKB [51]. These findings suggest that the frequency of cyclic tension force is one of the key determinants of chondrocyte metabolism.

Using confocal microscopy and fluorescent techniques it is possible to monitor and measure intracellular calcium ion concentration in isolated articular chondrocytes subjected to controlled deformation with the edge of a glass micropipette [52]. Intracellular calcium ion concentration reaches a peak within 5 sec following 25% deformation of the cells and returns to baseline levels in 3-5 minutes. The immediate and transient increase of intracellular calcium waves is abolished by removing Ca^{2+} from the culture medium and is significantly reduced by the presence of gadolinium and amiloride, agents known to block mechanosensitive ion channels [53-56]. Inhibitors of intracellular Ca^{2+} release or agents known to cause cytoskeletal disruption including cytochalasin D and colchicine had no significant effect on the Ca^{2+} waves. The results indicate that mechanosensitive ion channels are upstream in the mechanotransduction signaling pathway, consistent with results obtained using electrophysiological parameters in the assessment of the cell response to cyclical mechanical strain [56].

The effects of fluid-induced shear stress on articular chondrocyte morphology and metabolism in vitro have also been investigated [57]. Fluid-induced shear stress (1.6 Pa = 16 dynes/cm^2) was applied by cone viscometer to both normal human and bovine articular chondrocytes. Shear stress for 48 and 72 hours caused individual chondrocytes to elongate and align tangential to the direction of cone rotation. Glycosaminoglycan synthesis was increased 2-fold. After 48 hours of shear stress, the release of prostaglandin E2 (PGE2) was increased 10 to 20-fold. In human articular chondrocytes, mRNA levels for tissue inhibitor of metalloproteinase (TIMP) increased 9-fold in response to shear stress compared to controls. In contrast, mRNA levels for the neutral metalloproteinases, collagenase, stromelysin, and gelatinase, did not show significant changes [57].

5. Chondrocyte mechanoreceptors

The mechanisms by which chondrocytes recognize and respond to the various mechanical stresses encountered in mechanically loaded cartilage continue to be elaborated. A number of potential mechanoreceptors, sensory receptors that respond to vibration, stretching, pressure, or other mechanical stimuli have been identified in chondrocytes. In cartilage the extracellular matrix (ECM) transmits mechanical signals to the cell interior through changes in tension on the cell membrane. Integrins, stretch-activated ion channels, connexins, and primary cilia have each been identified as candidate mechanoreceptors [58-61].

5.1. Integrins

Integrins were first isolated, characterized, and sequenced from chick embryo fibroblast cDNA clones which encoded one subunit of the complex of membrane glycoproteins [62]. The name 'integrin' was proposed as the consequence of its role as an integral membrane complex involved in the transmembrane association between the ECM and the cytoskeleton. Integrins are a large family of α/β heterodimeric cell surface adhesion receptors that can bind a wide variety of ECM and cell surface ligands [63-69]. Most integrins bind ligands that are components of ECM, e.g. fibronectin, collagen, and vitronectin [70]; certain integrins can bind to soluble ligands (such as fibrinogen) or to counter receptors (such as intercellular adhesion molecules) on adjacent cells, leading to homo- or heterotypic aggregation [71,72]. Some of the integrin recognition sites in the ligands and counter receptors have been defined [73,74]. The first binding site to be defined was the Arg-Gly-Asp (RGD) containing sequence present in fibronectin, vitronectin, and a variety of other adhesive proteins [75,76].

Integrin expression by human chondrocytes has been investigated utilizing several techniques including immunohistochemistry, flow cytometry, immunoprecipitation, and northern blotting [77-79]. Normal adult human articular chondrocytes express $\alpha1\beta1$, $\alpha3\beta1$, $\alpha5\beta1$, $\alpha V\beta5$, $\alpha V\beta3$, $\alpha6\beta1$, $\alpha10\beta1$, and $\alpha2\beta1$, in which the $\alpha1\beta1$ (receptor for collagen), $\alpha5\beta1$ (receptor for fibronectin) and the $\alpha V\beta5$ (receptor for vitronectin) heterodimers are consistently expressed. In cartilage, integrin-ECM interactions are thought to be important in many aspects, physiological and pathological, of chondrocyte function, including adhesion, spreading, proliferation, signal transduction, biomechanical regulation, chondrogenesis, and gene expression [80]. Chondrocyte $\beta1$ integrin-ECM interactions are required for chondrocyte survival, matrix deposition and differentiation in models of chondrocyte development [81]. Integrins mediate chondrocyte adhesion to many ECM proteins including type II collagen, type VI collagen, fibronectin, laminin, and osteopontin [82-85]. Chondrocyte spreading and migration on type II collagen, type VI collagen, or fibronectin substrates in vitro is mediated by interactions with $\beta1$ integrins [86,87]. The interaction of the $\alpha5\beta1$ integrin with fibronectin is necessary for adhesion, spreading, and proliferation of both chicken and rabbit chondrocytes [88,89]. *In vitro* chondrogenesis (the differentiation of blastemal cells to chondroblasts and the formation of cartilage matrix) is inhibited by the function blocking anti-$\beta1$ integrin antibodies [90]. Laminin-$\alpha3\beta1/\alpha6\beta1$ interactions are regulated by the ligand trend (depletion/reconstitution or competition experiments) during early chondrocyte differentiation [89]. Other integrin-mediated chondrocyte-matrix interactions include $\beta1$-matrix Gla protein, $\beta3$-bone sialoprotein II, $\beta3$-osteopontin, and $\alpha2\beta1$-chondroadherin associations [84,86].

Integrins are involved in regulation of both cartilage matrix synthesis and integrity. Loss of integrin function inhibits type II collagen synthesis by chondrocytes in culture [91]. However, integrins are also involved in cartilage breakdown processes. Fibronectin fragments stimulate chondrolysis and decrease proteoglycan synthesis in cartilage explants through fibronectin-integrin dependent interactions [92]. Ligation of $\alpha5\beta1$ integrin with fibronectin in cultured chondrocytes results in the formation of focal adhesion complexes comprising actin, focal adhesion kinase (FAK) and the G protein Rho [93]. Nitric oxide (NO), a potential mediator of events occurring in osteoarthritis, can inhibit the assembly of the intracellular activation complex and the subsequent upregulation of proteoglycan synthesis that occurs following ligation of $\alpha5\beta1$ integrin to fibronectin [93].

Integrins also act as mechanoreceptors and transmit mechanical signals from the extracellular environment to the cytoskeleton [94-96]. Integrins can provide a gating function for signal transduction, by either supporting or prohibiting force transmission between ECM and the cytoskeleton [94]. Wang et al. [97], using a magnetic twisting device applied mechanical forces directly to cell surface receptors. They showed that the integrin subunit $\beta1$ induced focal adhesion formation and supported a force-dependent stiffening response, whereas nonadhesion receptors did not [97]. Maniotis et al. [98] reported that living cells and nuclei are hardwired. When integrins were stimulated by micromanipulating bound microbeads or micropipettes, cytoskeletal filaments reoriented, nuclei distorted, and nucleoli redistributed along the axis of the applied tension field. These effects were specific for integrins, independent of cortical membrane distortion, and were mediated by direct linkages between the cytoskeleton and nucleus [98]. Using a similar magnetic drag force device, intracellular Ca^{2+} concentration was shown to increase when the $\alpha2$ or the $\beta1$ integrin subunits were stressed, whereas mechanical loading of the transferrin receptor produced a significantly reduced effect [99]. An increase in tyrosine phosphorylation was observed as a reaction to mechanical stress on the $\beta1$-subunits of the integrin family, whilst stress to the transferrin or low density lipoprotein receptors which have no connection to the cytoskeleton did not produce this reaction [100,101].

Integrins are also modulated by mechanical stress [102]. When chondrosarcoma cells were exposed to mechanical stimulation, mRNA expression of the $\alpha5$ integrin subunit was found to increase whilst expression of the $\beta1$, $\alpha2$, and αV did not increase significantly [102]. The effect of mechanical stress on integrin subunit expression has also been investigated in cells cultured on type II collagen-coated dishes with a flexible base. Mechanical stress increased mRNA expression of the $\alpha2$ integrin subunit whilst the levels of mRNA for integrin subunits $\beta1$, $\alpha1$, $\alpha5$, and αV showed no or only small changes [102]. It is likely that mechanical induced regulation of integrins is closely regulated and may be dependent on the nature of the mechanical force acting on the cell and specific mechanoreceptor stimulated.

5.2. Stretch-activated Ion channels

Stretch-activated or stretch-sensitive ion channels (SACs) open as a consequence of mechanical deformation of the cell membrane [103]. SACs are directly activated by mechanical forces applied along the plane of the cell membrane that induce membrane tension and distortion of the lipid bilayer. These result in conformational changes which alter opening or closing rates of the channels permitting ion flux [104]. Application of mechanical forces perpendicular to the cell membrane, as seen with hydrostatic pressure, appears to be less effective in activating SACs [103]. Activation of calcium permeable SACs leads to local increase in intracellular calcium levels and stimulation of downstream calcium-dependent intracellular signal cascades. SACs sensitive to gadolinium are necessary for load and fluid flow related cellular responses in both chondrocytes and bone cells.

5.3. Connexins

Connexins are widely expressed in connective tissue where networks of cells are seen such as in bone, tendon and, meniscus. They probably act to allow propagation of a mechanical stimulus through a tissue. They are a superfamily of twenty-one transmembrane proteins that form gap junctions and hemichannels [105]. Gap junctions allow continuity between cells permitting diffusion of ions, metabolites and small signaling molecules such as cyclic nucleotides and inositol derivatives. Cx43 is the most abundant connexin present in skeletal tissue. Conditional deletion of Cx43 reduces mineral apposition rate to mechanical loading and Cx43 hemichannels are important for fluid shear induced PGE2 and ATP release in osteocytic cells [106]. Connexins and gap junctions are present at the tip of osteocyte dendritic processes and between these processes and osteoblasts indicating their potential importance in permitting cell–cell communication among the osteocytic network although propagation may be only directed from osteocytes to osteoblasts [107]. Cx43 hemichannels are activated and mediate small molecule exchange between cells and matrix under mechanical stimulation in rat temporomandibular joint (TMJ) chondrocytes [108]. Cx32 and Cx43 are important in tenocyte mechanotransduction [109]. Cx32 junctions form a communication network arranged along the line of principal loading and stimulate collagen production in response to strain. Connexin dependent mechanotransducation may be important in adaptation of subchondral bone to mechanical loading of joints rather than having a major role in chondrocyte dependent mechanotransduction. Nevertheless recent studies suggest that primary cilia associated connexins may be functional in responses of chondrocytes to mechanical loading.

5.4. Primary Cilia

Primary cilia are solitary, immotile cilium present in most cells including chondrocytes and bone cells. They are microtubule-based organelles, growing from the centrosome to extend from the cell surface and contain large concentrations of cell membrane receptors, including integrins [110]. They function both as chemosensors and mechanosensors [111,112]. Bending of the cilium upon matrix deformation or with fluid flow is thought to cause cilium bending, pulling on associated matrix receptors and activation of the mechanoreceptors [113]. In addition to integrins, Cx43 hemichannels are also present on primary cilia and by regulating ATP release cilia and activation of purine receptors cilia-associated connexins may also be involved in mechanotransduction.

6. Chondrocyte mechanotransduction

Mechanoresponsiveness is a fundamental feature of all living cells [94,114,115]. Studies with cultured cells confirm that mechanical stresses can directly alter many cellular processes, including signal transduction, gene expression, growth, differentiation, and survival [116]. Wright et al. [117] investigated the effects of applied hydrostatic pressure on the transmembrane potentials of articular chondrocytes. These studies have been pivotal in identifying potential mechanotransduction pathways in both normal and osteoarthritic human chondrocytes. In this system cells in monolayer culture were exposed to an increase in hydrostatic pressure by placing culture dishes in a sealed perspex pressure chamber with a gas inlet and outlet. Nitrogen or helium gas was used to pressurize the cultures. A hyperpolarization of the chondrocyte plasma membrane was induced by cyclic pressurization (0.33 Hz, 120 mmHg for 20 min) whilst depolarization was induced by continuous pressure (120 mmHg, 20 min). For the frequencies tested, the maximum values for chondrocyte hyperpolarization occurred at approximately 0.3-0.4 Hz. The mechanical stimulation regime (0.33 Hz, 120 mmHg, 20 min), similar to that used by Veldhuijzen et al. [35], allowed identification of a number of integral components of the electrophysiological response providing insight into molecules and pathways activated in chondrocyte upon mechanical stimulation. By the use of pharmacological inhibitors, it was shown that the hyperpolarization response in cultured human chondrocytes induced by cyclic pressurization involved Ca^{2+} activated K^+ channels and L-type calcium channels. Hyperpolarization was also produced by addition of the calcium ionophore A23187 to the culture medium showing that a rise in intracellular Ca^{2+} concentration within the cell could induce the response. Plasma membrane histamine H1 and H2 receptors, and β-adrenoreceptors did not appear to be involved in the hyperpolarization response. The studies also showed that the actin cytoskeleton, but not microtubules, was involved in the chondrocyte hyperpolarization response [117].

Subsequent studies identified that the electrophysiological response to cyclical pressurization was the result of deformation of the base of the culture dishes to which the chondrocytes were attached and therefore deformation (strain) on the chondrocytes rather than a direct effect of the increased hydrostatic pressure on chondrocytes [56]. The hyperpolarization response was proportional to the microstrain to which cells were subjected and did not occur when chondrocytes were subjected to cyclical pressurization in rigid glass culture dishes or when the plastic dishes were positioned in the pressurization chamber so as to avoid deformation of the base of the culture dish [56].

Experiments undertaken to identify the source of intracellular calcium that activated the SK channels leading to hyperpolarization demonstrated a requirement for extracellular calcium and activity of L-type calcium channels [118-120]. Thapsigargin which raises intracellular Ca^{2+} by inhibition of Ca^{2+}-ATPase in endoplasmic reticulum [121-123] caused hyperpolarization independent of mechanical strain but further hyperpolarization of the cells occurred after cyclical pressurization further supporting the idea that mechanically induced chondrocyte hyperpolarization is dependent on intracellular free Ca^{2+} levels [56]. In addition, TRPV4-mediated Ca^{2+} signaling has been demonstrated to play a central role in the transduction of mechanical signals to support cartilage extracellular matrix maintenance [124].

6.1. Intracellular signal cascades activated by mechanical stimulation

Stimulation of connective tissue cell mechanoreceptors is followed by generation of the secondary messenger molecules and activation of a cascade of downstream signaling events that regulate gene expression and cell function. Many intracellular signaling pathways are known to be activated by mechanical forces applied to tissues and cells including heterotrimeric guanine nucleotide binding proteins (G-proteins), protein kinases and transcription factors. These pathways that regulate tissue modelling/remodelling may be activated directly as a consequence of mechanoreceptor signaling or indirectly following production of autocrine/paracrine acting molecules.

PKB/Akt is a protein family of serine/threonine kinases that have multiple roles including inhibition of apoptosis by phosphorylation and inactivation of pro-apoptotic factors. Integrin-dependent activation of phosphoinositide3 kinase (PI3 kinase) by mechanical forces regulates PKB activity and can inhibit cell death. Inactivation of the PI3-K/PKB pathway may be important in deleterious effects of mechanical overloading of cartilage and bone loss in response to withdrawal of loading [125]. The activity of mammalian target of rapamycin (mTOR) may be an essential mechanotransduction component modulated by SH2-containing protein tyrosine phosphatase 2 and is required for cartilage development [126].

Mitogen-activated protein kinases (MAPKs) regulate multiple cellular activities, such as gene expression, mitosis, differentiation, and cell survival/apoptosis. ERK1/2, JNK and p38, of critical importance in regulation of matrix protein and protease gene expression have each been shown to be activated in chondrocytes following mechanical stimulation [127]. Mechanical stimuli may activate different MAPKs and through this mechanism differential cellular responses may occur. MAPK responses may also be cell type dependent. Mechanical stimulation induced ERK1/2 activation in bone cells requires calcium-dependent ATP release whilst in cartilage activation, under certain circumstances, is dependent on FGF-2 rather than through integrin mechanoreceptors [128]. Tyrosine phosphorylation of focal adhesion kinase (pp125FAK), beta-catenin, and paxillin following mechanical stimulation is also recognized in human articular chondrocytes [129].

In bone cells NF-κB, a protein complex that acts as a transcription factor, is directly stimulated by mechanical stimulation is dependent on intracellular calcium release [130]. In chondrocytes biomechanical signals within the physiological range block NF-κB activity and proinflammatory chondrocyte responses [131]. Mechanical stimuli that induce catabolic rather than anabolic responses in chondrocytes induce rapid nuclear translocation of NF-κB subunits p65 and p50 in a similar manner to IL-1β [132].

6.2. Growth factors and autocrine/paracrine signaling in mechanotransduction

As part of the cellular response to mechanical stimulation mechanosensitive connective tissue cells release a range of soluble mediators. These may be present in the cell and available for immediate release, or secretion may depend de novo synthesis by enzymatic activity or transcriptional activation and protein production. These mediators, including prostaglandins, nitric oxide, cytokines, growth factors, and neuropeptides are involved in downstream tissue modelling and remodelling responses initiated by the mechanosensitive cells or other effector cells. Production of soluble mediators by connective tissue cells in response to mechanical stimulation however may also be intrinsic to mechanotransduction pathways. Autocrine and paracrine activity allows increased regulation of the cellular response to mechanical stimuli by permitting cross talk between different components of a mechanotransduction cascade. As the cellular responses to mechanical stimuli and soluble mediators activate similar signal cascades inducing either anabolic or catabolic responses, it would be expected that they may be antagonistic, additive or synergistic. Anabolic cytokines and growth factors enhance production of matrix under mechanical loading conditions whilst anabolic mechanical stimuli antagonize the effects of catabolic cytokines such as IL-1β [133].

Prostaglandins, predominantly PGE2, NO and ATP are produced when bone cells and chondrocytes are mechanically stimulated. Prostaglandin production is integrin dependent requiring an intact cytoskeleton and activation of SACs, PKC, and PLA2. In cartilage PGE2 induced by mechanical loads is catabolic. Mechanical loading of chondrocytes by physiological stimuli inhibits production of PGE2 and NO whereas damaging loading induces PGE2 release [134]. Following mechanical stimulation bone cells and chondrocytes release ATP which can bind and activate purinergic receptors on these and adjacent cells. Both metabotropic P2Y receptors and ionotropic P2X receptors, have been shown to be involved in mechanical load activated signal cascades in chondrocytes and bone cells and may have physiological roles [135].

IL-4 and IL-1β autocrine/paracrine activity is seen in the integrin-dependent mechanotransduction cascade of chondrocytes (IL-4 and IL-1β) and bone cells (IL-1β) to mechanical stimulation [136,137]. These molecules are secreted within 20 minutes of the onset of mechanical stimulation, suggesting release from preformed stores. IL-4 release relies on secretion of the neuropeptide substance P which binds to its NK1 receptor. Both IL-4 and substance P are necessary but not sufficient for the increased expression of aggrecan mRNA and decrease in MMP3 mRNA induced by the mechanical stimulus suggesting cross talk with other mechanosensitive signaling pathways. IL-1β is involved in the early mechanotransduction pathway of both osteoarthritic chondrocytes and human trabecular bone derived cells [138]. Mechanical loading may also induce release or activation of sequestered growth factors in extracellular matrix which will then act on near-by resident connective tissue cells. Basic fibroblast growth factor (FGF2) is a possible mediator of mechanical signaling in cartilage through such a mechanism [128]. Dynamic compression of porcine cartilage induces release of FGF2 with activation of ERK MAP kinase, synthesis and secretion of TIMP-1. In contrast FGF2 production by bovine cartilage is inhibited by 1 hour of compressive stress of 20 MPa [139]. This mechanical induced suppression of FGF2 is blocked by IL-4 indicating further roles for this pleiotropic cytokine in the regulation of chondrocyte responses to mechanical stimulation.

7. Mechanical loading and osteoarthritis

Abnormal mechanical loading is associated with osteoarthritis [140]. Most animal models of OA are mechanically induced, for example, by introducing joint instability by anterior cruciate ligament section [22] or by altering the loading across the joint by menisectomy [141]. These changes in joint loading affect cartilage structure and chondrocyte activity within days of the procedure, and may eventually result in complete loss of cartilage [142]. When cartilage matrix is lost or made deficient as a consequence of direct physical effects or proteolytic digestion the articular cartilage loses its mechanical function. The tensile modulus has been shown to decrease by as much as 90%, reflecting damage to the cartilage matrix network [26]. Animal studies, for example, have shown that the tensile modulus of canine knee articular cartilage was reduced after one month of immobilization [143]. In the dog, severe OA lesions in the knee joint have been produced by treadmill exercise after the limb was immobilized for several weeks [144]. The compressive modulus also decreases with increasing severity of degeneration [27]. Other joint tissues (e.g., anterior cruciate ligament) also undergo similar changes of tensile and compressive modulus in an experimental OA model [145].

Mechanical loading out with that which joint tissues can normally withstand or are required to maintain a healthy state is central to the development of OA. OA arises when there is an imbalance between the mechanical forces within a joint and the ability of the cartilage to withstand these forces. This arises in two situations. In the first normal articular cartilage is exposed to abnormal mechanical loads whereas in the other the articular cartilage is fundamentally defective with biomaterial properties that are insufficient to withstand normal load bearing. Risk factors associated with development of OA may have influences in either one or both of these scenarios. The accumulation of advanced glycation end products (AGEs) in ECM with age results in a more brittle collagen network that is less able to withstand normal loads, again leading to cartilage degeneration.

The mechanisms by which abnormal mechanical loading may influence chondrocyte function to promote cartilage breakdown are beginning to be understood. Chondrocytes from osteoarthritic cartilage share mechanoreceptors with chondrocytes from normal chondrocytes [146,147]. Whilst activation of these receptors and downstream signaling cascades such as FAK, PKC, JAK/STAT and MAP kinases[148,149] result in pro-anabolic activity in normal chondrocytes activity through release of locally acting mediators that include the anti-inflammatory cytokine IL-4 and the neuropeptide substance P [136,150]. However the response of chondrocytes is aberrant with production of proinflammatory cytokines such as IL-1 and TNF-α which increase production of MMPs and aggrecanases, further accelerating disease progression and attenuating cartilage repair [151-156].

7.1. Altered responses to mechanical stimulation in osteoarthritic chondrocytes

Chondrocytes from osteoarthritic cartilage show a membrane depolarization response to IL-4 that is inhibited by functional receptor antibodies. It is unclear why chondrocytes from osteoarthritic cartilage should show differences in their response to 0.33 Hz mechanical stimulation and recombinant IL-4. This may be result of a general phenotypic change seen in OA chondrocytes in which the cells are resident in a pro-inflammatory, catabolic environment. Indeed the observation that mechanical stimulation in osteoarthritis may result in production of proinflammatory mediators is supported by the findings that $\alpha5\beta1$ integrin ligation increases production of IL-1β by osteoarthritic human chondrocytes with subsequent induction of nitric oxide, PGE2, IL-6, and IL-8 [157]. These cytokines will inhibit anabolic responses and increase cartilage matrix breakdown by MMPs. This may be through direct mechanisms or by interfering with integrin signaling. Expression and function of molecules such as members of the SOCS (suppressors of cytokine signaling) which regulate cytokine signaling pathways [158] may also be implicated. These molecules modulate intracellular signals stimulated by IL-4 including JAK/STAT activation. SOCS-1 has been shown to bind to and inhibit kinase activity of JAK family members and inhibit IL-4 induced activation of JAK1 and STAT6. SOCS-3 has been shown mediate IL-1β inhibition of STAT5 activity. These and other regulators of STAT transcription factor signaling may be responsible for modulation of IL-4 dependent responses of chondrocytes in osteoarthritic cartilage to mechanical stimulation.

8. Summary

A healthy synovial joint requires exposure to mechanical loads within a physiological range. Osteoarthritis develops when joints are subjected to mechanical loads which they are not biomechanically conditioned to withstand. This may be because the loads are excessive due to obesity or joint malalignment or a consequence of intrinsic or acquired biomechanical weakness of joint tissues such as seen when cartilage proteoglycans are depleted secondary to synovial inflammation. Abnormal mechanical loads may have direct physical effects on joint tissues including cartilage but increasingly knowledge of the pathological process within the osteoarthritic joint indicate that chondrocytes regulated catabolic processes are of prime importance in cartilage degradation. The mechanisms by which chondrocytes recognize mechanical loads and how these mechanical stimuli are transduced into biochemical responses which subsequently lead to altered gene expression and cell function is being increasing understood (Figure 1). Knowledge of how anabolic and catabolic signaling cascades are differentially regulated in response to physiological and pathological mechanical stimuli will enable future strategies to be developed to prevent and treat the progression of cartilage pathology in osteoarthritis.

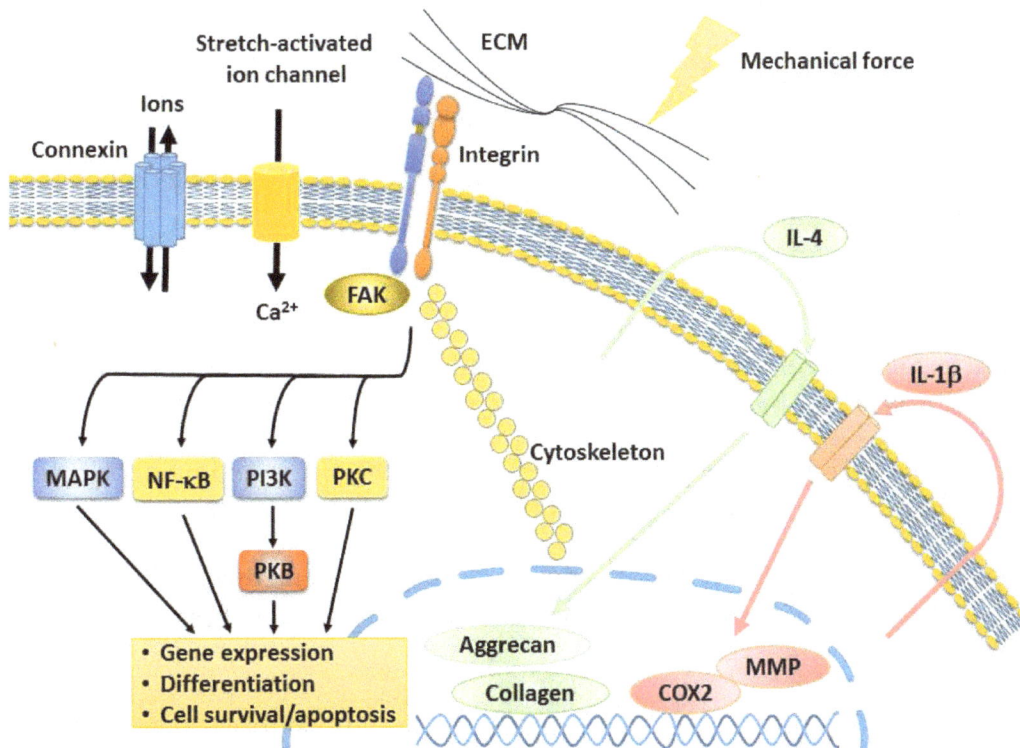

Figure 1. The major mechanotransduction components in chondrocytes. The integrin, connexin, and stretch-activated ion channel mechanoreceptors are stimulated by the mechanical forces transduced via the extracellular matrix (ECM). Downstream transduction pathways involve the cytoskeleton and signaling molecules, including FAK, PKC, PI3K,

PKB, NF-kB, and MAPK, which act to regulate gene expression, cell function and survival/apoptosis. The release and paracrine/autocrine activity of the anti-inflammatory cytokine IL-4 has beneficial effects in regulating an anabolic response with enhanced expression of aggrecan and inhibition of MMP expression. In contrast production of IL-1β, as seen in OA, has a catabolic outcome with activation of pathways resulting in increased expression of COX2 and MMPs.

Author details

Herng-Sheng Lee[1] and Donald M. Salter[2]

1 Department of Pathology and Laboratory Medicine, Kaohsiung Veterans General Hospital, Zuoying Dist., Kaohsiung City, Taiwan

2 Center for Genomics and Experimental Medicine, MRC IGMM, University of Edinburgh, Western General Hospital, Edinburgh EH4 2XU, United Kingdom

References

[1] Brand R A. Joint lubrication. In: Brand R A, Albright J A (eds) The Scientific basis of orthopaedics. Appleton & Lange: Norwalk, Conn.; 1987. 373-389.

[2] McCutchen C E. Lubrication of joints. In: Sokoloff L (ed.) The Joints and synovial fluid. Academic Press: New York; 1987. 437-483.

[3] Harris E D, Parker H G, Radin E L, Krane S M. Effects of proteolytic enzymes on structural and mechanical properties of cartilage. Arthritis and rheumatism 1972;15(5): 497-503.

[4] Kempson G E, Muir H, Pollard C, Tuke M. The tensile properties of the cartilage of human femoral condyles related to the content of collagen and glycosaminoglycans. Biochimica et biophysica acta 1973;297(2): 456-472.

[5] Kempson G. The mechanical properties of articular cartilage. In: Sokoloff L (ed.) The Joints and synovial fluid. Academic Press: New York; 1978. 177-238.

[6] Mayne R, Irwin M H. Collagen types in cartilage. In: Kuettner K E, Schleyerbach R, Hascall V C (eds) Articular cartilage biochemistry. Raven Press: New York; 1986. 23-38.

[7] Comper W D, Laurent T C. Physiological function of connective tissue polysaccharides. Physiological reviews 1978;58(1): 255-315.

[8] Greenwald R A, Moy W W, Seibold J. Functional properties of cartilage proteoglycans. Seminars in arthritis and rheumatism 1978;8(1): 53-67.

[9] Hascall V C. Interaction of cartilage proteoglycans with hyaluronic acid. Journal of supramolecular structure 1977;7(1): 101-120.

[10] Paul J. Joint kinetics. In: L S (ed.) The joints and synovial fluid. Academic press: New-York; 1980. 139-176.

[11] Seireg A, Arvikar. The prediction of muscular lad sharing and joint forces in the lower extremities during walking. Journal of biomechanics 1975;8(2): 89-102.

[12] van Kampen G, van de Stadt R. Cartilage and chondrocyte responses to mechanical loading in vitro. In: HJ H, I K, M T, AM S, K P, J J (eds) Joint Loading: biology and health of articular structures; 1987. 112-125.

[13] Helminen H, Jurvelin J, Kiviranta I, Paukkonen K, Saamanen A, Tammi M. Joint loading effects on articular cartilage: a historical review. In: Helminen H, Kiviranta I, Tammi M, Sasmanen A, Paukkonen K, Jurvelin J (eds) Joint Loading: biology and health of articular structures; 1987. 1-46.

[14] Jurvelin J, Helminen H J, Lauritsalo S, Kiviranta I, Saamanen A M, Paukkonen K, Tammi M. Influences of joint immobilization and running exercise on articular cartilage surfaces of young rabbits. A semiquantitative stereomicroscopic and scanning electron microscopic study. Acta anatomica 1985;122(1): 62-68.

[15] Eggli P S, Hunziker E B, Schenk R K. Quantitation of structural features characterizing weight- and less-weight-bearing regions in articular cartilage: a stereological analysis of medial femoral condyles in young adult rabbits. The Anatomical record 1988;222(3): 217-227.

[16] Kiviranta I, Tammi M, Jurvelin J, Saamanen A M, Helminen H J. Moderate running exercise augments glycosaminoglycans and thickness of articular cartilage in the knee joint of young beagle dogs. Journal of orthopaedic research : official publication of the Orthopaedic Research Society 1988;6(2): 188-195.

[17] Guilak F, Bachrach N M. Compression-induced changes in chondrocyte shape and volume determined in situ using confocal microscopy. Trans Orthopaedic Research Society 1993;18: 619.

[18] Bjelle A. Content and composition of glycosaminoglycans in human knee joint cartilage. Variation with site and age in adults. Connective tissue research 1975;3(2): 141-147.

[19] Roberts S, Weightman B, Urban J, Chappell D. Mechanical and biochemical properties of human articular cartilage in osteoarthritic femoral heads and in autopsy specimens. The Journal of bone and joint surgery. British volume 1986;68(2): 278-288.

[20] Slowman S D, Brandt K D. Composition and glycosaminoglycan metabolism of articular cartilage from habitually loaded and habitually unloaded sites. Arthritis and rheumatism 1986;29(1): 88-94.

[21] Palmoski M, Perricone E, Brandt K D. Development and reversal of a proteoglycan aggregation defect in normal canine knee cartilage after immobilization. Arthritis and rheumatism 1979;22(5): 508-517.

[22] Muir H, Carney S. Pathological and biochemical changes in cartilage and other tissues of the canine knee resulting from induced joint instability. In: Helminen H, Kiviranta I, Tammi M, Sasmanen A, Paukkonen K, Jurvelin J (eds) Joint Loading: biology and health of articular structures; 1987. 47-63.

[23] Caterson B, Lowther D A. Changes in the metabolism of the proteoglycans from sheep articular cartilage in response to mechanical stress. Biochimicaet Biophysica Acta 1978: 412-422.

[24] O'Conor C J, Case N, Guilak F. Mechanical regulation of chondrogenesis. Stem cell research & therapy 2013;4(4): 61.

[25] Hodge W A, Fijan R S, Carlson K L, Burgess R G, Harris W H, Mann R W. Contact pressures in the human hip joint measured in vivo. Proceedings of the National Academy of Sciences of the United States of America 1986;83(9): 2879-2883.

[26] Akizuki S, Mow V C, Muller F, Pita J C, Howell D S, Manicourt D H. Tensile properties of human knee joint cartilage: I. Influence of ionic conditions, weight bearing, and fibrillation on the tensile modulus. Journal of orthopaedic research : official publication of the Orthopaedic Research Society 1986;4(4): 379-392.

[27] Armstrong C G, Mow V C. Variations in the intrinsic mechanical properties of human articular cartilage with age, degeneration, and water content. The Journal of bone and joint surgery. American volume 1982;64(1): 88-94.

[28] Athanasiou K A, Agarwal A, Dzida F J. Comparative study of the intrinsic mechanical properties of the human acetabular and femoral head cartilage. Journal of orthopaedic research : official publication of the Orthopaedic Research Society 1994;12(3): 340-349.

[29] Zhu W, Mow V C, Koob T J, Eyre D R. Viscoelastic shear properties of articular cartilage and the effects of glycosidase treatments. Journal of orthopaedic research : official publication of the Orthopaedic Research Society 1993;11(6): 771-781.

[30] Spirt A A, Mak A F, Wassell R P. Nonlinear viscoelastic properties of articular cartilage in shear. Journal of orthopaedic research : official publication of the Orthopaedic Research Society 1989;7(1): 43-49.

[31] Setton L A, Mow V C, Howell D S. Changes in the shear properties of canine knee cartilage resulting from anterior cruciate transection. Journal of Orthopaedic Research 1995.

[32] Mow V C, Wang C C, Hung C T. The extracellular matrix, interstitial fluid and ions as a mechanical signal transducer in articular cartilage. Osteoarthritis and cartilage / OARS, Osteoarthritis Research Society 1999;7(1): 41-58.

[33] Rodan G A, Mensi T, Harvey A. A quantitative method for the application of compressive forces to bone in tissue culture. Calcified tissue research 1975;18(2): 125-131.

[34] Rodan G A, Bourret L A, Harvey A, Mensi T. Cyclic AMP and cyclic GMP: mediators of the mechanical effects on bone remodeling. Science 1975;189(4201): 467-469.

[35] Veldhuijzen J P, Bourret L A, Rodan G A. In vitro studies of the effect of intermittent compressive forces on cartilage cell proliferation. Journal of cellular physiology 1979;98(2): 299-306.

[36] Palmoski M J, Brandt K D. Effects of static and cyclic compressive loading on articular cartilage plugs in vitro. Arthritis and rheumatism 1984;27(6): 675-681.

[37] Schaffer J L, Rizen M, L'Italien G J, Benbrahim A, Megerman J, Gerstenfeld L C, Gray M L. Device for the application of a dynamic biaxially uniform and isotropic strain to a flexible cell culture membrane. Journal of orthopaedic research : official publication of the Orthopaedic Research Society 1994;12(5): 709-719.

[38] Banes A, Gilbert J, Taylor D, Monbureau O. A new vacuum-operated stress-providing instrument that applies static or variable duration cyclic tension or compression to cells in vitro. Journal of cell science 1985;75: 35-42.

[39] Gilbert J, Banes A, Link G. Characterization of the surface strain applied to cyclically stretched cells in vitro. Trans Orthopaedic Research Society 1989;14: 249.

[40] Vandenburgh H H. A computerized mechanical cell stimulator for tissue culture: effects on skeletal muscle organogenesis. In vitro cellular & developmental biology : journal of the Tissue Culture Association 1988;24(7): 609-619.

[41] Hasegawa S, Sato S, Saito S, Suzuki Y, Brunette D M. Mechanical stretching increases the number of cultured bone cells synthesizing DNA and alters their pattern of protein synthesis. Calcified tissue international 1985;37(4): 431-436.

[42] Andersen K L, Norton L A. A device for the application of known simulated orthodontic forces to human cells in vitro. Journal of biomechanics 1991;24(7): 649-654.

[43] Brighton C T, Strafford B, Gross S B, Leatherwood D F, Williams J L, Pollack S R. The proliferative and synthetic response of isolated calvarial bone cells of rats to cyclic biaxial mechanical strain. The Journal of bone and joint surgery. American volume 1991;73(3): 320-331.

[44] Williams J L, Chen J H, Belloli D M. Strain fields on cell stressing devices employing clamped circular elastic diaphragms as substrates. Journal of biomechanical engineering 1992;114(3): 377-384.

[45] Belloli D M, Williams J L, Park J Y. Calculated strain fields on cell stressing devices employing circular diaphragms as substrates. Trans Orthopaedic Research Society 1991;16: 399.

[46] Hung C T, Williams J L. A method for inducing equi-biaxial and uniform strains in elastomeric membranes used as cell substrates. Journal of biomechanics 1994;27(2): 227-232.

[47] Schaffer J, Newman N, Gray M, Gerstenfeld L. Osteoblast phenotypic expression after mechanical perturbation with a dynamic and isotropic and biaxially uniform strain. Journal of Bone and Mineral Research 1993;8: S367.

[48] Lee R C, Rich J B, Kelley K M, Weiman D S, Mathews M B. A comparison of in vitro cellular responses to mechanical and electrical stimulation. The American surgeon 1982;48(11): 567-574.

[49] De Witt M T, Handley C J, Oakes B W, Lowther D A. In vitro response of chondrocytes to mechanical loading. The effect of short term mechanical tension. Connective tissue research 1984;12(2): 97-109.

[50] Fujisawa T, Hattori T, Takahashi K, Kuboki T, Yamashita A, Takigawa M. Cyclic mechanical stress induces extracellular matrix degradation in cultured chondrocytes via gene expression of matrix metalloproteinases and interleukin-1. Journal of biochemistry 1999;125(5): 966-975.

[51] Chano T, Tanaka M, Hukuda S, Saeki Y. Mechanical stress induces the expression of high molecular mass heat shock protein in human chondrocytic cell line CS-OKB. Osteoarthritis and cartilage / OARS, Osteoarthritis Research Society 2000;8(2): 115-119.

[52] Guilak F, Zell R A, Erickson G R, Grande D A, Rubin C T, McLeod K J, Donahue H J. Mechanically induced calcium waves in articular chondrocytes are inhibited by gadolinium and amiloride. Journal of orthopaedic research : official publication of the Orthopaedic Research Society 1999;17(3): 421-429.

[53] Jorgensen F, Ohmori H. Amiloride blocks the mechano-electrical transduction channel of hair cells of the chick. The Journal of physiology 1988;403: 577-588.

[54] Yang X C, Sachs F. Block of stretch-activated ion channels in Xenopus oocytes by gadolinium and calcium ions. Science 1989;243(4894 Pt 1): 1068-1071.

[55] Hamill O P, Lane J W, McBride D W, Jr. Amiloride: a molecular probe for mechanosensitive channels. Trends in pharmacological sciences 1992;13(10): 373-376.

[56] Wright M, Jobanputra P, Bavington C, Salter D M, Nuki G. Effects of intermittent pressure-induced strain on the electrophysiology of cultured human chondrocytes: evidence for the presence of stretch-activated membrane ion channels. Clinical science 1996;90(1): 61-71.

[57] Smith R L, Donlon B S, Gupta M K, Mohtai M, Das P, Carter D R, Cooke J, Gibbons G, Hutchinson N, Schurman D J. Effects of fluid-induced shear on articular chondrocyte morphology and metabolism in vitro. Journal of orthopaedic research : official publication of the Orthopaedic Research Society 1995;13(6): 824-831.

[58] Roemer F W, Guermazi A, Niu J, Zhang Y, Mohr A, Felson D T. Prevalence of magnetic resonance imaging-defined atrophic and hypertrophic phenotypes of knee osteoarthritis in a population-based cohort. Arthritis and rheumatism 2012;64(2): 429-437.

[59] Zeng Q Y, Chen R, Darmawan J, Xiao Z Y, Chen S B, Wigley R, Le Chen S, Zhang N Z. Rheumatic diseases in China. Arthritis research & therapy 2008;10(1): R17.

[60] Lin J, Li R, Kang X, Li H. Risk factors for radiographic tibiofemoral knee osteoarthritis: the wuchuan osteoarthritis study. International journal of rheumatology 2010;2010: 385826.

[61] Pai Y C, Rymer W Z, Chang R W, Sharma L. Effect of age and osteoarthritis on knee proprioception. Arthritis and rheumatism 1997;40(12): 2260-2265.

[62] Tamkun J W, DeSimone D W, Fonda D, Patel R S, Buck C, Horwitz A F, Hynes R O. Structure of integrin, a glycoprotein involved in the transmembrane linkage between fibronectin and actin. Cell 1986;46(2): 271-282.

[63] Albelda S M, Buck C A. Integrins and other cell adhesion molecules. FASEB journal : official publication of the Federation of American Societies for Experimental Biology 1990;4(11): 2868-2880.

[64] Arnaout M A. Structure and function of the leukocyte adhesion molecules CD11/CD18. Blood 1990;75(5): 1037-1050.

[65] Hemler M E. VLA proteins in the integrin family: structures, functions, and their role on leukocytes. Annual review of immunology 1990;8: 365-400.

[66] Springer T A. Adhesion receptors of the immune system. Nature 1990;346(6283): 425-434.

[67] Springer T A. The sensation and regulation of interactions with the extracellular environment: the cell biology of lymphocyte adhesion receptors. Annual review of cell biology 1990;6: 359-402.

[68] Ruoslahti E. Integrins. The Journal of clinical investigation 1991;87(1): 1-5.

[69] Aplin A E, Howe A, Alahari S K, Juliano R L. Signal transduction and signal modulation by cell adhesion receptors: the role of integrins, cadherins, immunoglobulin-cell adhesion molecules, and selectins. Pharmacological reviews 1998;50(2): 197-263.

[70] Humphries M J, Newham P. The structure of cell-adhesion molecules. Trends in cell biology 1998;8(2): 78-83.

[71] Kuhn K, Eble J. The structural bases of integrin-ligand interactions. Trends in cell biology 1994;4(7): 256-261.

[72] Gahmberg C G, Valmu L, Fagerholm S, Kotovuori P, Ihanus E, Tian L, Pessa-Morika-
       wa T. Leukocyte integrins and inflammation. Cellular and molecular life sciences :
       CMLS 1998;54(6): 549-555.

[73] Komoriya A, Green L J, Mervic M, Yamada S S, Yamada K M, Humphries M J. The
       minimal essential sequence for a major cell type-specific adhesion site (CS1) within
       the alternatively spliced type III connecting segment domain of fibronectin is leucine-
       aspartic acid-valine. The Journal of biological chemistry 1991;266(23): 15075-15079.

[74] Newham P, Craig S E, Seddon G N, Schofield N R, Rees A, Edwards R M, Jones E Y,
       Humphries M J. Alpha4 integrin binding interfaces on VCAM-1 and MAdCAM-1. In-
       tegrin binding footprints identify accessory binding sites that play a role in integrin
       specificity. The Journal of biological chemistry 1997;272(31): 19429-19440.

[75] Pierschbacher M D, Ruoslahti E. Cell attachment activity of fibronectin can be dupli-
       cated by small synthetic fragments of the molecule. Nature 1984;309(5963): 30-33.

[76] Hynes R O. Integrins: versatility, modulation, and signaling in cell adhesion. Cell
       1992;69(1): 11-25.

[77] Salter D M, Hughes D E, Simpson R, Gardner D L. Integrin expression by human ar-
       ticular chondrocytes. British journal of rheumatology 1992;31(4): 231-234.

[78] Woods V L, Jr., Schreck P J, Gesink D S, Pacheco H O, Amiel D, Akeson W H, Lotz
       M. Integrin expression by human articular chondrocytes. Arthritis and rheumatism
       1994;37(4): 537-544.

[79] Camper L, Hellman U, Lundgren-Akerlund E. Isolation, cloning, and sequence anal-
       ysis of the integrin subunit alpha10, a beta1-associated collagen binding integrin ex-
       pressed on chondrocytes. The Journal of biological chemistry 1998;273(32):
       20383-20389.

[80] Hering T M. Regulation of chondrocyte gene expression. Frontiers in bioscience : a
       journal and virtual library 1999;4: D743-761.

[81] Hirsch M S, Lunsford L E, Trinkaus-Randall V, Svoboda K K. Chondrocyte survival
       and differentiation in situ are integrin mediated. Developmental dynamics : an offi-
       cial publication of the American Association of Anatomists 1997;210(3): 249-263.

[82] Durr J, Goodman S, Potocnik A, von der Mark H, von der Mark K. Localization of
       beta 1-integrins in human cartilage and their role in chondrocyte adhesion to colla-
       gen and fibronectin. Experimental cell research 1993;207(2): 235-244.

[83] Enomoto M, Leboy P S, Menko A S, Boettiger D. Beta 1 integrins mediate chondro-
       cyte interaction with type I collagen, type II collagen, and fibronectin. Experimental
       cell research 1993;205(2): 276-285.

[84] Camper L, Heinegard D, Lundgren-Akerlund E. Integrin alpha2beta1 is a receptor for the cartilage matrix protein chondroadherin. The Journal of cell biology 1997;138(5): 1159-1167.

[85] Enomoto-Iwamoto M, Iwamoto M, Pacifici M, Boettiger D, Kurisu K, Suzuki F. The interaction of alpha 5 beta 1 integrin with fibronectin is required for proliferation of chondrocytes. Trans Orthopaedic Research Society 1995;20: 396.

[86] Loeser R F. Integrin-mediated attachment of articular chondrocytes to extracellular matrix proteins. Arthritis and rheumatism 1993;36(8): 1103-1110.

[87] Loeser R F, Sadiev S, Tan L, Goldring M B. Integrin expression by primary and immortalized human chondrocytes: evidence of a differential role for alpha1beta1 and alpha2beta1 integrins in mediating chondrocyte adhesion to types II and VI collagen. Osteoarthritis and cartilage / OARS, Osteoarthritis Research Society 2000;8(2): 96-105.

[88] Enomoto-Iwamoto M, Iwamoto M, Nakashima K, Mukudai Y, Boettiger D, Pacifici M, Kurisu K, Suzuki F. Involvement of alpha5beta1 integrin in matrix interactions and proliferation of chondrocytes. Journal of bone and mineral research : the official journal of the American Society for Bone and Mineral Research 1997;12(7): 1124-1132.

[89] Tavella S, Bellese G, Castagnola P, Martin I, Piccini D, Doliana R, Colombatti A, Cancedda R, Tacchetti C. Regulated expression of fibronectin, laminin and related integrin receptors during the early chondrocyte differentiation. Journal of cell science 1997;110 (Pt 18): 2261-2270.

[90] Shakibaei M. Inhibition of chondrogenesis by integrin antibody in vitro. Experimental cell research 1998;240(1): 95-106.

[91] Beekman B, Verzijl N, Bank R A, von der Mark K, TeKoppele J M. Synthesis of collagen by bovine chondrocytes cultured in alginate; posttranslational modifications and cell-matrix interaction. Experimental cell research 1997;237(1): 135-141.

[92] Homandberg G A, Hui F. Arg-Gly-Asp-Ser peptide analogs suppress cartilage chondrolytic activities of integrin-binding and nonbinding fibronectin fragments. Archives of biochemistry and biophysics 1994;310(1): 40-48.

[93] Clancy R M, Rediske J, Tang X, Nijher N, Frenkel S, Philips M, Abramson S B. Outside-in signaling in the chondrocyte. Nitric oxide disrupts fibronectin-induced assembly of a subplasmalemmal actin/rho A/focal adhesion kinase signaling complex. The Journal of clinical investigation 1997;100(7): 1789-1796.

[94] Ingber D. Integrins as mechanochemical transducers. Current opinion in cell biology 1991;3(5): 841-848.

[95] Davies P F. Flow-mediated endothelial mechanotransduction. Physiological reviews 1995;75(3): 519-560.

[96] Shyy J Y, Chien S. Role of integrins in cellular responses to mechanical stress and adhesion. Current opinion in cell biology 1997;9(5): 707-713.

[97] Wang N, Butler J P, Ingber D E. Mechanotransduction across the cell surface and through the cytoskeleton. Science 1993;260(5111): 1124-1127.

[98] Maniotis A J, Chen C S, Ingber D E. Demonstration of mechanical connections between integrins, cytoskeletal filaments, and nucleoplasm that stabilize nuclear structure. Proceedings of the National Academy of Sciences of the United States of America 1997;94(3): 849-854.

[99] Pommerenke H, Schreiber E, Durr F, Nebe B, Hahnel C, Moller W, Rychly J. Stimulation of integrin receptors using a magnetic drag force device induces an intracellular free calcium response. European journal of cell biology 1996;70(2): 157-164.

[100] Bierbaum S, Notbohm H. Tyrosine phosphorylation of 40 kDa proteins in osteoblastic cells after mechanical stimulation of beta1-integrins. European journal of cell biology 1998;77(1): 60-67.

[101] Schmidt C, Pommerenke H, Durr F, Nebe B, Rychly J. Mechanical stressing of integrin receptors induces enhanced tyrosine phosphorylation of cytoskeletally anchored proteins. The Journal of biological chemistry 1998;273(9): 5081-5085.

[102] Holmvall K, Camper L, Johansson S, Kimura J H, Lundgren-Akerlund E. Chondrocyte and chondrosarcoma cell integrins with affinity for collagen type II and their response to mechanical stress. Experimental cell research 1995;221(2): 496-503.

[103] Martinac B. Mechanosensitive ion channels: molecules of mechanotransduction. Journal of cell science 2004;117(Pt 12): 2449-2460.

[104] Ingber D E. Cellular mechanotransduction: putting all the pieces together again. FASEB journal : official publication of the Federation of American Societies for Experimental Biology 2006;20(7): 811-827.

[105] Muller U. Cadherins and mechanotransduction by hair cells. Current opinion in cell biology 2008;20(5): 557-566.

[106] Civitelli R. Cell-cell communication in the osteoblast/osteocyte lineage. Archives of biochemistry and biophysics 2008;473(2): 188-192.

[107] Yellowley C E, Li Z, Zhou Z, Jacobs C R, Donahue H J. Functional gap junctions between osteocytic and osteoblastic cells. Journal of bone and mineral research : the official journal of the American Society for Bone and Mineral Research 2000;15(2): 209-217.

[108] Zhang J, Zhang H Y, Zhang M, Qiu Z Y, Wu Y P, Callaway D A, Jiang J X, Lu L, Jing L, Yang T, Wang M Q. Connexin43 hemichannels mediate small molecule exchange between chondrocytes and matrix in biomechanically-stimulated temporomandibu-

lar joint cartilage. Osteoarthritis and cartilage / OARS, Osteoarthritis Research Society 2014;22(6): 822-830.

[109] Waggett A D, Benjamin M, Ralphs J R. Connexin 32 and 43 gap junctions differentially modulate tenocyte response to cyclic mechanical load. European journal of cell biology 2006;85(11): 1145-1154.

[110] Ruhlen R, Marberry K. The chondrocyte primary cilium. Osteoarthritis and cartilage / OARS, Osteoarthritis Research Society 2014;22(8): 1071-1076.

[111] Whitfield J F. The solitary (primary) cilium--a mechanosensory toggle switch in bone and cartilage cells. Cellular signalling 2008;20(6): 1019-1024.

[112] Poole C A, Jensen C G, Snyder J A, Gray C G, Hermanutz V L, Wheatley D N. Confocal analysis of primary cilia structure and colocalization with the Golgi apparatus in chondrocytes and aortic smooth muscle cells. Cell biology international 1997;21(8): 483-494.

[113] Malone A M, Anderson C T, Tummala P, Kwon R Y, Johnston T R, Stearns T, Jacobs C R. Primary cilia mediate mechanosensing in bone cells by a calcium-independent mechanism. Proceedings of the National Academy of Sciences of the United States of America 2007;104(33): 13325-13330.

[114] Ingber D E. Tensegrity: the architectural basis of cellular mechanotransduction. Annual review of physiology 1997;59: 575-599.

[115] Chicurel M E, Chen C S, Ingber D E. Cellular control lies in the balance of forces. Current opinion in cell biology 1998;10(2): 232-239.

[116] Chen C S, Ingber D E. Tensegrity and mechanoregulation: from skeleton to cytoskeleton. Osteoarthritis and cartilage / OARS, Osteoarthritis Research Society 1999;7(1): 81-94.

[117] Wright M O, Stockwell R A, Nuki G. Response of plasma membrane to applied hydrostatic pressure in chondrocytes and fibroblasts. Connective tissue research 1992;28(1-2): 49-70.

[118] Tsunoo A, Yoshii M, Narahashi T. Block of calcium channels by enkephalin and somatostatin in neuroblastoma-glioma hybrid NG108-15 cells. Proceedings of the National Academy of Sciences of the United States of America 1986;83(24): 9832-9836.

[119] Narahashi T, Tsunoo A, Yoshii M. Characterization of two types of calcium channels in mouse neuroblastoma cells. The Journal of physiology 1987;383: 231-249.

[120] Bers D M. A simple method for the accurate determination of free [Ca] in Ca-EGTA solutions. The American journal of physiology 1982;242(5): C404-408.

[121] Thastrup O. Role of Ca2(+)-ATPases in regulation of cellular Ca2+ signalling, as studied with the selective microsomal Ca2(+)-ATPase inhibitor, thapsigargin. Agents and actions 1990;29(1-2): 8-15.

[122] Thastrup O, Cullen P J, Drobak B K, Hanley M R, Dawson A P. Thapsigargin, a tumor promoter, discharges intracellular Ca2+ stores by specific inhibition of the endoplasmic reticulum Ca2(+)-ATPase. Proceedings of the National Academy of Sciences of the United States of America 1990;87(7): 2466-2470.

[123] Lytton J, Westlin M, Hanley M R. Thapsigargin inhibits the sarcoplasmic or endoplasmic reticulum Ca-ATPase family of calcium pumps. The Journal of biological chemistry 1991;266(26): 17067-17071.

[124] O'Conor C J, Leddy H A, Benefield H C, Liedtke W B, Guilak F. TRPV4-mediated mechanotransduction regulates the metabolic response of chondrocytes to dynamic loading. Proceedings of the National Academy of Sciences of the United States of America 2014;111(4): 1316-1321.

[125] Dufour C, Holy X, Marie P J. Transforming growth factor-beta prevents osteoblast apoptosis induced by skeletal unloading via PI3K/Akt, Bcl-2, and phospho-Bad signaling. American journal of physiology. Endocrinology and metabolism 2008;294(4): E794-801.

[126] Guan Y, Yang X, Yang W, Charbonneau C, Chen Q. Mechanical activation of mammalian target of rapamycin pathway is required for cartilage development. FASEB journal : official publication of the Federation of American Societies for Experimental Biology 2014.

[127] Fitzgerald J B, Jin M, Chai D H, Siparsky P, Fanning P, Grodzinsky A J. Shear- and compression-induced chondrocyte transcription requires MAPK activation in cartilage explants. The Journal of biological chemistry 2008;283(11): 6735-6743.

[128] Vincent T, Saklatvala J. Basic fibroblast growth factor: an extracellular mechanotransducer in articular cartilage? Biochemical Society transactions 2006;34(Pt 3): 456-457.

[129] Lee H S, Millward-Sadler S J, Wright M O, Nuki G, Salter D M. Integrin and mechanosensitive ion channel-dependent tyrosine phosphorylation of focal adhesion proteins and beta-catenin in human articular chondrocytes after mechanical stimulation. Journal of bone and mineral research : the official journal of the American Society for Bone and Mineral Research 2000;15(8): 1501-1509.

[130] Chen N X, Geist D J, Genetos D C, Pavalko F M, Duncan R L. Fluid shear-induced NFkappaB translocation in osteoblasts is mediated by intracellular calcium release. Bone 2003;33(3): 399-410.

[131] Anghelina M, Sjostrom D, Perera P, Nam J, Knobloch T, Agarwal S. Regulation of biomechanical signals by NF-kappaB transcription factors in chondrocytes. Biorheology 2008;45(3-4): 245-256.

[132] Agarwal S, Deschner J, Long P, Verma A, Hofman C, Evans C H, Piesco N. Role of NF-kappaB transcription factors in antiinflammatory and proinflammatory actions of mechanical signals. Arthritis and rheumatism 2004;50(11): 3541-3548.

[133] Chowdhury T T, Bader D L, Lee D A. Dynamic compression counteracts IL-1 beta-induced release of nitric oxide and PGE2 by superficial zone chondrocytes cultured in agarose constructs. Osteoarthritis and cartilage / OARS, Osteoarthritis Research Society 2003;11(9): 688-696.

[134] Jeffrey J E, Aspden R M. Cyclooxygenase inhibition lowers prostaglandin E2 release from articular cartilage and reduces apoptosis but not proteoglycan degradation following an impact load in vitro. Arthritis research & therapy 2007;9(6): R129.

[135] Ke H Z, Qi H, Weidema A F, Zhang Q, Panupinthu N, Crawford D T, Grasser W A, Paralkar V M, Li M, Audoly L P, Gabel C A, Jee W S, Dixon S J, Sims S M, Thompson D D. Deletion of the P2X7 nucleotide receptor reveals its regulatory roles in bone formation and resorption. Molecular endocrinology 2003;17(7): 1356-1367.

[136] Salter D M, Millward-Sadler S J, Nuki G, Wright M O. Integrin-interleukin-4 mechanotransduction pathways in human chondrocytes. Clinical orthopaedics and related research 2001;(391 Suppl): S49-60.

[137] Millward-Sadler S J, Wright M O, Lee H, Nishida K, Caldwell H, Nuki G, Salter D M. Integrin-regulated secretion of interleukin 4: A novel pathway of mechanotransduction in human articular chondrocytes. The Journal of cell biology 1999;145(1): 183-189.

[138] Salter D M, Wallace W H, Robb J E, Caldwell H, Wright M O. Human bone cell hyperpolarization response to cyclical mechanical strain is mediated by an interleukin-1beta autocrine/paracrine loop. Journal of bone and mineral research : the official journal of the American Society for Bone and Mineral Research 2000;15(9): 1746-1755.

[139] Fujiwara Y, Uesugi M, Saito T. Down-regulation of basic fibroblast growth factor production from cartilage by excessive mechanical stress. Journal of orthopaedic science : official journal of the Japanese Orthopaedic Association 2005;10(6): 608-613.

[140] Woo S, Kwan M, Coutts R, Akeson W. Biomechanical considerations. In: Moskowitz R, Howell D, Goldberg V, Mankin H (eds) Osteoarthritis: Diagnosis and medical/ surgical management. Philadelphia: WB Saunders; 1992. 191-211.

[141] Hoch D H, Grodzinsky A J, Koob T J, Albert M L, Eyre D R. Early changes in material properties of rabbit articular cartilage after meniscectomy. Journal of orthopaedic research : official publication of the Orthopaedic Research Society 1983;1(1): 4-12.

[142] Burton W N, Todhunter R J, Lust G. Animal models of osteoarthritis. In: JF W, DS H (eds) Joint cartilage degradation: basic and clinical aspects. Marcel Dekker: New York; 1993. 347-384.

[143] Setton L, Zimmerman J, Mow V, Muller F, Pita J, Howell D. Effects of disuse on the tensile properties and composition of canine knee joint cartilage. Trans Orthopaedic Research Society 1990;15: 155.

[144] Palmoski M J, Brandt K D. Running inhibits the reversal of atrophic changes in canine knee cartilage after removal of a leg cast. Arthritis and rheumatism 1981;24(11): 1329-1337.

[145] Setton L A, Elliott D M, Mow V C. Altered mechanics of cartilage with osteoarthritis: human osteoarthritis and an experimental model of joint degeneration. Osteoarthritis and cartilage / OARS, Osteoarthritis Research Society 1999;7(1): 2-14.

[146] Wright M O, Nishida K, Bavington C, Godolphin J L, Dunne E, Walmsley S, Jobanputra P, Nuki G, Salter D M. Hyperpolarisation of cultured human chondrocytes following cyclical pressure-induced strain: evidence of a role for alpha 5 beta 1 integrin as a chondrocyte mechanoreceptor. Journal of orthopaedic research : official publication of the Orthopaedic Research Society 1997;15(5): 742-747.

[147] Orazizadeh M, Lee H S, Groenendijk B, Sadler S J, Wright M O, Lindberg F P, Salter D M. CD47 associates with alpha 5 integrin and regulates responses of human articular chondrocytes to mechanical stimulation in an in vitro model. Arthritis research & therapy 2008;10(1): R4.

[148] Millward-Sadler S J, Khan N S, Bracher M G, Wright M O, Salter D M. Roles for the interleukin-4 receptor and associated JAK/STAT proteins in human articular chondrocyte mechanotransduction. Osteoarthritis and cartilage / OARS, Osteoarthritis Research Society 2006;14(10): 991-1001.

[149] Lee H S, Millward-Sadler S J, Wright M O, Nuki G, Al-Jamal R, Salter D M. Activation of Integrin-RACK1/PKCalpha signalling in human articular chondrocyte mechanotransduction. Osteoarthritis and cartilage / OARS, Osteoarthritis Research Society 2002;10(11): 890-897.

[150] Millward-Sadler S J, Mackenzie A, Wright M O, Lee H S, Elliot K, Gerrard L, Fiskerstrand C E, Salter D M, Quinn J P. Tachykinin expression in cartilage and function in human articular chondrocyte mechanotransduction. Arthritis and rheumatism 2003;48(1): 146-156.

[151] Fitzgerald J B, Jin M, Dean D, Wood D J, Zheng M H, Grodzinsky A J. Mechanical compression of cartilage explants induces multiple time-dependent gene expression patterns and involves intracellular calcium and cyclic AMP. The Journal of biological chemistry 2004;279(19): 19502-19511.

[152] Murata M, Bonassar L J, Wright M, Mankin H J, Towle C A. A role for the interleukin-1 receptor in the pathway linking static mechanical compression to decreased proteoglycan synthesis in surface articular cartilage. Archives of biochemistry and biophysics 2003;413(2): 229-235.

[153] Fanning P J, Emkey G, Smith R J, Grodzinsky A J, Szasz N, Trippel S B. Mechanical regulation of mitogen-activated protein kinase signaling in articular cartilage. The Journal of biological chemistry 2003;278(51): 50940-50948.

[154] Li K W, Wang A S, Sah R L. Microenvironment regulation of extracellular signal-regulated kinase activity in chondrocytes: effects of culture configuration, interleukin-1, and compressive stress. Arthritis and rheumatism 2003;48(3): 689-699.

[155] Salter D M, Millward-Sadler S J, Nuki G, Wright M O. Differential responses of chondrocytes from normal and osteoarthritic human articular cartilage to mechanical stimulation. Biorheology 2002;39(1-2): 97-108.

[156] Millward-Sadler S J, Wright M O, Lee H S, Caldwell H, Nuki G, Salter D M. Altered electrophysiological responses to mechanical stimulation and abnormal signalling through alpha5beta1 integrin in chondrocytes from osteoarthritic cartilage. Osteoarthritis and cartilage / OARS, Osteoarthritis Research Society 2000;8(4): 272-278.

[157] Attur M G, Dave M N, Clancy R M, Patel I R, Abramson S B, Amin A R. Functional genomic analysis in arthritis-affected cartilage: yin-yang regulation of inflammatory mediators by alpha 5 beta 1 and alpha V beta 3 integrins. Journal of immunology 2000;164(5): 2684-2691.

[158] Boisclair Y R, Wang J, Shi J, Hurst K R, Ooi G T. Role of the suppressor of cytokine signaling-3 in mediating the inhibitory effects of interleukin-1beta on the growth hormone-dependent transcription of the acid-labile subunit gene in liver cells. The Journal of biological chemistry 2000;275(6): 3841-3847.

10

Hand Osteoarthritis —Clinical Presentation, Phenotypes and Management

Nidhi Sofat and Sharenja Jeyabaladevan

1. Introduction

Osteoarthritis (OA) is the most common arthritic disorder, affecting increasing numbers of people in an ageing population [1]. Nearly 27 million people are estimated to have OA among US adults [2]. OA of the hand is known to cause significant morbidity and can have a severe impact on patients' functional capacity. For example, the US Framingham study found that 27% of adults aged over 26 have hand OA (HOA) [2]. In addition, a large European study of 7983 people demonstrated that 25% of participants with hand pain showed significant hand disability [3]. Hand OA can lead to the development of chronic pain, causing significant emotional and financial burden to those affected, impacting on carers and on society as a whole [4]. Treatment of HOA currently comprises analgesia with analgesic drugs including topical or oral nonsteroidal anti-inflammatory agents (NSAIDs), opioid analgesics and rehabilitative hand physiotherapy [5]. However, large numbers of people continue to experience impaired hand function and pain.

Pathologically, OA is typified by cartilage degradation, osteophyte formation and underlying subchondral sclerosis. More recently, imaging-detected synovitis and bone marrow lesions have also been found to correlate with OA inflammation and pain. In this chapter we discuss the recognised clinical phenotypes of hand OA, typical features of hand OA, including Heberden's nodes, radiographic correlates of the clinical features observed and new insights into treatments for this chronic painful arthritic condition.

2. Clinical phenotypes of hand OA

2.1. Nodal hand OA

Nodal hand OA characteristically involves the distal interphalangeal (DIP) and proximal interphalangeal (PIP) joints of both hands. A typical swelling of the interphalangeal joints evolves, which can enlarge to a maximum size during its development (Figure 1). At the early to mid-stages when enlargement occurs, DIP joints can become painful, erythematous and difficult to mobilise. The underlying pathogenesis of this process includes bony enlargement of the underlying interphalangeal joints, synovitis and soft tissue swelling of the region affected [6]. When involving the DIP joints, the enlargement may give rise to an often typical feature described as a 'Heberden's node'. The historical context of the description of Heberden's nodes is given further below. The PIP joints are also a recognised feature of nodal hand OA. They can be associated with a very similar pathological process to the joints described in DIPs as above and are sometimes called 'Bouchard's nodes' [7]. The radiographic features of nodal hand OA are demonstrated in Figure 2. Interestingly, the presence of Heberden's and Bouchard's nodes can occur with or sometimes without associated symptoms of pain, stiffness and disability.

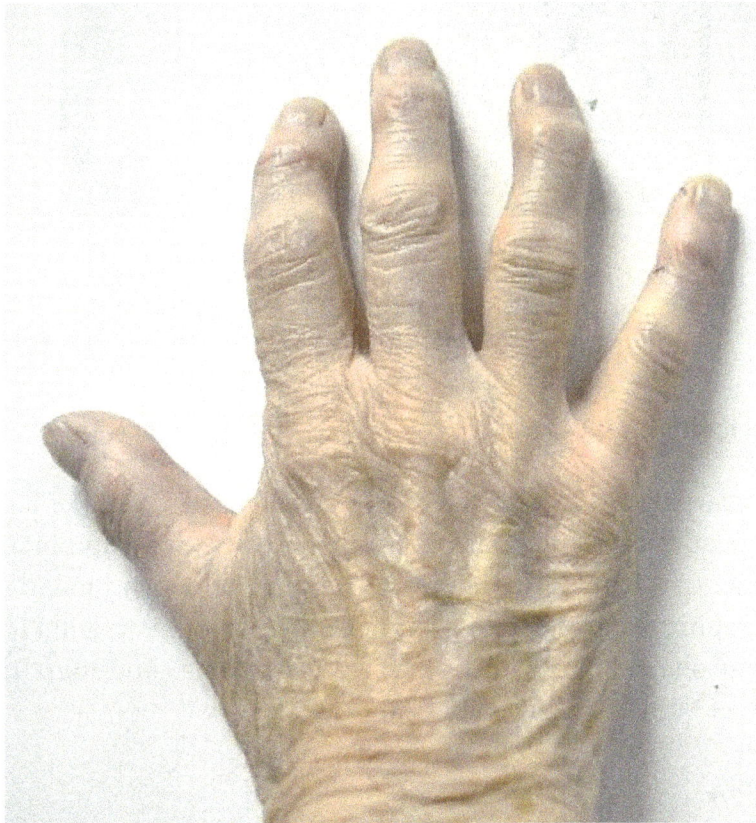

Figure 1. Distal interphalangeal (DIP) joint swelling of the index, middle and ring fingers demonstrating Heberden's nodes in a patient with hand OA. The patient also has involvement of the proximal interphalangeal joints (PIP) of the index, middle and ring fingers (Bouchard's nodes).

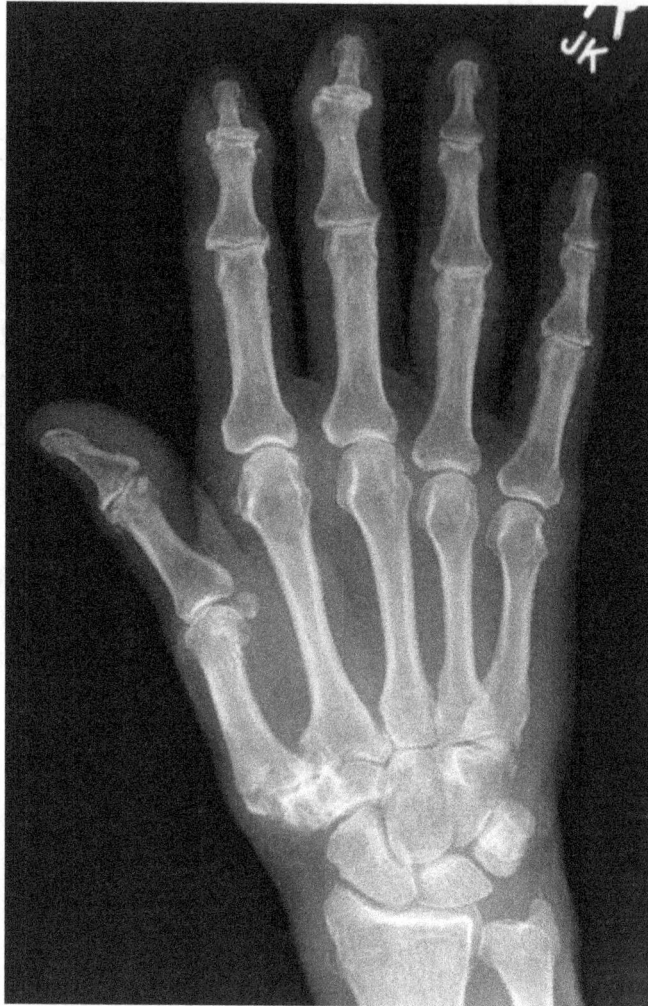

Figure 2. Radiographic features of nodal hand OA demonstrating DIP joint involvement (index and ring fingers especially) with joint space narrowing and osteophyte formation. This patient also has involvement of the first carpometacarpal (CMC) joint of the thumb. The metacarpophalangeal joints are spared, which is often a characteristic finding.

2.2. First carpometacarpal joint OA

The first carpometacarpal (CMC) joint is a distinct recognised feature of hand OA. It is often seen bilaterally in people affected and is often a major cause of symptomatic joint pain. Risk factors for first CMC joint hand OA include mechanical factors and manual occupations [8]. The typical radiographic features of CMC joint OA are demonstrated in Figure 2. They often give rise to a 'square-shaped' hand in people affected by this condition. Interestingly nodal hand OA can co-exist with first CMC joint OA.

2.3. Erosive hand OA

The erosive phenotype of hand OA is a particularly aggressive form of hand involvement. It is associated with erosions particularly in the DIP and PIP joints [9]. It is important to exclude other forms of inflammatory arthritis in its management. Typical radiographic features of this condition are shown in Figure 3. Historically, clinicians have considered the use of disease-modifying anti-rheumatic drugs (DMARDs) in this variant to avert the progression of this erosive form of the disease [10].

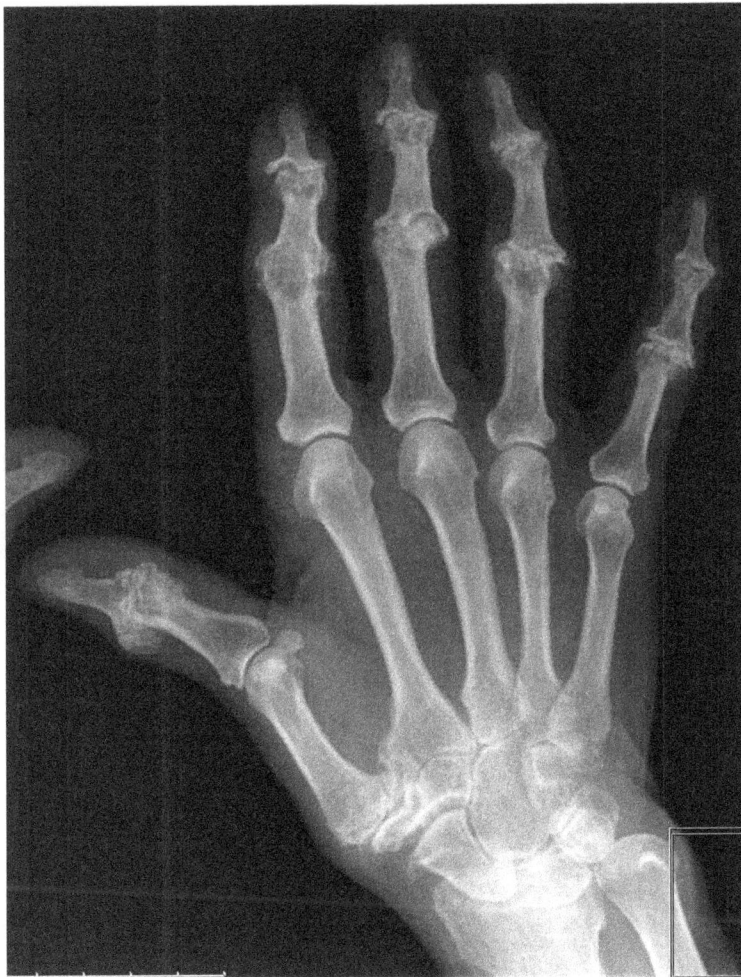

Figure 3. Typical radiographic features of erosive hand OA are shown. There has been aggressive erosive damage to the proximal and distal interphalangeal joints (PIPs) and (DIPs) respectively. A central erosion is observed in several of these joints with a corresponding characteristic 'gull-wing' deformity and osteophytes observed laterally on either side. The interphalangeal (IP) joint of the thumb is also involved and characteristic joint space narrowing at the first carpometacarpal (CMC) joint is observed. The metacarpophalangeal joints are characteristically spared.

Other rarer forms of hand OA are also observed in the context of underlying conditions e.g. inflammatory arthritides, where hand OA can be a secondary phenomenon. The may include rheumatoid arthritis or the crystal arthropathies including gout and pseudogout. In the crystal arthropathies, clinical and radiographic appearances can be very similar and may also respond to similar therapies [11], giving prolonged episodes of joint inflammation and pain. Other underlying conditions which may give rise to chronic OA of the hands include genetic conditions such as Stickler's syndrome, and others such as haemochromatosis, hyperparathyroidism and acromegaly.

3. Risk factors for hand OA development

The risk of OA rises with increasing age, with the prevalence of OA increasing over the age of 50 [4]. With respect to the question of whether heavy physical work is associated with hand OA, some researchers have suggested that heavy occupational work was not associated with the presence of OA [12] and other studies have favoured a positive correlation of manual work with OA [13]. Obesity has also been investigated as an independent risk factor for hand OA with occasionally conflicting results. Hochberg *et al.* previously suggested that age and not obesity, were the main risk factor for hand OA [14]. In contrast, Denisov *et al.* suggested that obesity was associated with the progression of knee and hand OA in a cohort of almost 300 patients [15]. Cicutinni *et al.* have also suggested that there is a 9 to 13% increase in knee and hand OA for every kilogram increase in body weight [16].

Since the range of presentation of hand OA is varied, with several clinical phenotypes recognised, it is perhaps not surprising that a number of genes have been identified as risk factors for hand OA. These have been summarised in a recent review [17]. The main themes which have arisen from genetic studies include the observation that the genetic associations for hand OA cover a broad nature of genes, perhaps reflecting the multifactorial risk factors in this condition. Reported genetic associations include a female preponderance carried in many family cohorts, OA susceptibility loci mapping to chromosome 6 for hip and knee OA. Recently a group reported a significant association between hand OA and susceptibility loci on chromosome 6 [18]. In a UK cohort, Zhang *et al.* have investigated four putatively functional genetic variants in the KLOTHO gene, which is a strong ageing-related gene [19]. The group suggested that one variant in the KLOTHO gene was associated with hand OA susceptibility and especially with osteophyte formation rather than cartilage damage. Further studies have reported four SNPs in the IL-1R1 gene suggesting an association between the gene encoding the IL-1R1 and hand OA. Since IL-1 is a cytokine that has catabolic effects on cartilage, this may be particularly relevant in human disease [20]. Recent work has also focused on the extracellular matrix protein found in cartilage: aggrecan. Kamareinen *et al.* [21] showed that patients homozygous for the most common aggrecan VTNR (variable number of tandem repeats) allele, A27, had a significantly lower risk of hand OA. People who carried 2 copies of the aggrecan alleles with less than 27 repeats or more than 27 repeats demonstrated a higher risk of hand OA. The link between hand OA and extracellular matrix proteins found in cartilage has received further attention with the recent reports that single nucleotide polymorphisms (SNPs) in the asporin (ASPN) gene are associated with hand OA progression [22]. A recent genome-wide association study in an Icelandic population has shown that variants within the ALDH1A2 gene was associated with hand OA. The variants within the ALDH1A2 gene were confirmed in replication sets from The Netherlands and UK [23].

Although the studies above suggest a strong familial association with hand OA, the broad nature of clinical presentation and phenotypes suggests that strong genetic associations with hand OA are difficult to identify. In future it would be useful to accumulate larger populations of specific phenotypes to establish genetic associations in greater detail.

4. Mechanisms of pain in hand osteoarthritis

Osteophytes, which are a pathognomonic feature of OA, are often observed to create a physical barrier to optimal range of movement and can give rise to severe joint pain as well. Recently, inflammatory changes have been found to relate to higher risk of structural damage in a study which looked at 2 years follow-up [6]. Kortekaas and colleagues showed that inflammatory features, defined by synovial thickening, effusion and increased power Doppler signal on ultrasound scan (demonstrated in Figure 4), when they persisted, were related to increased radiographic progression of OA after 2 years. The presence of synovitis by ultrasound may therefore guide treatment decisions such as corticosteroid-guided intra-articular injection in hand joints affected by OA.

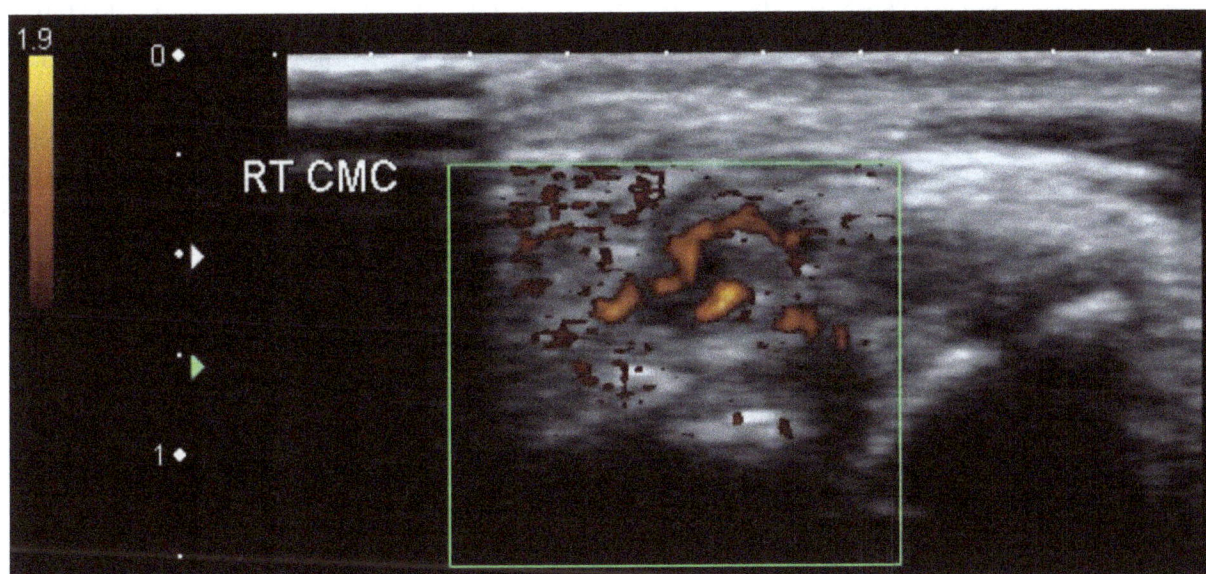

Figure 4. Ultrasound image of the right first carpometacarpal joint, showing evidence of synovial thickening and increased vascularity on power Doppler imaging.

Recent work has demonstrated the evidence of bone marrow lesions (BML), which are defined as high density signal lesions on MRI with T2-weighted imaging, especially in the knee [24], have also been observed in people with hand OA [25]. In their study, Haugen *et al.* showed that bone marrow lesions, synovitis and erosions were associated with joint tenderness. It is therefore possible that synovitis and bone marrow lesions could be future targets for therapeutic interventions in hand OA.

5. Heberden's nodes: A historical perspective

"What are those little hard knobs, about the size of a small pea, which are frequently seen upon the fingers, particularly a little below the top, near the joint? They have no connection with the gout, being found in persons who never had it; they continue for life; and being hardly ever attended with pain, or disposed to become sores, are rather unsightly, than inconvenient, though they must be some little hindrance to the free use of the fingers." [26]. These were the observations of William Heberden whose philosophy in medicine was that one must always be guided by their own direct observations. Heberden's nodes, which are classical lesions of osteoarthritis, were initially described as 'digitorum nodi' in Latin by Heberden himself, which led him to make the important distinction between gout and osteoarthritis [27]. OA remains a common disabling condition worldwide and the most common form of arthritis [28]. However, there are few diagnostic tests and unfortunately current treatments for OA have not been able to successfully eliminate pain from the clinical manifestations of the disease [5].

In addition to Heberden's description further observation of the nodes have led them to be classified according to the location (Figure 1). Nodes either appear on the lateral aspect on the dorsolateral margins or in the central midline where occasionally they fuse with the lateral nodes to form a ridge. They can also be classified as idiopathic or traumatic, with the latter most commonly resulting in a solitary Heberden node [29]. Idiopathic nodes are easily identifiable from the clinical history, which usually consists of a node, which slowly and gradually increases in size on one finger and then spreads to other fingers. Reports from patients about pain associated with the nodes are inconsistent, with some reporting painful growth of the nodes whereas others report the growth as painless [30]. Stecher [29] described the progression of Heberden's nodes having observed around 7,000 individuals with Heberden's nodes. He noted that the progression could be divided into three stages. The initial stage consists of a visible enlargement of the joint; this enlargement is also palpable at the proximal end of the distal phalanx as two spherical nodules or as prominent ridge. In some people it was noted that the enlargement was so severe that the nodules were palpable at the sides of the joint and on the palmar surface. The second stage consists of palmar flexion of the distal phalanx in addition to the enlargement. In addition to the previous two stages the third stage consists of lateral deviation of the distal phalanx from the midline (see Figure 1) [29].

It is well established that Heberden's nodes are associated with underlying radiographic changes [30]. More recent studies have shown that Heberden's nodes, which are more developed and affecting both sides of the joint show joint space narrowing as opposed to Heberden's nodes in their initial stages. This can be attributed to the slow growth of Heberden's nodes and that joint space narrowing is possibly a late manifestation of the disease [31]. With this knowledge it can be assumed that Heberden's nodes affecting both aspects of the joint can be used as a clinical marker for radiographic change [31].

OA is a process of cartilage and bone damage in which changes are eventually irreversible. However it seems that Heberden's nodes have a different process governing their formation and they are histologically different depending on the location on the joint. Midline nodes are traction spurs growing in the extensor tendon, this growth is usually found in athletes as a physiological response to excessive tension. It is important to note that this spur is not a true osteophyte and that it can be identified by its location and the lack of a cartilage cap. Conversely, the lateral node has shown to have a constant presence of osteophyte, which arises from one or both of the phalanges and is located lateral to the extensor tendon. These histological findings are supported by radiological observation. Radiography of Heberden's nodes shows that there is evidence of osteophyte formation in the lateral node and a traction spur in the middle node [31]. Osteophytes consist of both new bone and cartilage formation, which arise from progenitor cells, indicating that the sequelae of joint destruction induces a pluripotent cell response [32]. The exact function of osteophytes in osteoarthritis is yet be understood but can been seen as an adaptive mechanism against joint injury to stabilize the joint [33, 34]. Analysis of osteophytes at different developmental stages has shown a sequential process of differentiation and the presence of the anabolic factor transforming growth factor-beta (TGF-β) [32]. Osteophyte growth usually occurs in the direction of least resistance; in joints such as the shoulder and ankle the strong capsules restrict osteophyte growth. At the distal interphalangeal joint the only obstruction is a thin capsule, which holds in synovial fluid. This obstruction is not sufficient to restrict osteophyte growth hence the presence of such prominent Heberden's nodes. To what extent the osteophyte causes deviation of the distal phalanx is dependent on the strength of the collateral ligament, which is genetically determined [31]. Extensive research by Stecher has shown that there may be a single autosomal gene responsible for the inheritance of Heberden's nodes however it seems to exhibit a sex-linked pattern as it is dominant in females and recessive in males [29].

Although Heberden's nodes were first described over 150 years ago and despite extensive research their exact mechanism and purpose has not been fully understood. They are part of the clinical picture of osteoarthritis but it seems that their pathophysiology and genetic inheritance somewhat differs to our current understanding of generalised osteoarthritis.

6. Treatments for hand osteoarthritis

A range of treatments have been used in hand OA, including physical techniques such as taping and splinting to reduce pain and improve function [35, 36]. Such treatment is often administered through physiotherapy and/or occupational therapy units and can be repeated during flares.

Pharmacological treatments are often focused around symptomatic pain relief including paracetamol, topical and oral non-steroidal anti-inflammatory drugs such as ibuprofen, naproxen and others, which have been shown to be efficacious over and above other analgesic treatments in large scale meta-analyses [4]. Such treatments are now recommended within several international guidelines for the treatment of OA [36]. Recent imaging studies which have shown synovitis and bone marrow lesions to correlate with painful progressive hand OA have led to renewed interest in considering disease-modifying anti-rheumatic agents for hand OA.

Previous studies have shown that intra-articular injections of corticosteroid can be particularly beneficial in hand OA, particularly at the first CM joint [37]. However, repeated injections are not without significant side-effects, including local tissue damage and skin atrophy. The general consensus is that, if not straightforward, local injections may best be performed under ultrasound guidance. Some reports have suggested intra-articular hyaluronic acid may also be a potential therapeutic option, but such studies have not yet been subjected to large scale clinical trials [38]. With respect to systemic steroid, a recent study showed improvement in synovitis following intramuscular depomedrone injection of steroid for hand OA, which was sustained for 4 weeks [39]. However, the effects of systemic corticosteroid treatment were relatively short-lived and synovitis returned by ultrasound measures after 12 weeks of treatment.

With respect to the use of other disease-modifying agents, a recent trial of hydroxychloroquine has been conducted for the treatment of hand OA [40] and the results of this study are now awaited. Other groups have investigated the use of bisphosphonates e.g. intravenous clodronate in the treatment of hand OA with beneficial outcome for pain in their study [41]. However, a recent meta-analysis by our group did not show overall significant benefit overall for pain and function after use of bisphosphonates across several phenotype of OA, including hip, knee and hand [42]. Future studies targeted at specific stages of disease with proven synovitis and bone marrow lesions may be more helpful in establishing the potential future therapeutic use of bone-modulating agents in the clinic.

Author details

Nidhi Sofat* and Sharenja Jeyabaladevan

*Address all correspondence to: nsofat@sgul.ac.uk

Institute for Infection and Immunity, St George's, University of London, Cranmer Terrace, London, UK

References

[1] Hunter, D.J and Felson, D.T. (2006) 'Osteoarthritis'. *British Medical Journal.* 18(332): 640-642

[2] Lawrence, D. J. et al. (2008) 'Estimates of the prevalence of arthritis and other rheumatic conditions in the United States. Part II.' *Arthritis and Rheumatism* 58(1): 26-35.

[3] Dahaghin, S. et al. (2005) 'Prevalence and determinants of one month hand pain and hand related disability in the elderly (Rotterdam study)'. *Annals of the Rheumatic Diseases.* 64(1): 99-104

[4] Zhang, W. et al. (2007) 'EULAR evidence based recommendations for the management of hand osteoarthritis: report of a task force of the EULAR Standing Committee

for International Clinical Studies Including Therapeutics (ESCISIT)' *Annals of the Rheumatic Diseases.* 66(3):377–388.

[5]   Sofat, N., Ejindu, V. and Kiely, P. (2011) 'What makes osteoarthritis painful? The evidence for local and central pain processing', *Rheumatology (Oxford, England), 50 (12),* pp. 2157-2165.

[6]   Kortekaas, M.C., et al. (2014) 'Inflammatory ultrasound features show indepdendent associations with progression of structural damage after 2 years of follow-up in patients with hand osteoarthritis'. *Ann Rheum Dis.* Doi: 10.1136/annrheumdis-2013-205003

[7]   Rees, F. et al. (2012). 'Distribution of finger nodes and their association with underlying radiographic features of osteoarthritis. *Arthritis Care Res (Hoboken)* 64(4): 533-8

[8]   Jensen J.C., Sherson, D. (2007) 'Work-related bilateral osteoarthritis of the first carpometacarpal joints'. *Occup Med (Lond)* 57(6): 456-60

[9]   Marshall, M. et al. (2013) 'Erosive osteoarthritis: a more severe form of radiographic hand osteoarthritis rather than a distinct entity?' *Ann Rheum Dis.* doi: 10.1136/annrheumdis-2013-203948

[10] Bryant LR, et al. (1995) 'Hydroxychloroquine in the treatment of erosive osteoarthritis'. *J Rheumatol.* 22(8): 1527-31

[11] Rothschild, B.M. (2013) 'Distinguishing erosive osteoarthritis and calcium pyrophosphate deposition disease. *World J Orthop.* 4(2): 29-31

[12] Goekoop, R.J et al. (2011) 'Determinants of absence of osteoarthritis in old age'. *Scan J Rheum.* 40(1): 68-73

[13] Snodgrass SJ, Rivett DA, Chiarelli P, Bates AM, Rowe LJ, Aust J Physio 2003; 49(4): 243-50

[14] Hochberg, M.C. et al. (1993) 'Obesity and osteoarthritis of the hands in women'. *Osteoarthritis Cartilage* 1(2): 129-35

[15] Denisov, L.N. et al. (2011) 'Role of obesity in the development of osteoarthrosis and concomitant diseases'. *Ter Arkh,* pp 34-7

[16] Cicuttini, et al. (1996) 'The association of obesity with osteoarthritis of the hand and knee in women: a twin study. *J Rheumatol* 23: 1221-6

[17] Gabay, O and Gabay, C. (2013) 'Hand osteoarthritis: new insights'. *Joint Bone Spine.* 80(2): 130-4

[18] Jakowlev, K. et al. 'Search for hand osteoarthritis susceptibility locus on chromosome 6p12.3-p12.1'. *Human Biol.* 79(1): 1-14

[19] Zhang F, et al. 'Association between KLOTHO gene and hand osteoarthritis in a female Caucasian population'. *Osteoarthritis Cartilage* 2007; 15: 624-9

[20] Nakki, A. et al. (2011) 'Allelic variants of IL1RI gene associated with sever hand osteoarthritis'. *BMC Med Genet* 11: 50

[21] Kamarainen, O.P. (2006) 'Aggrecan core protein of a certain length is protective against hand osteoarthritis'. *Osteoarthritis Cartilage*, 14: 1075-8

[22] Bijsterbosch, J. et al. (2013) 'Association study of candidate genes for the progression of hand osteoarthritis'. *Osteoarthritis Cartilage* 21(4); 565-9

[23] Styrkarsdottir, U. et al. (2014) 'Severe osteoarthritis of the hand associates with common variants within the ALDH1A2 gene and with rare variants at 1p31. *Nat. Genet.* 46(5): 498-502.

[24] Crema, M. D. et al. (2013) 'Prevalent cartilage damage and cartilage loss over time are associated with bone marrow lesions in the tibiofemoral compartments: the MOST study'. *Osteoarthritis Cartilage* 21(2):306-13

[25] Haugen, I.K. et al. (2012) 'Associations between MRI-defined synovitis, bone marrow lesions and structural features and measures of pain and physical function in hand osteoarthritis'. *Ann Rheum Dis.* 71(6): 899-904

[26] Heberden, W. (1818) 'Commentaries on the History and Cure of Diseases', pp. 119

[27] Lian, T. Y. and Lim, K. K. (2004) 'The legacy of William Heberden the Elder (1710-1801)', *Rheumatology (Oxford, England)*, 43 (5), pp. 664-665.

[28] WHO (2014) *Chronic diseases and health promotion.* Available at: http://www.who.int/chp/topics/rheumatic/en/ (Accessed: 3/13 2014).

[29] Stecher, R. M. (1948) 'Heberden's Nodes: The Clinical Characteristic Of Osteo-Arthritis Of The Fingers', *Annals of the Rheumatic Diseases*, 7 (1), pp. 1-8.

[30] Swanson, A. B. and de Groot Swanson, G. (1985) 'Osteoarthritis in the hand', *Clinics in Rheumatic Diseases*, 11 (2), pp. 393-420

[31] Alexander, C. J. (1999) 'Heberden's and Bouchard's nodes', *Annals of the Rheumatic Diseases*, 58 (11), pp. 675-678

[32] Sandell, L. J. and Aigner, T. (2001) 'Articular cartilage and changes in Arthritis: Cell biology of osteoarthritis', *Arthritis Research*, 3 (2), pp. 107-113

[33] Pottenger, L. A., et al. 'The effect of marginal osteophytes on reduction of varus-valgus instability in osteoarthritic knees', *Arthritis and Rheumatism*, 33 (6), pp. 853-858

[34] Fassbender, H., G (2002) *Pathology and Pathobiology of Rheumatic Diseases.* 2nd edn. Germany: Springer.

[35] Brandt KD. Diagnosis and Nonsurgical Management of Osteoarthritis

[36] Hochberg, M.C. et al. (2012). 'American College of Rheumatology 2012 recommendations for the use of nonpharmacologic and pharmacologic therapies in osteoarthritis of the hand, hip and knee'. *Arthritis Care Res (Hoboken)* 64(4): 465-74

[37] Maarse, W. et al. (2009) 'Medium-term outcomes following intra-articular corticosteroid injection in first CMC joint arthritis using fluoroscopy'. *Hand Surg* 14(2-3): 99-104

[38] Fuchs, S. et al. (2006) 'Intra-articular hyaluronic acid compared with corticosteroid injections for the treatment of rhizarthrosis'. *Osteoarthritis Cartilage* 14(1); 82-8

[39] Wenham, C.Y. (2012). 'A randomized, double-blind, placebo-controlled trial of low-dose oral prednisolone for treating painful hand osteoarthritis. *Rheumatology (Oxford)* 51(12): 2286-94

[40] Kingsbury, S.R. et al. (2013). 'Hydroxychloroquine effectiveness in reducing symptoms of hand osteoarthritis (HERO): study protocol for a randomized controlled trial'. *Trials* 14:64

[41] Saviola, G. et al.(2012) 'Clodronate and hydroxychloroquine in erosive osteoarthritis: a 24-month open randomized pilot study'. *Mod Rheumatol.* 22(2): 256-63

[42] Davis AJ, et al. (2013) 'Are bisphosphonates effective in the treatment of osteoarthritis pain? A research synthesis and meta-analysis'. PLOS ONE, 8(9):e72714

11

Superficial Heat and Cold Applications in the Treatment of Knee Osteoarthritis

Çalışkan Nurcan and Mevlüde Karadağ

1. Introduction

There is information related to the need to perform heat and cold applications as non-pharmacological methods for the pain control in patients with knee osteoarthritis available in the literature. However, the basis of scientific data supporting the therapeutic effect of the superficial heat and cold application in knee osteoarthritis is weak. The purpose of this study is to consider the basic information about the evidence for the superficial heat and cold application in the treatment of knee osteoarthritis.

2. Body

Heat and cold applications for the purpose of treatment are applied to a part or whole of the body and cause local or systemic effects [1]. In general, the physiological effects of heat are vasodilatation, increased capillary permeability, acceleration of cell metabolism, muscle relaxation, acceleration of inflammation, pain reduction by relaxing muscles, sedative effect, and reducing the viscosity of the synovial fluid to decrease joint stiffness. The physiological effects of cold are generally the opposite of warm effects. The effects of cold are vasoconstriction, a slowdown in cell metabolism, local anesthesia, decrease in blood flow, reduction of the arrival of oxygen and metabolites to the area and the reduction of residuum removal (Table 1) [1-4].

When applying heat to a local and large area of the body, low blood pressure can be seen due to the excessive peripheral vasodilation. This reduction in blood pressure can cause fainting if it is serious. This effect of heat application in individuals with heart, lung or circulatory system diseases, such as arteriosclerosis, develops more frequently than healthy individuals.

Heat Application Effects	Therapeutic Benefits
Vasodilatation	Accelerates the transport of nutrients and the removal of the residuum by increasing blood flow to the injured area of the body. It reduces the accumulation of venous blood in the region.
Decrease in blood viscosity.	Accelerates the transport of leucocyte and antibody to the injured area
Decrease in blood spasm	Reduces the pain caused by muscle relaxation, muscle spasm or stiffness
Increase in tissue metabolism	Blood flow increases due to the increased local temperature
Increase in capillary permeability	Transition of nutrients and residuum increases
Cold Application Effects	Therapeutic Benefits
Vasoconstriction	Blood flow to the injured area decreases, edema formation is prevented, inflammation reduces
Local anesthesia	Reduces the localized pain
Slowdown in cell metabolism	Decreases the oxygen requirement of the tissues
Increase of blood viscosity	Increases blood coagulation in injured area
Decrease the blood spasm	Reduce the pain

Table 1. The effects of heat and cold application [4]

The prolonged cold application and vasoconstriction may cause an increase in the blood pressure. Because, the way of blood flow changes towards the internal blood vessels from the surface (cutaneous) due to the vasoconstriction. Shivering is another general effect of long stay in the cold and a response of the body to warm itself [5].

3. Physiological tolerance to heat and cold

The tolerations to the heat and cold applications of individuals are quite different (See Table 2). In some cases, when performing the heat and cold applications, precautions are required to reduce the risk of injury. Conditions that increase the risk of injury are given in Table 3.

Condition	Risk factors
Part of the body where the application is done	Back of the hands and feet are not very sensitive to temperature changes. The inner face of the forearm and wrist, neck and perineum are sensitive to temperature changes.
The size of the body area where the application is done	When the areas exposed to heat or cold tolerance grows, tolerance decreases When the areas exposed to heat or cold tolerance get smaller, tolerance increases
Individual tolerance	Tolerance in infants and elderlies are generally very low. Tolerance to heat or cold is high in individuals with Sensory and nervous system disorders. However, warm or cold damage risks of these people are too much.
The duration of administration	Individual feels heat or cold severely until the skin temperature changes, however, later tolerance increases.
The integrity of the skin	Impaired skin integrity is more sensitive to temperature changes.

Table 2. Factors affecting physiological tolerance to heat and cold [5]

Condition	Risk factors
Age (infants, children and elderly individuals)	Having a thin skin layer in children, decreasing the sensitivity to pain in the elderly increases the risk of burns
Disruption of skin integrity, open wound, stoma	Subcutaneous and deep tissues are more sensitive to temperature changes. Because they do not contain the heat receptors and their pain receptors are few.
Edema or scar regions	Intracellular accumulation of fluid or thickening caused by scar tissue reduces the sensitivity to heat.
Peripheral vascular disease (diabetes mellitus, arteriosclerosis, etc.).	Sensitivity to temperature and pain in the extremities decrease due to the circulatory disorders and local tissue damage. Cold application further reduces the blood flow.
Confusion, loss of consciousness	Sensory stimuli or the perception of pain decrease
Spinal cord injury	Sensory stimuli and the perception of pain is prevented due to the changes in the nerves transmit pathway

Table 3. Situations enhancing the injury risk in heat and cold applications [4]

4. The adaptation of heat and cold receptors

Heat and cold receptors (thermo receptors) are attuned to the changes of temperatures. Receptors are initially and strongly stimulated when exposed to sudden temperature changes. This stimulation is strong at the first few seconds, and stimulation continues more slowly during the following half an hour. Thus, receptors are adapted to the new temperature. This adaptation explains why an individual feels very cold when suddenly comes out of a cold environment to a warm room, or vice a versa, why the individual feels so hot when suddenly comes out of a warm environment to a cold room.

An understanding of this adaptation mechanism is very important when heat and cold applications are performed. Patients cannot evaluate the temperature of the heat or cold applications developed right after adaptation. When heat applications are performed, serious burns after performing adaptation can develop. On the contrary, when the cold application is performed, this may result in pain, or blood circulation may be impaired in the area of application [5].

4.1. Rebound phenomenon

Rebound phenomenon is a situation that is developed by exceeding the maximum time of therapeutic effect in heat and cold applications, and in which an opposite effect of the practice other than the desired effect occurs. The heat generates vasodilation maximum 20-30 minutes. If the application continues more than 30-45 minutes, the congestion occurs in tissue, and the blood vessels react to this case by constricting. The reason of this reaction is unknown. If heat applications further extend, burn risks are likely to occur, since the constricted blood vessels cannot deliver the heat application to the other parts of the body by circulation enough [5].

In cold applications, when the skin temperature falls to 15 °C (60 °F), vasoconstriction gets the maximum level, and vasodilatation starts below 15 °C. In normal conditions, this is a protective mechanism that prevents the body tissues such as the nasal and ear from freezing when exposed to cold. This is due to this mechanism that a person's skin becomes red when walking at cold weather. Heat and cold applications must be completed before a rebound phenomenon initiates [5].

5. Heat and cold applications

The use of hot and cold applications in medicine history goes back to the ancient times. For example, Hippocrates, in his book titled "Management of Acute Disease ", recommended the application of the hot water -filled caps made of clay or metal for the pain in the costal joints, and to place a soft material between skin and cap to prevent the burns. In addition, he mentioned the dry and heat applications that consisted of a heated corn in the blanket made of wool [6].Different types of materials related to general and local heat and cold applications have been produced by the medical technology since Hippocrates.

Patients should be considered before performing heat or cold applications. The application area should be checked for the tolerance of application, skin integrity of the patient, bleeding, and circulatory disorder, and the information about the application to the patient should be provided. The conditions in which heat application must be avoided are shown in Box 1.

Box 1. The conditions in which heat and cold applications must be avoided:

The conditions in which heat applications must be avoided [5]:

- *Within the first 24 hours after traumatic injury.* Temperature increases bleeding and edema.

- *In active bleedings.* Temperature causes vasodilation and increases bleeding.

- *Edema not caused by inflammation.* Temperature increases capillary permeability and edema.

- *In localized malignant tumors.* Temperature increases the risk of metastasis by accelerating the cell metabolic rate, cell growth and circulation.

- *In the skin problems characterized by redness and blistering.* Temperature can cause severe damage or skin burns.

The conditions in which cold applications must be avoided:

- *In an open wound.* Cold decreases the blood flow, so the tissue damage may increase.

- *In the patients with circulatory disorders.* Cold disrupts the nutrition of the tissue and can cause tissue damage. In patients with Raynaud's disease, cold increases arterial spasm.

- *In the patients with cold allergy or hypersensitivity to cold.* Inflammatory response begins in some patients that have cold allergy. Erythema, urticaria, edema, joint pain, and muscle spasms may occur. If individuals have hypersensitivity, some of the inflammatory responses may cause a sudden rise of the blood pressure.

6. Selecting wet or dry applications

Heat and cold applications can be applied in two ways: dry and wet. The type of wound or injury, the part of the body that application will be carried out, and the presence of inflammation are the factors affecting the choice of dry or wet application (Table 4).

Multiple treatment options are available for patients with OA of the knee including the use of superficial heat or cold, transcutaneous electrical nerve stimulation (TENS), oral medications, the injection of hyaluronic acid or a corticosteroid, or ultimately knee joint replacement surgery. Common ways of superficial heat-cold application are thermoforms, electrical heating pads, aquathermia pads, hot-cold packs, hot water bath, ice bags or collars, and warm – cold soaks, combined cold compression system [1, 3 -5, 7-10].

Advantages	Disadvantages
Wet applications	*Wet applications*
Wet applicationprevents drying of the skin and softens the wound exudates.	Softening of the skin (maceration) occurs in the long-term application.
Wet compresses are suitable for many part of the body.	Quick cooling appears due to the evaporation in wet heat applications.
Wet heat applications affect the deep tissues.	
Slightly wet and heat application does not increase the perspiration and insensible fluid loss.	Burn risk is high because moisture transmits the temperature in wet heat applications.
Dry applications	*Dry applications*
Dry heat application has less risk of burns than Wet heat application.	Dry heat increases fluid loss by perspiration.
	Dry application is not effective in deep tissues.
Dry application does not cause the skin softening (maceration).	Dry heat can cause drying of the skin.
Temperature is retained longer because there is no evaporation of water in dry heat application.	

Table 4. Selecting Wet or Dry Application[4]

6.1. Thermophore

Thermophore (hot water bag) is widely used, especially for dry heat application at home. It is cheap and easy to use, but there are some disadvantages. Leaking of the bag of hot water or using the bag in appropriate circumstances can cause burns. The temperature of the water in adults and children 2 years of age should be 46-52 °C (115-125 °F). The temperature of the water in unconscious, weak persons and the children under the age of 2 should be 40.5 - 46 °C (105-115 °F) [5, 9].

6.2. Aquathermic pad (Pillow)

Aquatermic or aquamatic (also named K-pad) pads consist of tubes that provide water circulation inside (See Figure 1). Some pads are water-resistant, and some pads have absorbent surface that allows applying wet application. There are various sizes of pads depending on the body parts to be treated. Pads should be applied to the skin in a cover. If pads are directly applied to the skin, they can cause burns. Patients should never lie down on the pad and should be observed for the signs of skin burns during application. While aquatermic pad is applied, the temperature should be 40.5 - 43 ° C (105-110 °F) for adults, and the application period is usually 20 - 30 minutes [4, 5].

6.3. Electric heating pad

Electric Heating Pads are utilized for the purpose of local heat application. They are easy to use, relatively reliable, and provide warmth of the same value and can easily get shape of the body part they are applied to. There are a variety of sizes depending on the body area to be treated. There are water resistant covers to make application to the wet dressing in some models [1, 5].

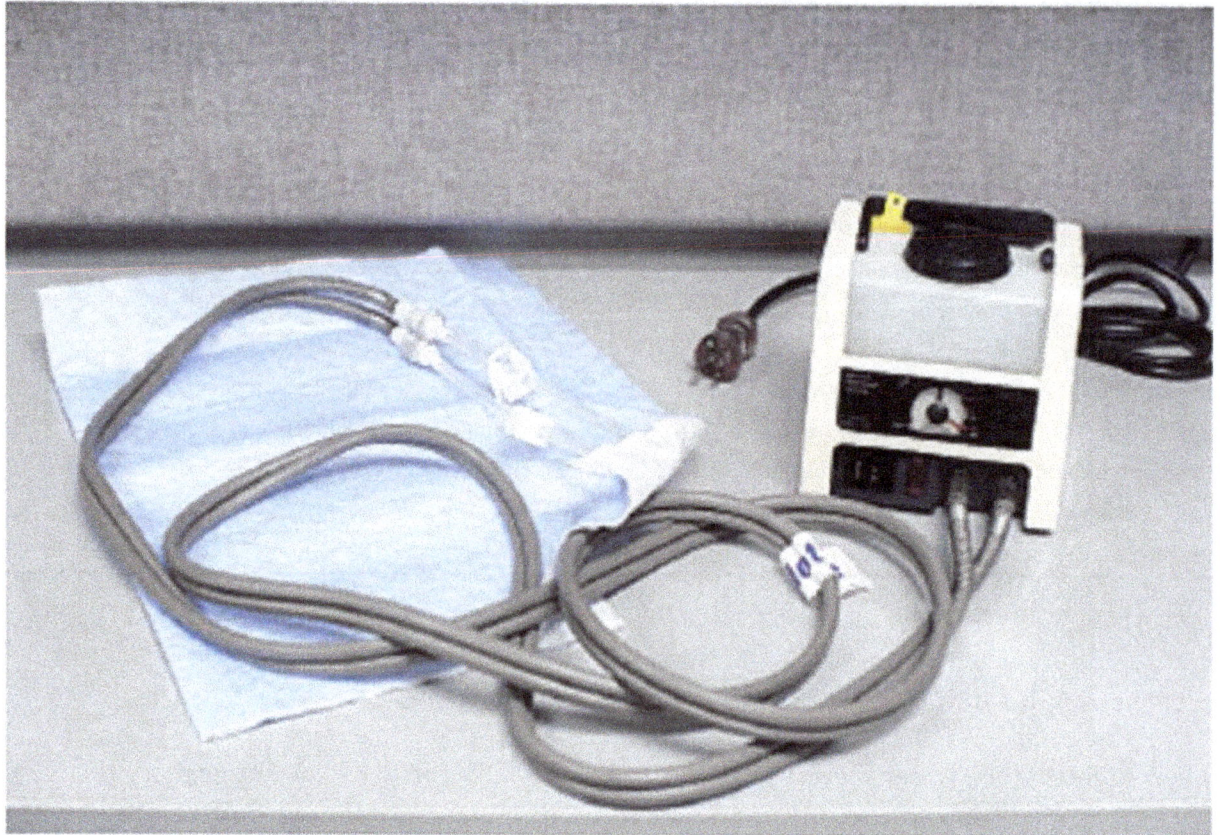

Figure 1. Aquatermic pad [1]

Electric heating pads provide as much temperature as the heat packs with silicondioxyte (hot packs) do. They do not require reheating between the applications, and can be used more than 20 minutes. Furthermore, it has been emphasized that electric heating pads are more suitable for the home use [11].

There are some rules that should be attended by the practitioner when electric heating pad application is performed, otherwise serious burns can occur. These rules are;

• Do not stich the drilling tools such as needle to the pad. The needle may damage the electrical system of the pad and may cause electric shock.

• Application area should be dry if pad does not have a water resistant coating. The presence of water may cause an electric shock.

• Pad should be applied with heating pad key to prevent the patient from increasing the temperature of the pad.

• The patient should not lie on the pad. Burns can occur if the temperature is not spread [5].

The utilization of electric heating pad is limited in hospitals due to the security problems caused by not paying attention to these rules in crowded places such as hospitals [1, 12].

6.4. Hot – Cold pack

Hot - cold packs are used for heat or cold applications and are the bags filled with the silicate gel (Figure 2). The use and preparation of hot and cold packs varies according to the manufacturing company. Therefore, the preparation of the pack and the application time must done as specified in the user guide. The pack should be prepared by waiting in hot water or microwave if it will be used for the purpose of heat application. Otherwise, the pack should be prepared by waiting in the fridge at least 1.5 hours if it will be used for the purpose of cold application. When disposable quick hot or cold packs are pressurized, the chemical mixture in the package and the heat are released and warming / cooling begins. These packages cannot be used again. These packages should not be tightened, and should be protected from kneaded and shock until the time of use [4, 5, 13].

Hot packs are used for the purpose of dry heat applications, however there are some varieties that are used for wet heat applications. These packages are made of impermeable fabric, and there are special heating units to heat (Figure 3). Silica gel in the fabric bag swells by absorbing large amounts of heat and water. Therefore, the extra water must be filtered; dry towel should be wrapped to the package, and the package should not be placed under the patients, but should be placed over the patients [10, 14].

Hot - cold packs are also utilized by wrapping in a wet towel. Water-resistant treatment cloth or plastic wrap should be used during application to prevent the loss of temperature as in the compressed application [5]. Steps for the application of hot packs:

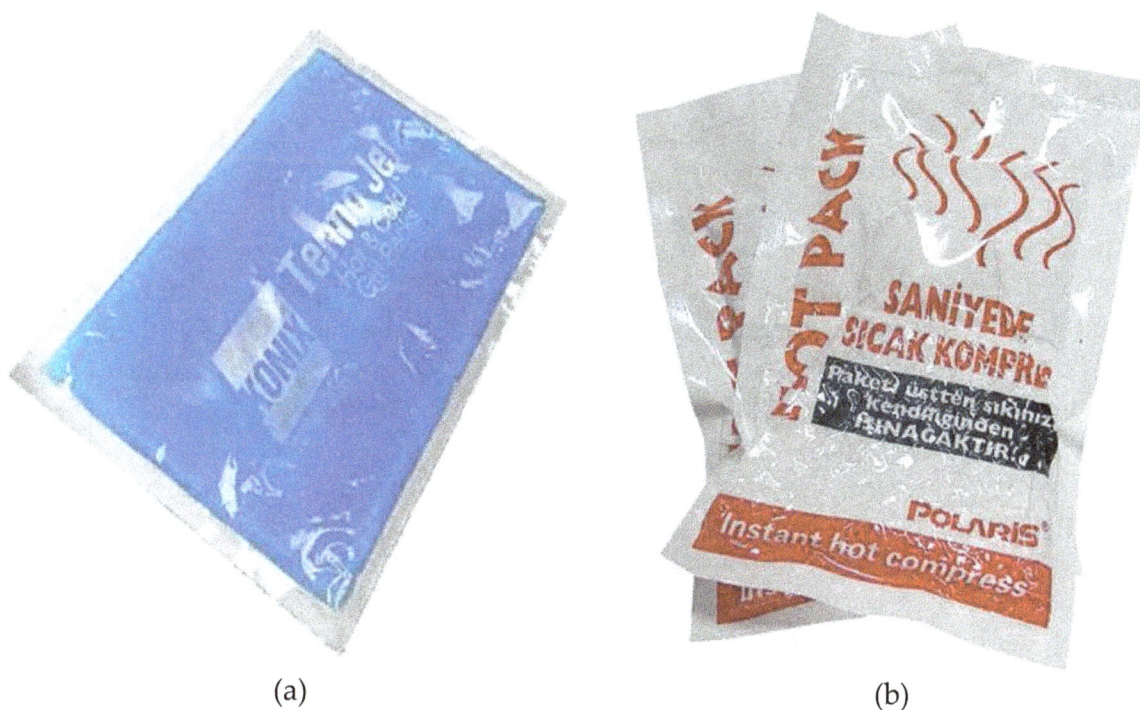

(a)   (b)

Figure 2. Hot Packs A. Commercial Hot pack B. Single Use Hot pack

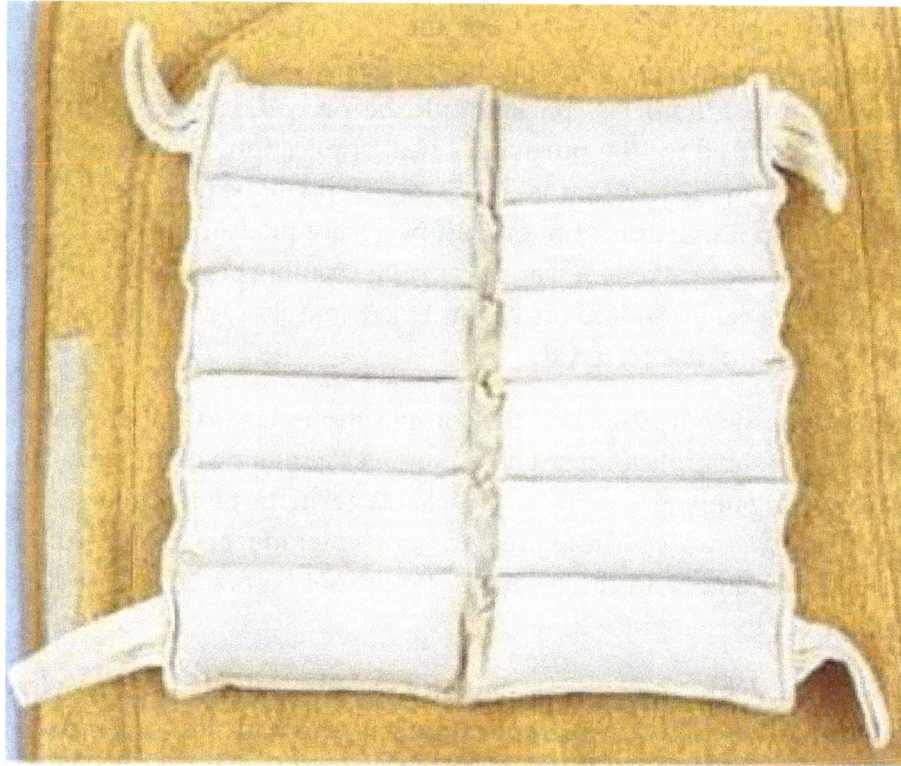

Figure 3. Hot Pack (used for wet heat applications)[13]

6.5. Hot compress

Sterile wet hot compress improves circulation in open wounds, helps to solve the edema, provides drainage and prevents the spread of infections. The temperature of the water in the hot compress applications varies according to the purpose, and it is sufficient to be 40.5 - 43 ° C (105-110 °F). During the applications heat disperses quickly. Compresses should be changed frequently for the purpose of keeping the temperature at the same level, and compresses should be wrapped with a plastic cover or a dry towel. Wetness causes Vasodilatation and evaporates the heat from the skin's surface; therefore the patient may feel cold. The room temperature should be controlled [4, 5, 9].

6.6. Hot immersion bath

Hot immersion bath is performed by immersing a part of the body in a heated solution. Hot immersion bath accelerates the circulation, decreases the edema, and provides muscle relaxation. Immersion bath can also be applied to an area that is closed by dressing, and the bath is available with a heated solution. The position of the patient should be comfortable during the application and the solution should be heated up to 40.5 – 43 °C (105 - 110 °F) [4]. Surgical asepsis principles must be complied if the bath is applied with an open wound [5].

6.7. Sitz bath

Sitz bath is an operation by immersing the pelvic part into hot water or in some cases cold water. Sitz bath is useful in patients with painful hemorrhoids, vaginal inflammation, a history of rectal surgery, and opened episiotomy (incision made between the vagina and rectum to facilitate the birth and to prevent the tearing of the vagina) during childbirth. Application should take 15 - 20 minutes and the temperature of the water should be 40.5 - 43 ° C (105-110 °F). However, the time and temperature vary depending on the patient's health status. The patient sits in a tub or a special chair. A large part of the body is exposed to heat during the sitz bath so that the patient should be evaluated in terms of changes in consciousness, nausea, pallor in face, and increase in patient pulse rate [4, 5].

6.8. Cold compress

The application should take 20 minutes to reduce the edema and inflammation and the temperature should be 15 °C (59 °F). Surgical aseptic technique should be used for open wounds. When a cold compress is applied, some unwanted side effects such as burning or numbness, mottling of the skin, redness, extreme pallor, and bluish - purple mottled appearance on the skin can be observed. The procedure for the application of cold compress are the same as hot compress applications [4].

6.9. Cold immersion bath

The procedure for application of cold immersion bath are the same as hot immersion bath applications. The application should take 20 minutes and the temperature should be 15 °C (59 °F) [4].

6.10. Ice bag

Ice bag is made of plastic or rubber, and its mouth is wide enough to contain ice. The ice bag is used for sprains, localized bleeding or hematoma, preventing edema after dental surgery, controlling the bleeding, and creating a local anesthetic effect in the area [4]. An ice bag must be applied by wrapping with a towel or blanket [5].

6.11. Combined cold compress system

Combined Cold Compress System is capable of performing both compression and cold application. It consists of cuffs in the appropriate size of each body region, a refrigerator that is placed in into ice-water, a connecting pipe that provides ice water flows to cuff (Figure 4). Compression allows conductance by increasing the contact between the skin and ice water and reduces blood flow. Thus, it has been indicated that the co-administration of cold with compression in the therapy is more effective than only implementing cold. Combined Cold Compress System is preferred in the control of postoperative pain and the swelling after acute trauma [15].

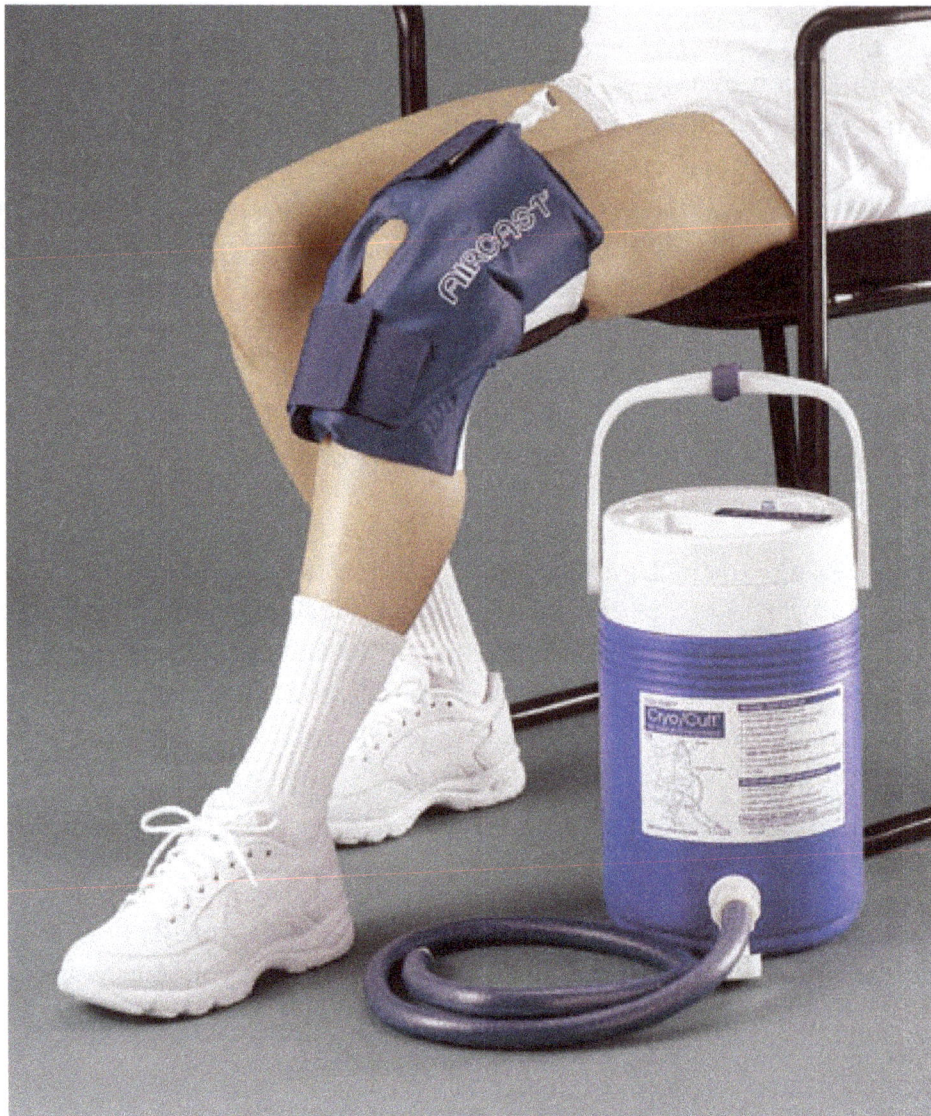

Figure 4. Combined Cold Compress System

7. Superficial heat and cold application in the treatment of knee osteoarthritis: Is the evidence enough?

Rakel and Barr (2003) have stated that nurses/physicians, traditionally apply heat and cold applications and some massages, thus they should be informed about the strength of the evidence for the efficiency of these applications. The authors have expressed that the methodological evidence for the effect of heat and cold applications on chronic pain is limited [16]. Wright and Sluka (2001) have claimed that the information about the effect of superficial heat application on depressing the pain or improving the physical function are contradictory, and that there are different studies stating that heat application increased, decreased or did not change arthritis pain and other symptoms [17].

Brosseau et al. (2003) investigated the literature in The Cochrane Library for the purpose of determining the effectiveness of heat and cold applications in knee OA, and they found 3 randomized controlled trial involving 179 patients. In one of these studies, ice massage did not have a significant impact on the increase the quadriceps muscle strength (29% relative difference) for 20 minutes for 5 times a week, totally for three weeks compared with the clinical control group. However, ice massage in patients with knee OA was statistically significant different compared with the control group in physical function in and ROM. The role of ice in reducing the pain is uncertain. In another study, ice packs were applied to three days a week for three weeks and there was no positive effect of the treatment compared with the control group. It was suggested that cold packs could be used for reducing knee edema. Heat application had no significant effect compared with the control group or alternative application. Hot pack had no effect on edema compared with placebo or cold packs. The authors stated that a greater number of participants and well-planned researches should be required to determine heat and cold applications in the treatment of knee OA [18]. Jamtvedt et al. (2008) indicated that the above-mentioned studies had small samples and low quality of the work. Furthermore, the authors concluded that the effects of heat and cold applications were unclear [19].

Yıldırım et al. (2010) studied the effect of superficial local heat application that was performed with digital moist heating pad for 20 minutes every other day for 4 weeks. The results showed that heat application reduce pain and increase physical function in patients with knee OA, however it had no effect on stiffness. In this study, patients were followed for routine treatment plan suggested by the physician [20].

Mazzuca et al. (2004) investigated the comparison of warm maintaining kneepad and an elastic kneepad made of cotton. The difference between them was insignificant. The patients in this study continued to pharmacological treatment [21].

Shereif and Hassa (2011) determined that when therapeutic exercise and heat application performed together, pain and stiffness reduced, and physical function improved. However, objective measurement criteria were not used in the evaluation. The patients in this study continued to pharmacological treatment, as well [22].

According to Brandt (1998), although the effect of heat or cold application was not well-researched, approximately 60% of patients diagnosed with rheumatoid arthritis (RA) and OA preferred heat application on their aching joints, while 20% of the patients preferred cold application [23]. Veitiene & Tamulaitiene (2005) studied the applications preferred by the patients diagnosed with OA and RA and benefits obtained. They found that patients with OA specified exercise (55 7%), the use of assistive devices like walking sticks and walkers (29 6%), and heat application (25 9%) as the most effective; splint (3 7%), resting (3 7%) and joint protection (3 7%) as the least effective; and cold application (0%), not effective at all [24].

Davis and Atwood (1996) stated that the current knowledge on the therapeutic benefits of heat application is insufficient and the expected benefit from heat application is low in conditions of severe pain, but in their study with 82 patients with RA and OA, 70% expressed that they applied heat application [25].

Chandler et al. (2002) have found limited scientific evidence for the analgesic effects of heat although heat has been used to relieve pain for years. They attributed this to the lack of well-organized studies [12]. Similarly, Öneş et al. (2006) have mentioned that although heat application has been used extensively on outpatient treatment, the randomized controlled studies were limited in number and were not scientifically conducted [26].

As a result of the meta-analysis study by Philadelphia Panel (2001), which was randomized controlled and depended on the findings of observation studies; it was found that no evidence was present neither for the usage / not usage nor for the clinical usefulness of the physical rehabilitation applications like heat, cold, ultrasound, and massage in practical life [27].

The responsibility for providing better quality care requires decisions based on evidence. Evidence-based applications are important for the results such as improving quality of care and care outcomes, making a difference in the results in clinical practices and patient care results, and standardizing the care [28]. Application guidance is directive for the evidence-based practice. Osteoarthritis Research Society International (OARSI), which is the most comprehensive guide published on hip and knee OA treatment so far, has referred to the study by Brosseau et al. in 2003 as the first systematic review published regarding heat and cold applications [18]. Kirazlı (2011) stated that research evidences supporting the treatment of localized heat and cold applications were less, however this treatment method was widely used by the patients with OA, and it was recommended as a simple and reliable method for the relief of pain in most guidelines [29].

8. Conclusion

As discussed above, there is some information in the literature that heat and cold applications should be superficially performed in patients with knee OA as a non-pharmacological method for controlling pain. However, the basis of scientific data that supports heat and cold applications could be effective on chronic pains such as the knee OA is weak [16, 30]. Today, although the need for quality care based on evidence exists, the existing studies on the effectiveness of heat and cold applications on knee OA are not sufficient to cover it. As a result, in spite of the need for further research to determine the effectiveness of the superficial heat and cold applications, superficial heat and cold applications are available to help treatment due to the presence of very few side effects, ease of implementation, and their non-invasiveness [31].

Author details

Çalışkan Nurcan* and Mevlüde Karadağ

*Address all correspondence to: nurcany@gazi.edu.tr

Gazi University, Faculty of Health Sciences, Nursing Department, Ankara, Turkey

References

[1] Taylor C., Lillis C., LeMone P. Fundamentals of Nursing The Art & science of Nursing Care. (4th ed.), Philadelphia: Lippincott Williams & Wilkins: In Tech;2001.

[2] Berman A., Synder S., Kozier B., Erb G. Heat And Cold Measures techniques, Kozier and Erb's Techniques in Clinical Nursing. (5th ed.), New Jersey: Prentice Hall: In Tech;2002.

[3] Çalışkan N. Sıcak – Soğuk Uygulamalar In: Atabek Aştı T., Karadağ A. (ed.) Hemşirelik Esasları Hemşirelik Bilimi ve Sanatı. Akademi Basın ve Yayıncılık, İstanbul: In Tech;2012. p663-696.

[4] Potter PA., Perry AG. Fundamentals of Nursing. (7th ed.), St. Louis: Mosby Elsevier: In Tech;2009.

[5] Berman A., Synder S., Kozier B., Erb G. Kozier and Erb's Fundamentals of Nursing. (8th ed.), New Jersey: Prentice Hall: In Tech;2008.

[6] Smith RP. Heat therapy: the next hot topic. The Female Patient, 2003;27:25–31, http://www.femalepatient.com/html/arc/sel/march03/028_03_030.asp (accessed 10 August 2010).

[7] McHugh GA., Silman AJ., Luker KA. Quality of care for people with osteoarthritis: a qualitative study. Journal of Clinical Nursing 2007;16(7b) 168-176.

[8] Kozier B., Erb G., Berman AJ., Snyder SJ. Fundamentals of Nursing Concepts, Process, and Practice, seventh edition, New Jersey, Prentice Hall Health: In Tech;2004.

[9] Evans-Smith P. Taylor's Clinical Nursing Skills. Philadelphia: Lippincott Williams & Wilkins: In Tech;2005.

[10] Öztürk C., Akşit R. Tedavide Sıcak ve Soğuk. Tıbbi Rehabilitasyon. In: Oğuz H., Dursun E., Dursun N. (Ed.) İstanbul: Nobel Tıp Kitabevleri: In Tech;2004.

[11] Wood C., Dry and moist heat application and the subsequent rise in tissue temperatures. https://orca.byu.edu/content/jug/2002 reports/ _hhp /wood.pdf (accessed 01 October 2010).

[12] Chandler A., Preece J., Lister, S. Using heat therapy for pain management, Nursing Standard 2002;17(9):40-42.

[13] Rosdahl C., MaKowalski MT. Heat and Cold Applications. Textbook of Basic Nursing, (9th ed.), Philadelphia: Lippincott Williams & Wilkins: In Tech;2008. http://books.google.com.tr/books?id=tB1YiYj_kdkC&printsec=frontcover&dq=Textbook+of+Basic+Nursing+book&source=bl&ots=xBPJxx6NLx&sig=UYqzZ3aRbT-1YCnpN-XuBJCo71tk&hl=tr&ei=FXBqTJu5K9fPjAfV6bl2&sa=X&oi=book_result&ct=result&resnum=3&ved=0CCwQ6AEwAg#v=onepage&q&f=false (accessed 01 October 2010).

[14] Delisa J.A., (2007) Terapötik Fiziksel Ajanlar, Fiziksel Tıp ve Rehabilitasyon İlkeler ve Uygulamalar. In:T. Arasıl (Ed.) Ankara:Güneş Tıp Kitabevleri: In Tech;2007.

[15] Erek Kazan E. Soğuk Uygulamalar ve Hemşirelik Bakımı. Sağlık Bilimleri Fakültesi Hemşirelik Dergisi 2011; 73-82

[16] Rakel B., Barr JO. Physical modalities in chronic pain management. The Nursing Clinics of North America 2003;(38): 477-494.

[17] Wright A., Sluka KA. Nonpharmacological treatments for musculoskeletal pain. The Clinical Journal of Pain 2001; (17): 33-46.

[18] Brosseau L., Yonge KA., Robinson V., Marchand S., Judd M., Wells G. Et al. Thermotherapy for treatment of osteoarthritis. The Cochrane Database of Systematic Reviews 2003; 4, Art. No.: CDoo4522.

[19] Jamtvedt G, Dahm KT, Christie A, et al. Physical therapy interventions for patients with osteoarthritis of the knee: an overview of systematic reviews. Phys Ther 2008;88(1):123-135.

[20] Yıldırım N, Ulusoy MF, Bodur H. Effect of Heat Application on Pain, Stiffness, Physical Function and Quality of Life in Patients with Knee Osteoarthritis. J Clin Nurs 2010;19:1113-1120.

[21] Mazzuca SA, Page MC, Meldrum RS, Brandt KD, Petty-Saphon S. Pilot study of the effects of a heat-retaining knee sleeve on joint pain, stiffness, and function in patients with knee osteoarthritis. Arthritis Rheum 2004;51(5):716-721.

[22] Shereif WI, Hassanin AA. Comparison between Uses of Therapeutic Exercise and Heat Application on Relieve Pain, Stiffness and Improvement of Physical Function for Patient with Knee Osteoarthritis, Life Sci J 2011;8(3):388-396.

[23] Brandt KD. The importance of nonpharmacologic approaches in management of osteoarthritis. Am J Med 1998;105(1B):39S-44S.

[24] Veitiene D, Tamulaitiene M. Comparison of self-management methods for osteoarthritis and rheumatoid arthritis. J Rehabil Med 2005;37(1):58-60.

[25] Davis GC, Atwood JR. The development of the pain management inventory for patients with arthritis. Journal of Advanced Nursing. 1996;24 236-243.

[26] Öneş K, Tetik S, Tetik C, Öneş N. The effects of heat on osteoarthritis of the knee. Pain Clinic 2006;18(1):67-75.

[27] Philadelphia panel evidence-based clinical practice guidelines on selected. Physical Therapy 2001; 81(10): 1675-1700.

[28] Kocaman G. Hemşirelikte Kanıta Dayalı Uygulama. HEMAR-G 2003;5(2):61-69.

[29] Kirazlı Y. Osteoartrit Tanı ve Tedavi Kılavuzlarına Güncel Bakış. Türk J Geriatr 2011;14, Suppl 1:119-125.

[30] Hanada EY. Efficacy of rehabilitative therapy in regional musculoskeletal conditions. Best Pract Res Cl Rh 2003;17(1):151-166.

[31] Çalışkan N. Diz Osteoartriti Tedavisinde Yüzeysel Sıcak Soğuk Uygulama: Kanıtlar Yeterli mi? Journal of Contemporary Medicine 2013;3(2):144-147.

12

Spine Osteoarthritis

Elizabeth Pérez-Hernández,
Nury Pérez-Hernández and Ariel Fuerte-Hernández

1. Introduction

Osteoarthritis (OA) is a widespread disease and is considered the most common form of arthritis. The current OA prevalence is estimated at 15% of the population [1], but this rate is predicted to double by 2020 [2] and this increase is related with some lifestyle diseases like obesity [2]. OA affects the joints of the hand and the lower extremities such as knee and hip. OA of the spine occurs in approximately 40–85% of the adult population, but it is often omitted in prevalence studies. The rate disparities are due to the differences on the definition of the disease and to the variability between demographic groups studied [3]. Generally, the costs for OA care are high, as well as the economic implications for prolonged work disability [4, 5]. Symptomatically, it is considered that 80% of Americans suffer an episode of low back pain (LBP) in their lifetime [6, 7], thus care costs for LBP are estimated to be more than 100 billion dollars per year in the US [8], with a loss of 149 million workdays per year [9, 10].

OA of the lumbar spine is related with the degeneration of the intervertebral disc (ID) and bone formation, which is called spondylosis [11]. There has been a lack consensus on whether or not the combination of decreased disc space and osteophyte formation is a characteristic of OA or is a separate phenomenon. Clinically, the association between OA of the hand, knee and facet joint has been described, but no relationship was found between disc degeneration (DD) and OA of the hip, knee, or hand, or between the formation of osteophytes and OA of the hip and hand [12].

OA is defined as a disease resulting in structural and functional failure of synovial joints, which usually is characterized by progressive articular cartilage damage, involvement of the synovium and subchondral bone hypertrophy. OA affects the spinal zygapophyseal joints and is closely related to degenerative disc disease (DDD) despite the pathophysiological differences between the two disorders [13]. This degenerative cycle has mechanical impact with significant and progressive changes in the functional anatomy and mechanobiology, manifesting pain syndromes, destabilization, and impaired quality of life.

2. Anatomy and mechanics of the spinal joints

2.1. Normal facet joints

The vertebral joints are complex structures made up of posterior and anterior elements. The posterolateral spine consists of facet joints that are considered true synovial joint. One ID and two facet joints comprises a "three-joint complex." This complex binds two adjacent vertebrae, and the superior articular process of the inferior vertebra joins with the inferior articular processes of the overlying vertebra (Figure 1). The joint surfaces in the cervical and thoracic spinal regions are convex and concave, and the lumbar region of the facet joints shows a devastated form [14]. The orientation of the articular surfaces has a basic biomechanical role. The articular surfaces of the cervical and thoracic spinal segments are arranged horizontally [14, 15], favoring the axial rotation and lateral flexion [16, 17]. Comparatively, lower thoracic and lumbar spinal regions tend to adopt a more vertical orientation [18] that limits lateral flexion and rotation, protecting the IDs and spinal cord. Generally, the inclination angles of cervical facet joints in the sagittal plane ranges from 20° to 78° and in the axial plane from 70° to 96°, while the angle between the thoracic facet joints range from 55° to 80° and 85° to 120°, and the lumbar region range from 82° to 86° and 15° to 70° in both planes, respectively [14, 18].

Typically, facet synovial joints have a hyaline cartilage cover, subchondral bone, synovium, and a ligament system that envelops the entire joint [19, 20]. The cartilage layer is thinner at the edges of the joint surface and gradually thicker in the central portion thereof [21]. The composition of the articular cartilage does not differ from that observed in other diarthrodial surfaces, a cellular component, chondrocytes, and an abundant extracellular matrix (EM) composed of water, fibrillar proteins, glycosaminoglycans, and proteoglycans. The mechanical properties, such as load distribution and low-friction movement are dependent on the articular cartilage integrity [22, 23].

The subchondral bone has been considered as a morphological unit that provides a link between the articular cartilage and cancellous bone, which plays a key role in mitigate the impact of axial forces during dynamic joint load [24, 25]. It has been reported that the subchondral bone thickness is greater in asymptomatic males and increases with each successive lower spinal level, suggesting its association with the increased load [25].

Additionally, synovium and the ligament system facilitate movement with minimal friction and provide mechanical resistance, while synovial fluid lubricates and nourishes the joint surfaces [26]. The meniscoides or intraarticular synovial folds also protect the articular cartilage during movement [27], compensate the irregularities of the joint surface and increase the contact surface with the facets [28]. The meniscoides are formed by fatty, fibrous connective tissues and a lining of synovium [29, 28].

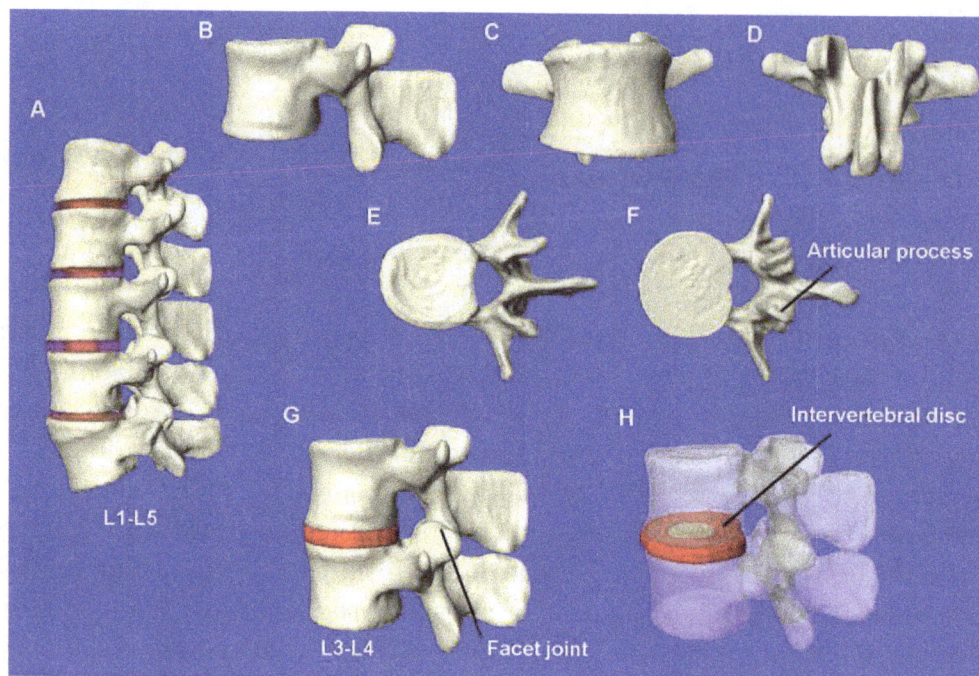

Figure 1. Normal anatomy of the facet joint and ID. A. Sagittal view of segments L1–L5; B. Sagittal view (L3); C–D. Coronal views (L3); E–F. Axial view (L3); G. Lumbar disc-facet unit (L3–L4); H. ID (L3–L4).

Moreover, the capsule comprises ligament fibroblasts, dense collagen fibers, elastic fibers, and proteoglycans [30, 31], and one of its main functions is to allow movement without provide mechanical resistance.

2.2. Normal intervertebral disc

In the anterior spine, the vertebral bodies are attached through the IDs. These structures provide support for load and flexibility during mechanical exposure; they also facilitate the movements of flexion, extension, and rotation. The typical composition of the ID consists of a central nucleus pulposus, which is contained in an outer annulus fibrous at the periphery, and the inferior and superior cartilage endplates [32].

Annulus fibers are agreed in concentric lamellae and consist predominantly of type I collagen [33]. In the early stages of life, these lamellae are arranged regularly, these are divide and interdigitate, and during aging they form an intricate and complex network in response to the load. Adult lumbar discs may contain up to 25 lamellae, thus lead to an increase in thickness toward the center portion thereof [34]. Annulus cells are small, elongated, disposed parallel to lamellae, and synthesize types I and II collagen [35], elastin [36], proteoglycans [37], and types III, IV, and VI collagens in various proportions [38, 39, 40, 41]. Other proteins with leucine-rich repeat, such as fibromodulin, decorin, and lumican, regulate the assembly of collagen fibers; similarly, the cartilage oligomeric matrix protein (COMP) is involved in regulation of the assembly of fibrillar proteins. Furthermore, chondroadherin, other protein with leucine-rich repeat without carbohydrate substituents and without the N-terminal binds to collagen participates in the maintenance of chondrocyte phenotype [41].

The center of the ID is the nucleus pulposus, which becomes gelatinous and more fibrous with aging. The nucleus pulposus is surrounded by a fibrous capsule and consists of round or oval chondrocyte-like cell with abundant cytoplasm and prominent cytoskeleton. These cells are called "physaliphorus" cells, which present large vacuoles. In this region, these cells are responsible in the synthesis of type II collagen [35]. The nucleus pulposus is rich in proteoglycan aggrecan, which consists of approximately chondroitin sulfate chains hundred, and each polysaccharide chain has about hundred negatively charged groups. Furthermore, the keratan sulfate chains are disposed in clusters located in a different area to that of chondroitin sulfate chains. Moreover, hundred molecules bind aggrecan and hyaluronate, as well as fibulin and tenascin proteins [41, 42]. These negatively charged macromolecular structures promote osmotic water retention.

The interface between the disc and the vertebral body consists of a thin layer of hyaline cartilage called endplate. This is extended across most of the vertebral body except at the outer rim, where the fibers of annulus fibrosus are inserted. In adults, this tissue is avascular, so the metabolites diffuse through it to the cells of the endplate and the center of the disc. During adulthood, the endplate thickness is reduced to approximately 0.6 mm [43]. Biochemically, the endplate contains type X collagen, which is involved in calcification processes [44].

It is well known that the main source of energy disc cells is derived from glycolysis [45]. Due to the low oxygen tension, protein synthesis and macromolecules, such as sulfated glycosaminoglycans is inhibited. Stimuli such as growth factors also come from the extracellular fluid [46], while the ATP production in disc cells depends on the local pH and nutrient availability. Most studies have reported that an acidic pH level significantly reduces the glycolytic metabolism and the rate of oxygen consumption, with concomitant decrease in ATP production [47, 48]. However, the effect of oxygen concentration in disc cells remains controversial, as some studies have described a positive effect [45, 46]. Protein synthesis is also a process affected by local oxygen and pH levels, which significant decrease if the low oxygen tension to less than 5% [46]. Similarly, extracellular pH affects protein synthesis, so an abrupt decrease in acidic environments [48]. Contrary to this event, the activity of matrix metalloproteinases is generally not inhibited at low pH, which may enhance the rate of matrix breakdown [49].

Dependent glucose supply (primary energy source), disc cells can die within 24 hours if glucose concentrations fall below 0.2 mM. Under these conditions, the intracellular glucose transport is also significantly reduced [50]. In this respect, it has been reported that the rate of cell death of the disc increases in acidic conditions (pH 6.0) despite of an adequate glucose intake [51, 52].

The avascular nature of the adult human ID is well known, with minimal penetration of capillaries and nerve endings in the outer regions of the annulus. This capillary network comes from the vertebral arteries which across the subchondral bone forming the loops of the interface between cartilage endplate and the bone [53, 54]. Thus, vascularity is protected by the cartilage endplate and promotes selective transport of molecules through the disc [55, 56].

Nutrients diffuse from capillary vascularity of the disc, through cartilage endplate, EM until the cells [57, 58, 59]. This solute movement is associated with load patterns to which it is usually subjected the disc. Apparently, the mechanical load on the disc is inversely proportional to nutrient transport. For example, during the redistribution of the load, the disc thickness is decreased, favoring the transport of nutrients from the cartilage endplate; however, if the proportion of fluid in the tissue matrix is decreased, diffusion is reduced, and this could affect the metabolic levels [60, 61]. This charge-nutrients ratio in the ID is still under investigation. Diffusion gradient, which is dependent on passive transport, leads to differences in the metabolic activity of the disc cells. Generally, the center of the disc contains lower concentrations of glucose and oxygen, and higher concentrations of lactic acid [45].

2.3. Mechanobiology

The mechanical load on the ID can cause multiple physical changes and mechanobiological effects. Volumetric changes, fluid flows, pressure changes, electrokinetic activity, and changes in cell shape are events that occur secondarily to tension, compression, or shear. Previous studies in vitro and in vivo on animal models have shown that the static compressive load or strain (0.2 to 0.4 MPa) [62] can induce anabolic cellular responses in the disc, with increased gene expression and synthesis of EM components such as proteoglycans and types I and II collagens [63].

Comparatively, during dynamic compression at low frequency (0.01 Hz, 1 MPa) in cells of rodent disc, induce an increase in the gene expression of macromolecules such as aggrecan and types I and II collagens. At higher frequencies of load an increase in expression of mRNA of proteases like MMP-3, MMP-13, ADAMTS-4 (a disintegrin and metalloproteinase with thrombospondin motifs) has been observed [64, 65]. Additionally, disc cell death occurred after exposure to high magnitudes (> 0.4 MPa) and low frequency (0.01 Hz) of dynamic load.

In response to moderate hydrostatic pressure (<3.0 MPa), the cells cultured or tissue explants of disc may increase the synthesis collagen, proteoglycans, and tissue inhibitor of metalloproteinase 1 (TIMP1), which applies to cells of the nucleus pulposus and annulus inner regions [66, 67, 68]. The inhibition of protein synthesis, the increase in the nitric oxide and the synthesis of MMP-3 have been shown in disc cells in extreme downward or high pressures [69].

Similarly, the metabolic activity of the disc cells has been influenced by changes in osmotic pressure. In vitro tests have shown high rates of proteoglycan synthesis at in situ extracellular osmolarity (~430 mOsm); however, when this concentration is increased or decreased, protein synthesis declines [70]. Another manifestation of compressive deformation of disc cells is the reorganization of the cytoskeleton, including the increase of early polymerization of vimentin [63]. Also depolymerization of actin filament calcium-dependent and the volume change on disc cells grown in hyper or hypo-osmotic media has also been shown [71, 72].

Moreover, disc cells exposed to stress in vitro undergo changes in the membrane potential associated with apoptosis. These cells increase nitric oxide production and decrease the proteoglycans synthesis [73, 74].

3. Epidemiology

3.1. Facet arthrosis

LBP is considered epidemic, and its prevalence varies in developed countries from 60% to 90% of patients undergoing orthopedic consultation [75, 76]. The cost of care for these patients varies from $100 to $200 billion annually [8]. One of the main causes of LBP is facet arthrosis. Since 1930, it has been called as facet syndrome [77, 78]; many studies on cadavers have described the presentation of facet arthrosis around the third decade of life [79, 80]. According to epidemiological studies based on imaging, the cervical facet OA has been reported in 19% of adults between 45 and 64 years of age and in 57% of adults over 65 years [81]. On severe lumbar facet OA diagnosed by computed tomography (CT) images, prevalence rates are estimated to be 36% in adults under 45 years of age, 67% in adults between 45 and 64 years, and 89% in individuals over 65 years [82]. Thus, it can be concluded that the prevalence of facet OA and its progression are dependent on age [81, 83].

The literature reports higher prevalence and degree of arthrosis at L4–L5 facet joints [79, 84, 85]. This was more prevalent at L4–L5 (from 45.1% to 79%), followed by L5–S1 (from 38.2% to 59%), and finally L3–L4 (from 30.6% to 72%) [79, 84]. These reports support the fact that the degenerative lumbar stenosis is related to the more mobile segments (L3–L4, L4–L5) of the lumbar spine [86, 87]. On the frequency of occurrence on the right or left side, an equal distribution has been reported [88].

With respect to gender, higher prevalence has been reported in males, and apparently, there is no significant difference in relation to race [79, 80]. However, in image studies using CT scans and planar radiography, women have been shown to have a higher prevalence of lumbar facet OA than men [12].

Moreover, the body mass index (BMI) has been found to be associated with an increased prevalence of cervical facet OA [83] and, even more, of the lumbar region [12, 82]. In this respect, the risk of lumbar facet OA is almost three times higher in overweight individuals (BMI 25–30 kg/m^2) and five times more associated with obesity (BMI 30–35 kg/m^2), in comparison with the normal-weight reference group (BMI ≤ 25 kg/m^2) [12].

Another risk factor for facet OA is the anatomy of the spine; for example, the changes in the orientation of the articular facet and facet joint asymmetry or "tropism" [89, 90, 91, 92] and simultaneously the disc-height narrowing represents the risk of contracting the disease [82]. Similarly, other factors such as the poor quality of the extensor muscles have been associated with facet OA of L4–L5 [93].

3.2. Disc degeneration

Although there is no standard definition of disc degeneration (DD), it is considered the product of the degradation and remodeling of the ID and adjacent vertebrae, with adaptive changes and/or consequential damage induced by physical load. Radiographic studies, particularly magnetic resonance imaging (MRI), have allowed qualitative assessment of disc degeneration (DD). Particular emphasis has been given on disc space narrowing, the disc-vertebra remodeling with formation of osteophytes and disc bulge peripherals, changes or loss of signal intensity with development of annular tears, herniations, Schmorl nodes, and endplate sclerosis [94, 95]. In this regard, the prevalence of disc-bulging has been described from 10% to over 80% in asymptomatic patients, and the prevalence of annular tears varies from 6% to 56% [3].

Age has been widely related to disc degeneration (DD). Degenerative changes have been described since childhood and young adulthood, such as the presence of annular tears between 3 and 10 years old [96, 97, 98]. Moreover, the water content of the nucleus pulposus shown by the disc signal intensity has been reported from 35 years of age [99].

It has also been proposed that mechanical load and nutritional states could contribute to the early development of DD, and it has found more severe in men than in women [100]. The association of heavy physical load and DD is still controversial and inconsistent. Similarly, relation to smoking has not been found [99].

Studies on the genetic influence in monozygotic male twins have shown a substantial familial influence on disc degenerative changes such as lumbar disc-height narrowing, bulging or herniation, and disc desiccation [99, 101, 102]. It seems likely that the DD is a multifactorial genetic condition, oligogenic. Some of the human gene forms reported as TaqI and FokI of the vitamin-D receptor gene have been associated with low intensity of magnetic resonance signal of thoracic and lumbar discs [103]. Two genotypes of MMP-3 gene have been related with degenerative disc changes in the elderly, and type IX collagen, alpha 2 (COL9A2), and 3 (COL9A3) gene forms have been linked with symptomatic disc pathology [104]. Nevertheless, research in this is still lacking.

4. Pathophysiology

4.1. Mechanical response and degeneration

DD is the manifestation of damage set caused by heavy physical load, posture or improper movement, and vibration. Therefore, it is extremely important to know the mechanical consequences of spinal motion segments under conditions of cyclic load, load magnitude, and frequency [105]. The investigations on degenerative mechanisms have been greatly supported in numerical models of the disc in animals, such as a finite element model [106]. One of the main advantages of the finite element model is the ability to parametrically manipulate one input factor and evaluate the resulting effects. These models have improved gradually, with the inclusion of poroelastic material properties of the motion segment facilitating the evaluation of physiological parameters related to cyclic load [107].

The application of the models in the evaluation of DD include analysis of disc geometry and mechanical properties of the nucleus, changes in permeability, porosity, and water content.

The decreased content of fluid that occurs in degenerative processes is known to affect not only the nucleus pulposus but also the annulus matrix resulting in disc stiffness [106, 108, 109]. Poroelastic finite models have allowed evaluation of the effect on the strain-dependent permeability and osmotic potential in cyclic compression and expansion [110, 111]. These studies have shown time-dependent deformation of a lumbar motion segment subjected to multiple creep-compression-expansion loads. Another study that used an asymmetric disc-body-disc poroelastic finite element model has shown that sustained compression maintains tensile stresses in the outer portion of the annulus but not in the middle and inner regions [108]. This correlates with the progressive disruption of the annulus fibrosus observed in vivo as well as the increase in apoptosis and the consequent decrease of cellularity. Similarly, other authors have demonstrated changes in the density and distribution of electric charges in healthy versus degenerated discs, which induced stress, water loss, and nutritional implications [59, 112].

A poroelastic finite element model determines the interaction of fluid with the proteoglycans in the nucleus. Using this model, it has been shown that normal discs are much more deformable that discs degenerate in response to cyclic load. The loss of healthy disc height in load cycle at a maximum load of 2000 N varied between 2.5 mm and 4.5 mm as opposed to between 1.0 mm and 1.8 mm in the degenerated disc [107, 113]. Similarly, stiffness of the disc was shown to be inversely proportional to the load cycles, while under higher compression loads (3000 N), loss of healthy disc height was demonstrated in 48% in comparison with 40% in degenerated discs [108].

Additionally, the poroelastic finite element model can predict the evolution of disc failure. A previous study showed that disc failure is propagated when the elastic modulus is decreased and the rate of disc failure associated with increase load was greater than that due to the decrease in elastic modulus [107].

4.2. Intervertebral disc aging and degeneration

DD is a process related to physiological conditions, such as aging in most asymptomatic individuals, and is associated with pathological processes involving pain and disability. The definition of DD has not been fully established; two possibilities have emerged: one in which degenerative disc changes correspond to premature aging, and the other in which there is similarity between DD: and age changes but at an accelerated rate [114, 115]. It is possible that changes in the spine associated with aging are genetically predetermined and/or are associated with exposure to heavy mechanical forces throughout life. Independent of the trigger mechanism, degenerative changes begin with biochemical alterations, followed by structural changes of the spinal functional units [116].

The notochordal cells constitute the primordium of the nucleus during the development of the ID and generally decrease in number rapidly after birth [117, 118]. Gradually, cellularity of the nucleus pulposus is replaced by chondrocyte-like cells, which may originate and migrate from the cartilaginous endplate and inner annulus [119]. Apparently, the Fas-mediated apoptosis plays an important role in this process [120]. The notochordal cells synthesize more proteoglycans than chondrocytes and might be responsible in maintaining the fluid gelatinous nucleus pulposus [121]. Due to the reduction of these cells, the nucleus pulposus becomes more solid cartilage, which also decreases the signal intensity on MRI. On cell density, some studies have suggested an increase in the proportion of cells in the inner annulus fibrosus and the nucleus pulposus [122, 123].

The normal ID maintains a balance between synthesis and degradation of EM components, but it is well known that the age-related early degenerative changes are loss of aggrecan, collagen, and water in the nucleus pulposus. In addition, the release of molecules, including proinflammatory cytokines such as interleukin 1 (IL-1) and tumor necrosis factor-α (TNF-α) [124, 125], increases the synthesis of metalloproteinases [126] contributes also to this degenerative process. However, it is noteworthy that annulus cells in the early stages of DD synthesize a larger amount of proteoglycans and collagen, probably in response to a repair process [127]. The progress of degeneration involves the reduction of production of most of the molecules of the EM, except for biglycan and fibronectin [127].

Generally, degenerative disc changes are of multifactorial origin. One of the most important determinants is the nutritional deficit secondary to decreased blood supply to the endplate. Apparently, this process could start early in the second decade of life [97]. Vascularization and innervation of the disc are also associated with aging and degeneration. Similarly, inflammatory cells and macrophages have been identified in degenerated discs and have been found responsible in the synthesis of cytokines and proteases by endogenous cells and by the vascular cells of the invading vessels [128]. The painful sensation that accompanies DD associated with aging is due to the presence of nociceptive nerve fibers in the annulus and inner nucleus [129].

Additionally, macroscopic changes can be observed, as well as concentric fissures and radial tears in the annulus from the third and fourth decades of life [130]. These modifications are due to increased synthesis of metalloproteinases that occurs as a result of the advance of age [130].

Besides, cell viability is also affected in aging due to thinning and calcification of the endplates, which impair the nutritional contribution of the disc [131]. Also, other factors like stress induced by overload or nonphysiological static compression and cyclic stretching are involved in cell death and DD [65, 74, 108, 132, 133, 134]. Furthermore, there are reports of cell proliferation in human degenerative discs especially in areas where cell clusters are integrated [135].

4.3. Facet articular OA and aging

The degenerative processes associated with age or other factors may also affect the facet joint indirectly. These changes are usually associated with variations in the load surfaces of the joint [136]. This can manifest macroscopically with osteophytes and bone overgrowth with stenosis of the foramen, lateral and central spinal canal [85, 88, 90, 137, 138, 139]. Previous studies reported that the subchondral cortex shows no significant morphological variation in different spinal levels as a result of aging, suggesting that it may be due to a slower rate of remodeling.

Moreover, the fraction of bone volume and trabecular thickness decrease is more frequent in women than in men during aging [140].

It is generally accepted that degenerative facet changes are preceded by DD [137, 141]. We already mentioned that the consequences of DD include segmental instability and increase in facet load, which could induce joint subluxation and damage the cartilage surface. The changes in the cartilage are characterized by progressive erosion and subchondral bone sclerosis. Degenerative changes of facet articular are identical to OA seen in other synovial articulations. In addition to facet hypertrophy, apophyseal misalignment and osteophyte formation may narrow the spinal canal. Also, involvement of the triple articulation can influence degenerative spondylolisthesis and scoliosis [116].

Bone also undergoes sclerosis with consequent redistribution of loads, which may progress and induce bone remodeling and subsequent rotatory deformities of the posterior elements [142].

5. Spinal pain

5.1. Lumbar facet syndrome and cervical facet pain

The facet joints are often associated with neck pain and LBP. The mechanical painful stimuli have been detected in sensory fibers, nociceptive endings, sensory afferent nerve endings, and types III/A and IV/C fibers located in the joint capsule, ligaments, periosteum, and subchondral bone [143, 144].

Neurophysiological studies have shown the involvement of small-diameter sensory neurons of the capsule, facet sensory neurons during inflammation and the effect of substance P in lumbar facet pain [145, 146, 147]. Furthermore, it has been demonstrated that substance P is also contained in nerve endings of subchondral bone in patients with facet OA [148].

The prevalence of cervical facet pain has been reported in about 55% of patients with chronic nonspecific pain [149]. Previous studies have suggested that the cervical facet pain signals are derived from the capsule, where the immunoreactivity of substance P and calcitonin gene-related peptides has been demonstrated [150]. Several mechanisms have been proposed in facet joint injury including facet-joint impingement, synovial pinching, and strain injury to the capsule [151, 152, 153, 154, 155]. In this regard, it was deduced that noxious and trigger nociceptive discharges from the capsule are transmitted to the central nervous system for pain sensation [155]. This response was seen not only as a result of the injury but also secondary to high-magnitude mechanical stimuli such as tension, compression, and rotation. This persistent discharge was related to nerve or capsular injury with the consequent release of inflammatory mediators, which could stimulate signaling pathways of pain in the spinal cord by central sensitization [156, 157].

5.2. Disc pain

Degenerative spinal disease is the condition most frequently associated with chronic LBP, particularly in older adults. As a definition, degenerative spinal disease includes DDD and degenerative facet disease or facet OA [158]. A study for the purpose analyze and compare the radiographic severity of DDD and facet degeneration of the lumbosacral spine in adult subjects with and without chronic LBP showed no association between them. This was despite the fact that the highest radiographic severity scores were associated with the presence of pain [159]. Usually, DD may result in radicular pain secondary to stenosis and nerve-root or cauda equina irritation, and discogenic pain derived from disc lesion [160].

Animal studies of healthy IDs have demonstrated the presence of mechanoreceptors in the outer portion of the annulus fibrosus. These nerve fibers correspond to small myelinated (group-III or A-delta fibers) and unmyelinated (group-IV or C fibers) fibers [161, 162, 163]. These fibers are classified into those containing neuropeptides, which express substance P and calcitonin gene-related peptides [164], and nociceptors fibers related to inflammatory pain. These fibers are also dependent on nerve growth factor and have high affinity with the tyrosine kinase A (TrkA) receptor [165]. Discal nerve fibers generally exhibit afferent axons, and cell bodies are located in the dorsal root ganglia [166].

6. System grading in DD and facet joint degeneration

Currently, MRI is considered as the gold standard in imaging of the spine; however, the diagnosis of facet OA remains a challenge for clinicians. For this purpose, different methods have been used such as the planar X-ray, CT and MRI scans, dynamic bending films, and planar radionuclide bone scanning [167].

Usually, the degree of DD is determined by macroscopic observation on MRI. Comparatively, facet OA may not be evaluated with precision by MRI as with CT scans [168, 169]. Commonly, conventional radiography (X-ray films) is used in the evaluation of arthritic changes of the spine, although CT shows joints with better resolution [170, 171]. It has been reported that CT can show the axial plane of the facet joint and the osteoarthritic changes with precision [171]. However, MRI provides axial and sagittal images of the facet, which are useful in assessing degenerative spinal joint disease [168]. Several studies have reported accuracy in the evaluation of the facet OA with MRI at the rate of between 93% and 95% [85, 172]. So far, it has been accepted that MRI is a useful method in the assessment of OA of the lumbar facet joints.

Different scoring systems have been described in evaluating the disc and facet degeneration. A previous study recommends intraobserver and interobserver reliability tests in the evaluation of lumbar degenerative changes [173]. One of these systems used lateral radiographic projections and was easy to apply [174]. However, one that used MRI showed high feasibility [175]. Comparatively, other systems cannot be applied to patients and have been used to evaluate DD in vitro based on detailed morphological studies [97, 176]. In cervical DD, a system based on lateral radiographs and easy to implement was the only one recommended [177].

Regarding grading systems for lumbar facet joint degeneration, recommendations were based solely on CT [170] or CT and MRI systems [178]. Differentially in cervical facet joint degeneration, a system based on lateral radiographs was recommended [177].

Lumbar DD is classified into five grades according to macroscopic characteristics such as fibrosis, mucinous degeneration, erosion of cartilage endplate, and osteophyte formation on sagittal sections [176]. Histologically, lumbar DD on sagittal paraffin sections contains parameters such as cell proliferation, mucinous degeneration, cell death, tear and cleft formation, and disc granular changes. Additional features include disorganization and cracks of cartilage, microfractures, bone neoformation, and endplate sclerosis [97].

Radiographically, a method for assessing the presence and severity of lumbar DD is based on joint space narrowing, anterior and posterior osteophyte formation, and subchondral sclerosis [174]. However, the best accepted grading system is based on the characteristics of the degenerative lumbar disc on MRI, such as the distinction of nucleus and annulus, the signal intensity, and height of ID [175]. Moreover, grading of lumbar facet joint degeneration appreciates the joint space narrowing, sclerosis, hypertrophy, and osteophyte formation on oblique conventional radiographs and CT scans [170] or CT and MRI scans [178].

Categorization of cervical DD is based on plain radiography and includes parameters such as osteophytosis, disc space narrowing, and sclerosis of vertebral plates [177]. Furthermore, grading of cervical facet joint degeneration on lateral radiographs determines the presence of osteophytes on the articular margins of facets of apophyseal joints and sclerosis [177].

Additionally, radionuclide bone scintigraphy with single photon emission CT (SPECT) has been used to detect microcalcification due to increased osteoblastic activity [179, 180]. More recently, it was reported that the hybrid SPECT/CT imaging identifies potential chronic spinal pain generators in 92% of cervical spine scans and 86% of lumbar spine scans [181].

Figures 2 and 3 show the MRI results of patients with cervical and lumbar OA.

7. Inflammatory cytokines and degenerative lumbar spinal disease

It is known that OA is associated with facet joint pain. The generation mechanisms of pain could be due to mechanical stress and joint instability or misalignment that often accompany DD and aging. In this regard, the presence of inflammatory mediators such as prostaglandins in facet joints of patients with lumbar spinal degenerative disorders were found [182]. These findings suggest that chemical factors besides mechanical factors arising from the facet joint could be related to pain in OA [183, 184, 185].

Another study demonstrated increase in the concentration of IL-6 in the synovium and cartilage of the facet joint by CLEIA method (Chemiluminescent Enzyme Immunoassay). The tissues analyzed in this study were obtained from patients with disc herniation and lumbar spinal stenosis [186]. The role of IL-6 in the spinal joint disease is controversial; it can facilitate the inflammation together with IL-1β and TNF-α in the early stages of the immune reaction, or may be involved in autoimmune states producing antibodies or act as an anti-inflammatory cytokine. According to these assertions, the authors proposed that IL-6 induces continuous local inflammation caused by mechanical stress on the facet joint [186]. Similarly, a significant increase was detected in IL-1β in patients with lumbar spinal canal stenosis than the lumbar herniated disc, which correlated with higher scores on scales of leg pain [187]. More recently, the overexpression of MMP-1 induced by IL-1β was revealed, suggesting an important role in the inflammation associated with lumbar facet joint degeneration [188].

Also were reported inflammatory chemical mediators such as prostaglandins and leukotrienes in facet cartilage and subchondral bone obtained from patients with degenerative lumbar spinal disorders. Here, it was suggested that these chemical mediators may be involved in inflammation and pain generation at the local lumbar facet joints [182].

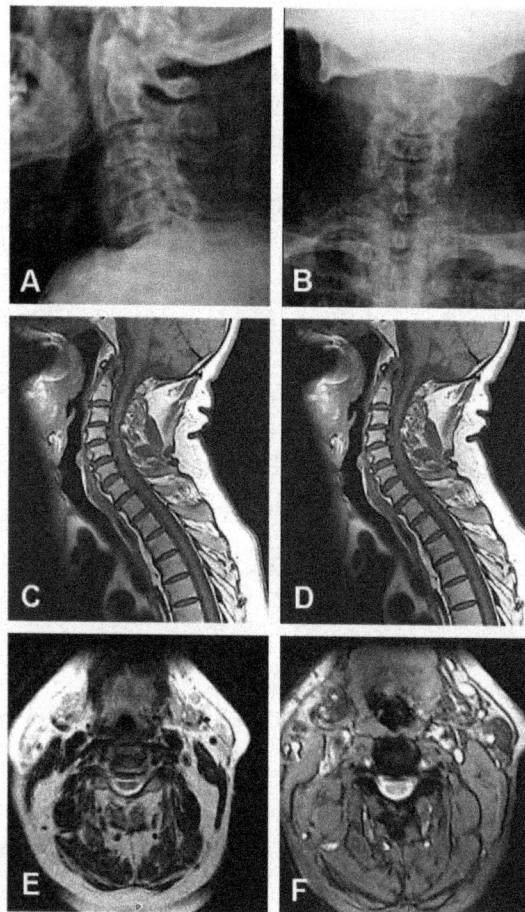

Figure 2. A. Lateral cervical spine radiograph with decreased general bone density; correction of the cervical lordosis; vertebral platforms sclerosis; decrease in intervertebral spaces at C3–C4, C4–C5, and C5–C6; syndesmophytes; reduction in diameter of intervertebral foramina at C2–C3, C3–C4, and C4–C5; decreased facet interface at C2–C3, C3–C4, and C4–C5; and spondylolisthesis at C4–C5. B. Anterior-posterior cervical spine radiograph with loss facet interface at C2–C3, C3–C4, and C4–C5; decreased vertebral space at C2–C3, C3–C4, and C4–C5. C. Sagittal MRI of cervical spine at stage T1 with vertebral platforms sclerosis, osteophyte formation, decreased height of IDs, and disc extrusion mainly in the intervertebral spaces at C4 and at C3–C4–C5. D. Sagittal MRI in T2 phase with decrease caliber medullary canal by the presence of posterior osteophytes, hypertrophy of posterior longitudinal ligament, and ID extrusion. E–F. MRI axial slices in T2 phase with reduced caliber of the cervical canal and compression of the spinal cord.

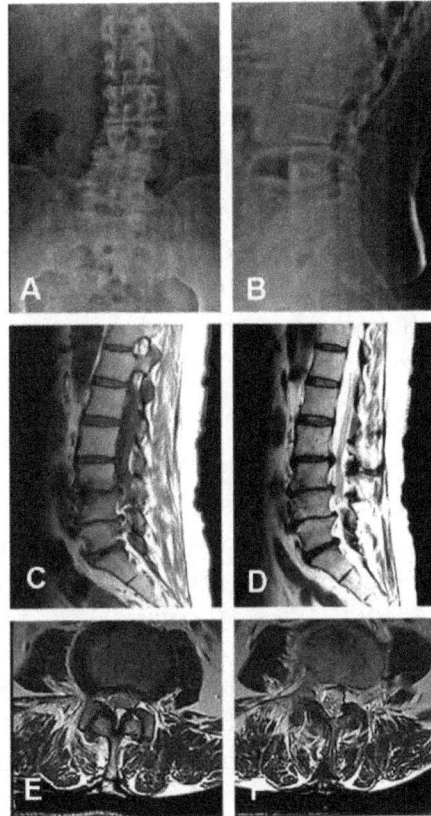

Figure 3. A. Antero-posterior radiograph with left lumbar scoliosis, plastic deformation of the last three lumbar verte-brae, vertebral platforms sclerosis, osteophytes, and decreased height of intervertebral spaces. B. Lateral radiograph of lumbar spine with spinal platform sclerosis, osteophytes, and reduced height of the L3–L4, L4–L5, and L5–S1 IDs. C. Sagittal MRI of lumbar spine in T1 phase with sclerosis of the vertebral platforms, Modic changes, osteophytes, de-creased height of IDs, and disc protrusion at L3–L4, L4–L5, and L5–S1 with narrow lumbar canal. D. Sagittal MRI of lumbar spine in T2 phase with vertebral platform sclerosis; osteophytes; decreased height of IDs; disc protrusion at L3–L4, L4–L5, and L5–S1 with lumbar canal narrowing; decreased spaces at L3–L4 and L4–L5; and bulging of IDs at L2–L3 and L5–S1. E–F. MRI axial slices of lumbar spine facet degenerative changes and hypertrophy of the ligamentum fla-vum and lumbar stenosis at different levels.

8. Angiogenesis, calcification, and programmed cell death in DD

As described above, degenerative changes of the ID involve processes such as neovasculari-zation, calcification, and cell death. Angiogenesis has been described in degenerated and herniated discs [189]. A degenerative disc is defined as a disc protruding into the spinal canal or neural foramens resulting in compression of the nerve roots [189]. The herniated nucleus pulposus develops fibrotic and angiogenic reactions [190, 191]. This process involves factors such as TGF-β, TNF-α, VEGF, MMP-1, and MMP-3 [191, 192].

Similarly, the intradiscal calcification has been significantly correlated with DD [193]. Disc calcification occurs in the annulus, fibrocartilaginous plate, and nucleus pulposus that appears as amorphous deposits of calcium salts [194] asymptomatic in most cases. The frequency of degenerative disc calcification varies from 3.1% to 65% as assessed by microscopy and MRI

[195, 196, 197]. Another study reported that microscopic calcification was significantly higher in degenerative discs than in those obtained from normal cadavers (54.4% vs. 6.7%), and it is also higher in Modic type III than in type I (95.0% and 13.0%, respectively). The same study also refers angiogenesis in degenerative discs (41.0%) and in calcified discs (59.2%) [198].

The etiology of disc calcification remains uncertain. Two possible mechanisms of calcification disc have been proposed: one in which inflammatory cytokines such as VEGF and MMPs released into the degenerative disc promote expression of osteopontin, induce differentiation of osteoprogenitor cells, and allow calcification; and the other through indirect mechanisms in which these molecular mediators promote angiogenesis, and this, in turn, stimulates macrophage infiltration, the formation of new osteoprogenitor cells, and finally the progressive calcification [198].

As we have mentioned in this review, in addition to mechanical and genetic factors, apoptotic cell death is another event type that contributes to the development of disc degeneration (DD) [74, 132, 134, 199, 200, 201, 202, 203]. Apoptosis in degenerative discs is described as that occurring through activation of the mitochondrial [74], death receptor [204], and the endoplasmic reticulum pathway [205, 206].

The static axial compressive load [74, 108, 134], the static bending compressive load [133], the dynamic axial compressive load [65, 207], and the imbalance of dynamic and/or static forces of the spine [199] have been considered in programmed cell death (PCD) on degenerative disc. Load effects increase lactate concentration, decline oxygen tension, decrease nutrient level, reduces tissue permeability and secondarily the water content [208, 209]. Biomechanical stimuli such as serum deprivation [210], nitric oxide [201], lipid peroxidation [132], hypoxia-inducible factor-1α [211], and even normal oxygen concentrations [212] have also been involved in the induction and increase of PCD.

The death of disc cells has been reported to be significant as age increases [97]. Elsewhere in the body, it is well established that apoptotic cells are removed by phagocytosis; however, macrophages or phagocytes are not cells that are normally present on the disc. In vitro studies have shown that nucleus pulposus cells are able to perform, as well as competent phagocytes and stimulate phagocytosis [213].

9. Conclusion

Spinal OA is a condition characterized by failure in motion segments, usually as a result of exposure to heavy physical load and aging. By definition, this disease induces degenerative changes in the facet joints and the IDs. One of the predominant symptoms of spinal OA is neck pain and LBP syndrome, which involves prolonged disability and high care costs. However there is controversy whether the prevalence, severity, and imaging findings are related to the pain sensation. The fields of molecular biology and mechanobiology of the degenerative process also require research to understand the pathophysiological mechanisms that lead to it and, thus, be able to contribute in the development of regenerative medicine and technological innovation with the improvement of prototypes for design of orthopedic components.

Acknowledgements

We thank M.D. Eulalio Elizalde Martínez, Chief of Orthopaedic Spine Surgery; M.D. Armando Fabio Ramos Guerrero, Spine Surgery Training of Hospital "Dr. Victorio de la Fuente Narváez", IMSS, Distrito Federal, Mexico; and M.D. Misael Vargas López of the Escuela Nacional de Medicina y Homeopatía-IPN for their valuable support in the preparation of this chapter. This work was supported by the SIP 20141449 project.

Author details

Elizabeth Pérez-Hernández[1*], Nury Pérez-Hernández[2] and Ariel Fuerte-Hernández[3]

*Address all correspondence to: perezheliza@aol.com

1 División de Educación e Investigación en Salud, UMAE "Dr. Victorio de la Fuente Narváez", Hospital de Ortopedia, Instituto Mexicano del Seguro Social, Distrito Federal, México

2 Escuela Nacional de Medicina y Homeopatía, Instituto Politécnico Nacional, Distrito Federal, México

3 Escuela Superior de Ingeniería Mecánica y Eléctrica, Instituto Politécnico Nacional, Distrito Federal, México

References

[1] Guccione AA, Felson DT, Anderson JJ, Anthony JM, Zhang Y, Wilson PW, et al. The effects of specific medical conditions on the functional limitations of elders in the Framingham Study. Am J Public Health. 1994; 84(3): 351-8.

[2] Lawrence RC, Felson DT, Helmick CG, Arnold LM, Choi H, Deyo RA, et al. Estimates of the prevalence of arthritis and other rheumatic conditions in the United States. Part II. Arthritis Rheum. 2008; 58(1): 26-35.

[3] Battié MC, Videman T, Parent E. Lumbar disc degeneration: epidemiology and genetic influences. Spine. 2004; 29(23): 2679-90. Review.

[4] Ethgen O, Bruyere O, Richy F, Dardennes C, Reginster JY. Health-related quality of life in total hip and total knee arthroplasty. A qualitative and systematic review of the literature. J Bone Joint Surg Am. 2004; 86-A(5): 963-74.

[5] Bitton R. The economic burden of osteoarthritis. Am J Manag Care. 2009; 15(8 Suppl): S230-5.

[6]   Borenstein D. Does osteoarthritis of the lumbar spine cause chronic low back pain? Curr Rheumatol Rep. 2004; 6(1): 14-9.

[7]   Rubin DI. Epidemiology and risk factors for spine pain. Neurol Clin. 2007; 25(2): 353-71.

[8]   Katz JN. Lumbar disc disorders and low back pain: socioeconomic factors and consequences. J Bone Joint Surg Am. 2006; 88(Suppl 2): 21-4.

[9]   Ricci JA, Stewart WF, Chee E, Leotta C, Foley K, Hochberg MC. Back pain exacerbations and lost productive time costs in United States workers. Spine. 2006; 31(26): 3052-60.

[10] Stewart WF, Ricci JA, Chee E, Morganstein D, Lipton R. Lost productive time and cost due to common pain conditions in the US workforce. Jama. 2003; 290(18): 2443-54.

[11] Muraki S, Akune T, Oka H, Ishimoto Y, Nagata K, Yoshida M, et al. Incidence and risk factors for radiographic lumbar spondylosis and lower back pain in Japanese men and women: the ROAD study. Osteoarthritis and cartilage. 2012; 20(7): 712-8.

[12] Goode AP1, Marshall SW, Renner JB, Carey TS, Kraus VB, Irwin DE, et al. Lumbar spine radiographic features and demographic, clinical, and radiographic knee, hip and hand osteoarthritis. Arthritis Care Res (Hoboken). 2012; 64(10): 1536-44.

[13] Gellhorn AC, Katz JN, Suri P. Osteoarthritis of the spine: the facet joints. Nat Rev Rheumatol. 2013; 9(4): 216-24.

[14] Pal GP, Routal RV, Saggu SK. The Orientation of the Articular Facets of the Zygapophyseal Joints at the Cervical and Upper Thoracic Region. J Anat. 2001; 198(4): 431-41.

[15] Pal GP, Routal RV. Mechanism of Change in the Orientation of the Articular Process of the Zygapophyseal Joint at the Thoracolumbar Junction. J Anat. 1999; 195(2): 199-209.

[16] Panjabi MM, Crisco JJ, Vasavada A, Oda T, Cholewicki J, Nibu K, et al. Mechanical Properties of the Human Cervical Spine as Shown by Three-Dimensional Load-Displacement Curves. Spine. 2001; 26(24): 2692-700.

[17] Kozanek M, Wang S, Passias PG, Xia Q, Li G, Bono CM, et al. Range of Motion and Orientation of the Lumbar Facet Joints in Vivo. Spine. 2009; 34(19): E689-96.

[18] Panjabi MM, Oxland T, Takata K, Goel V, Duranceau J, Krag M. Articular Facets of the Human Spine. Quantitative Three-Dimensional Anatomy. Spine. 1993; 18(10): 1298-310.

[19] Yoganandan N, Knowles SA, Maiman DJ, Pintar FA. Anatomic Study of the Morphology of Human Cervical Facet Joint. Spine. 2003; 28(20): 2317-23.

[20] Varlotta GP, Lefkowitz TR, Schweitzer M, Errico TJ, Spivak J, Bendo JA, et al. The Lumbar Facet Joint: a Review of Current Knowledge: Part 1: Anatomy, Biomechanics, and Grading. Skeletal Radiol. 2011; 40(1): 13-23.

[21] Womack W, Woldtvedt D, Puttlitz CM. Lower Cervical Spine Facet Cartilage Thickness Mapping. Osteoarthritis Cartilage. 2008; 16(9): 1018-23.

[22] Armstrong CG, Mow VC. Variations in the Intrinsic Mechanical Properties of Human Articular Cartilage with Age, Degeneration, and Water Content. J Bone Joint Surg Am. 1982; 64(1): 88-94.

[23] Adams MA, Dolan P, McNally DS. The Internal Mechanical Functioning of Intervertebral Discs and Articular Cartilage, and its Relevance to Matrix Biology. Matrix Biol. 2009; 28(7): 384-9.

[24] Eckstein F, Milz S, Anetzberger H, Putz R. Thickness of the subchondral mineralised tissue zone (SMZ) in normal male and female and pathological human patellae. J Anat 1998; 192(Pt 1): 81-90.

[25] Duan CY, Espinoza Orías AA, Shott S, An HS, Andersson GB, Hu JZ, et al. In vivo measurement of the subchondral bone thickness of lumbar facet joint using magnetic resonance imaging. Osteoarthritis Cartilage. 2011; 19(1): 96-102.

[26] Iwanaga T, Shikichi M, Kitamura H, Yanase H, Nozawa-Inoue K. Morphology and Functional Roles of Synoviocytes in the Joint. Arch Histol Cytol. 2000; 63(1): 17-31.

[27] Bogduk N, Engel R. The Menisci of the Lumbar Zygapophyseal Joints. A Review of Their Anatomy and Clinical Significance. Spine. 1984; 9(5): 454-60.

[28] Friedrich KM, Reiter G, Pretterklieber ML, Pinker K, Friedrich M, Trattnig S, et al. Reference Data for in Vivo Magnetic Resonance Imaging Properties of Meniscoids in the Cervical Zygapophyseal Joints. Spine. 2008; 33(21): E778–E83.

[29] Taylor JR, McCormick CC. Lumbar Facet Joint Fat Pads: Their Normal Anatomy and Their Appearance when Enlarged. Neuroradiology. 1991; 33(1): 38-42.

[30] Yahia LH, Garzon S. Structure on the Capsular Ligaments of the Facet Joints. Ann Anat. 1993; 175(2): 185-8.

[31] Yamashita T, Minaki Y, Ozaktay AC, Cavanaugh JM, King AI. A Morphological Study of the Fibrous Capsule of the Human Lumbar Facet Joint. Spine. 1996; 21(5): 538-43.

[32] Roberts S, Evans H, Trivedi J, Menage J. Histology and pathology of the human intervertebral disc. J Bone Joint Surg Am. 2006 Apr; 88(Suppl 2): 10-4. Review.

[33] Schollmeier G, Lahr-Eigen R, Lewandrowski KU. Observations on fiber-forming collagens in the anulus fibrosus. Spine. 2000; 25(21): 2736-41.

[34] Marchand F, Ahmed AM. Investigation of the laminate structure of lumbar disc anulus fibrosus. Spine. 1990; 15(5): 402-10.

[35] Chelberg MK, Banks GM, Geiger DF, Oegema TR Jr. Identification of heterogeneous cell populations in normal human intervertebral disc. J Anat. 1995 Feb; 186(Pt 1): 43-53.

[36] Yu J, Fairbank JC, Roberts S, Urban JP. The elastic fibre network of the annulus fibrosus of the normal and scoliotic human intervertebral disc. Spine. 2005; 30(16): 1815-20.

[37] Gruber HE, Hanley EN Jr. Ultrastructure of the human intervertebral disc during aging and degeneration: comparison of surgical and control specimens. Spine. 2002; 27(8): 798-805.

[38] Roberts S, Menage J, Duance V, Wotton S, Ayad S. Collagen types around the cells of the intervertebral disc and cartilage end plate: an immunolocalization study. Spine. 1991; 16(9): 1030-8.

[39] Roberts S, Menage J, Duance V, Wotton SF. Type III collagen in the intervertebral disc. Histochem J. 1991a; 23(11-12): 503-8.

[40] Roberts S, Ayad S, Menage PJ. Immunolocalisation of type VI collagen in the intervertebral disc. Ann Rheum Dis. 1991b; 50(11): 787-91.

[41] Feng H, Danfelter M, Strömqvist B, Heinegård D. Extracellular matrix in disc degeneration. J Bone Joint Surg Am. 2006; 88(Suppl 2): 25-9. Review.

[42] Heinegård D, Aspberg A, Franzén A, Lorenzo P. Glycosylated matrix proteins. In: Royce PM, Steinmann B, editors. Connective tissue and its heritable disorders: molecular, genetic, and medical aspects. 2nd ed. New York: Wiley-Liss. 2003; 271-91.

[43] Roberts S. Disc morphology in health and disease. Biochem Soc Trans. 2002; 30(Pt 6): 864-9. Review.

[44] Aigner T, Gresk-otter KR, Fairbank JC, von der Mark K, Urban JP. Variation with age in the pattern of type X collagen expression in normal and scoliotic human intervertebral discs. Calcif Tissue Int. 1998; 63(3): 263-8.

[45] Holm S, Maroudas A, Urban JP, Selstam G, Nachemson A. Nutrition of the intervertebral disc: solute transport and metabolism. Connect Tissue Res. 1981; 8(2): 101-19.

[46] Ishihara H, Urban JP. Effects of low oxygen concentrations and metabolic inhibitors on proteoglycan and protein synthesis rates in the intervertebral disc. J Orthop Res. 1999; 17(6): 829-35.

[47] Bibby SR, Jones DA, Ripley RM, Urban JP. Metabolism of the intervertebral disc: effects of low levels of oxygen, glucose, and pH on rates of energy metabolism of bovine nucleus pulposus cells. Spine. 2005; 30(5): 487-96.

[48] Ohshima H, Urban JP. The effect of lactate and pH on proteoglycan and protein syn-thesis rates in the intervertebral disc. Spine. 1992; 17(9): 1079-82.

[49] Razaq S, Wilkins RJ, Urban JP. The effect of extracellular pH on matrix turnover by cells of the bovine nucleus pulposus. Eur Spine J. 2003; 12(4): 341-9.

[50] Windhaber RA, Wilkins RJ, Meredith D. Functional characterisation of glucose trans-port in bovine articular chondrocytes. Pflugers Arch. 2003; 446(5): 572-7.

[51] Bibby SR, Urban JP. Effect of nutrient deprivation on the viability of intervertebral disc cells. Eur Spine J. 2004; 13(8): 695-701.

[52] Horner HA, Urban JP. 2001 Volvo Award Winner in Basic Science Studies: Effect of nutrient supply on the viability of cells from the nucleus pulposus of the interverte-bral disc. Spine. 2001; 26(23): 2543-9.

[53] Crock HV, Goldwasser M, Yoshizawa H. Vascular anatomy related to the interverte-bral disc. In: Ghosh P, editor. Biology of the intervertebral disc. Boca Raton, FL: CRC Press. 1991; 109-33.

[54] Crock HV, Yoshizawa H. The blood supply of the lumbar vertebral column. Clin Or-thop Relat Res. 1976; (115): 6-21.

[55] Roberts S, Menage J, Urban JP. Biochemical and structural properties of the cartilage end-plate and its relation to the intervertebral disc. Spine. 1989; 14(2): 166-74.

[56] Setton LA, Zhu W, Weidenbaum M, Ratcliffe A, Mow VC. Compressive properties of the cartilaginous end-plate of the baboon lumbar spine. J Orthop Res. 1993; 11(2): 228-39.

[57] Urban JP, Holm S, Maroudas A, Nachemson A. Nutrition of the intervertebral disc: effect of fluid flow on solute transport. Clin Orthop Relat Res. 1982; (170): 296-302.

[58] Katz MM, Hargens AR, Garfin SR. Intervertebral disc nutrition. Diffusion versus con-vection. Clin Orthop Relat Res. 1986; 210: 243-5.

[59] Ferguson SJ, Ito K, Nolte LP. Fluid flow and convective transport of solutes within the intervertebral disc. J Biomech. 2004; 37(2): 213-21.

[60] Mokhbi Soukane D, Shirazi-Adl A, Urban JPG. Nonlinear coupled diffusion of glu-cose, oxygen and lactic acid in the intervertebral disc. Presented as a poster exhibit at the 52nd Annual Meeting of the Orthopaedic Research Society; Chicago, IL. 2006 March 19-22.

[61] Boubriak OA, Lee RB, Urban JPG. Nutrient supply to cells of the intervertebral disc: effect of diurnal hydration changes. Presented as a poster exhibit at the 49th Annual Meeting of the Orthopaedic Research Society. New Orleans, LA. 2003 February 2-5.

[62] Ohshima H, Urban JP, Bergel DH. Effect of static load on matrix synthesis rates in the intervertebral disc measured in vitro by a new perfusion technique. J Orthop Res. 1995; 13(1): 22-9.

[63] Chen J, Yan W, Setton LA. Static compression induces zonal-specific changes in gene expression for extracellular matrix and cytoskeletal proteins in intervertebral disc cells in vitro. Matrix Biol. 2004; 22(7): 573-83.

[64] Maclean JJ, Lee CR, Alini M, Iatridis JC. Anabolic and catabolic mRNA levels of the intervertebral disc vary with the magnitude and frequency of in vivo dynamic compression. J Orthop Res. 2004; 22(6): 1193-200.

[65] Walsh AJ, Lotz JC. Biological response of the intervertebral disc to dynamic loading. J Biomech. 2004; 37(3): 329-37.

[66] Handa T, Ishihara H, Ohshima H, Osada R, Tsuji H, Obata K. Effects of hydrostatic pressure on matrix synthesis and matrix metalloproteinase production in the human lumbar intervertebral disc. Spine. 1997; 22(10): 1085-91.

[67] Hutton WC, Elmer WA, Boden SD, Hyon S, Toribatake Y, Tomita K, et al. The effect of hydrostatic pressure on intervertebral disc metabolism. Spine. 1999; 24(15): 1507-15.

[68] Ishihara H, McNally DS, Urban JP, Hall AC. Effects of hydrostatic pressure on matrix synthesis in different regions of the intervertebral disk. J Appl Physiol. 1996; 80(3): 839-46.

[69] Liu GZ, Ishihara H, Osada R, Kimura T, Tsuji H. Nitric oxide mediates the change of proteoglycan synthesis in the human lumbar intervertebral disc in response to hydrostatic pressure. Spine. 2001; 26(2): 134-41.

[70] Urban JP. The role of the physicochemical environment in determining disc cell behaviour. Biochem Soc Trans. 2002; 30(Pt 6): 858-64.

[71] Ishihara H, Warensjo K, Roberts S, Urban JP. Proteoglycan synthesis in the intervertebral disk nucleus: the role of extracellular osmolality. Am J Physiol. 1997; 272: C1499-506.

[72] Pritchard S, Erickson GR, Guilak F. Hyperosmotically induced volume change and calcium signaling in intervertebral disk cells: the role of the actin cytoskeleton. Biophys J. 2002; 83(5): 2502-10.

[73] Rannou F, Richette P, Benallaoua M, Francois M, Genries V, Korwin-Zmijowska C, et al. Cyclic tensile stretch modulates proteoglycan production by intervertebral disc annulus fibrosus cells through production of nitrite oxide. J Cell Biochem. 2003; 90(1): 148-57.

[74] Rannou F, Lee TS, Zhou RH, Chin J, Lotz JC, Mayoux-Benhamou MA, et al. Intervertebral disc degeneration: the role of the mitochondrial pathway in annulus fibrosus cell apoptosis induced by overload. Am J Pathol. 2004; 164(3): 915-24.

[75] Brodke DS, Ritter SM. Nonoperative management of low back pain and lumbar disc degeneration. Instr Course Lect. 2005; 54: 279-86.

[76] Bressler HB, Keyes WJ, Rochon PA, Badley E. The prevalence of low back pain in the elderly: a systematic review of the literature. Spine. 1999; 24(17): 1813-9.

[77] Mooney V, Robertson J. The facet syndrome. Clin Orthop Relat Res.1976; 115: 149-56.

[78] Eisenstein SM, Parry CR. The lumbar facet arthrosis syndrome. J Bone Joint Surg Br. 1987; 69(1): 3-7.

[79] Eubanks JD, Lee MJ, Cassinelli E, Ahn NU. Prevalence of lumbar facet arthrosis and its relationship to age, sex, and race: an anatomic study of cadaveric specimens. Spine. 2007; 32(19): 2058-62.

[80] Master DL, Toy JO, Eubanks JD, Ahn NU. Cervical endplate and facet arthrosis: an anatomic study of cadaveric specimens. J Spinal Disord Tech. 2012; 25(7): 379-82.

[81] Mikkelsen W, Duff I. Age-sex specific prevalence of radiographic abnormalities of the joints of the hands, wrists and cervical spine of adult residents of the Tecumseh, Michigan, Community Health Study area, 1962–1965. J Chronic Dis. 1970; 23(3): 151-9.

[82] Suri P, Miyakoshi A, Hunter DJ, Jarvik JG, Rainville J, Guermazi A, et al. Does lumbar spinal degeneration begin with the anterior structures? A study of the observed epidemiology in a community-based population. BMC Musculoskelet. Disord. 2011; 12: 202.

[83] Bernard TE, Wilder FV, Aluoch M, Leaverton PE. Job-related osteoarthritis of the knee, foot, hand, and cervical spine. J Occup Environ Med. 2010; 52(1): 33-8.

[84] Kalichman L, Li L, Kim DH, Guermazi A, Berkin V, O'Donnell CJ, et al. Facet joint osteoarthrosis and low back pain in the community-based population. Spine. 2008; 33(23): 2560-5.

[85] Fujiwara A, Tamai K, Yamato M, An HS, Yoshida H, Saotome K, et al. The relationship between facet joint osteoarthritis and disc degeneration of the lumbar spine: an MRI study. Eur Spine J. 1999; 8(5): 396-401.

[86] Abbas J, Hamoud K, Masharawi YM, May H, Hay O, Medlej B, et al. Ligamentum flavum thickness in normal and stenotic lumbar spines. Spine. 2010; 35(12): 1225-30.

[87] Kirkaldy-Willis WH, McIvor GW. Spinal stenosis. Clin Orthop Relat Res. 1976; (115): 2-144.

[88] Tischer T, Aktas T, Milz S, Putz R. Detailed pathological changes of human lumbar facet joints L1–L5 in elderly individuals. Eur Spine J. 2006; 15(3): 308-15.

[89] Kalichman L, Suri P, Guermazi A, Li L, Hunter DJ. Facet orientation and tropism: associations with facet joint osteoarthritis and degeneratives. Spine. 2009; 34(16): E579-85.

[90] Fujiwara A, Tamai K, An HS, Lim TH, Yoshida H, Kurihashi A, et al. Orientation and osteoarthritis of the lumbar facet joint. Clin Orthop Relat Res. 2001; 385: 88-94.

[91] Masharawi Y, Rothschild B, Dar G, Peleg S, Robinson D, Been E, et al. Facet orientation in the thoracolumbar spine: three-dimensional anatomic and biomechanical analysis. Spine 2004; 29(16): 1755-63.

[92] Abbas J, Hamoud K, Peleg S, May H, Masharawi Y, Cohen H, Peled N, Hershkovitz I. Facet joints arthrosis in normal and stenotic lumbar spines. Spine. 2011; 36(24): E1541-6.

[93] Kalichman L, Hodges P, Li L, Guermazi A, Hunter DJ. Changes in paraspinal muscles and their association with low back pain and spinal degeneration: CT study. Eur Spine J. 2010; 19(7): 1136-44.

[94] Battié MC, Videman T. Lumbar disc degeneration: epidemiology and genetics. J Bone Joint Surg Am. 2006; 88(Suppl 2): 3-9. Review.

[95] Videman T, Battié MC, Gill K, Manninen H, Gibbons LE, Fisher LD. Magnetic resonance imaging findings and their relationships in the thoracic and lumbar spine. Insights into the etiopathogenesis of spinal degeneration. Spine. 1995; 20(8): 928-35.

[96] Beneke R. Zur Lehre von der Spondylitis deformans. Versammlung deutscher Naturforscher und Arzte. Braunschweig. 1897.

[97] Boos N, Weissbach S, Rohrbach H, Weiler C, Spratt KF, Nerlich AG. Classification of age-related changes in lumbar intervertebral discs: 2002 Volvo Award in basic science. Spine. 2002; 27(23): 2631-44.

[98] Videman T, Nurminen M. The occurrence of anular tears and their relation to lifetime back pain history: a cadaveric study using barium sulfate discography. Spine. 2004; 29(3): 2668-76.

[99] Battié MC, Videman T, Gibbons LE, Fisher LD, Manninen H, Gill K. Determinants of lumbar disc degeneration. A study relating lifetime exposures and magnetic resonance imaging findings in identical twins. Spine. 1995; 20(24): 2601-12.

[100] Miller JA, Schmatz C, Schultz AB. Lumbar disc degeneration: correlation with age, sex, and spine level in 600 autopsy specimens. Spine. 1988; 13(2): 173-8.

[101] Battié MC, Haynor DR, Fisher LD, Gill K, Gibbons LE, Videman T. Similarities in degenerative findings on magnetic resonance images of the lumbar spines of identical twins. J Bone Joint Surg Am. 1995a; 77(11): 1662-70.

[102]   Sambrook PN, MacGregor AJ, Spector TD. Genetic influences on cervical and lumbar disc degeneration: a magnetic resonance imaging study in twins. Arthritis Rheum. 1999; 42(2): 366-72.

[103]   Videman T, Leppävuori J, Kaprio J, Battié MC, Gibbons LE, Peltonen L, et al. Intragenic polymorphisms of the vitamin D receptor gene associated with intervertebral disc degeneration. Spine. 1998; 23(23): 2477-85.

[104]   Solovieva S, Lohiniva J, Leino-Arjas P, Raininko R, Luoma K, Ala-Kokko L, et al. COL9A3 gene polymorphism and obesity in intervertebral disc degeneration of the lumbar spine: evidence of gene-environment interaction. Spine. 2002; 27(23): 2691-6.

[105]   Liu YK, Njus G, Buckwalter J, Wakano K. Fatigue response of lumbar intervertebral joints under axial cyclic loading. Spine. 1983; 8(8): 857-65.

[106]   Gilbertson LG, Goel VK, Kong WZ, Clausen JD. Finite element methods in spine biomechanics research. Crit Rev Biomed Eng. 1995; 23(5-6): 411-73.

[107]   Natarajan RN, Williams JR, Andersson GB. Modeling changes in intervertebral disc mechanics with degeneration. J Bone Joint Surg Am. 2006; 88(Suppl 2): 36-40. Review.

[108]   Lotz JC, Colliou OK, Chin JR, Duncan NA, Liebenberg E. Compression-induced degeneration of the intervertebral disc: an in vivo mouse model and finite-element study. Spine. 1998; 23(23): 2493-506.

[109]   Simon BR, Wu JS, Carlton MW, Evans JH, Kazarian LE. Structural models for human spinal motion segments based on a poroelastic view of the intervertebral disk. J Biomech Eng. 1985; 107(4): 327-35.

[110]   Riches PE, Dhillon N, Lotz J, Woods AW, McNally DS. The internal mechanics of the intervertebral disc under cyclic loading. J Biomech. 2002; 35(9): 1263-71.

[111]   Laible JP, Pflaster DS, Krag MH, Simon BR, Haugh LD. A poroelastic-swelling finite element model with application to the intervertebral disc. Spine. 1993; 18(5): 659-70.

[112]   Selard E, Shirazi-Adl A, Urban JP. Finite element study of nutrient diffusion in the human intervertebral disc. Spine. 2003; 28(17): 1945-53.

[113]   Natarajan RN, Williams JR, Andersson GB. Recent advances in analytical modeling of lumbar disc degeneration. Spine. 2004; 29(23): 2733-41.

[114]   Adams MA, Roughley PJ. What is intervertebral disc degeneration, and what causes it? Spine. 2006; 31(18): 2151-61.

[115]   Le Maitre CL, Freemont AJ, Hoyland JA. Accelerated cellular senescence in degenerate intervertebral discs: a possible role in the pathogenesis of intervertebral disc degeneration. Arthritis Res Ther. 2007; 9(3): R45.

[116] Benoist M. Natural history of the aging spine. Eur Spine J. 2003; 12(Suppl 2): S86-9. Review.

[117] Pazzaglia UE, Salisbury JR, Byers PD. Development and involution of the notochord in the human spine. J R Soc Med. 1989; 82(7): 413-5.

[118] Wolfe HJ, Putschar WG, Vickery AL. Role of the Notochord in human intervetebral disk. I. Fetus and infant. Clin Orthop Relat Res. 1965; 39: 205-12.

[119] Kim KW, Lim TH, Kim JG, Jeong ST, Masuda K, An HS. The origin of chondrocytes in the nucleus pulposus and histologic findings associated with the transition of a notochordal nucleus pulposus to a fibrocartilaginous nucleus pulposus in intact rabbit intervertebral discs. Spine. 2003; 28(10): 982-90.

[120] Kim KW, Kim YS, Ha KY, Woo YK, Park JB, Park WS, et al. An autocrine or paracrine Fas-mediated counterattack: a potential mechanism for apoptosis of notochordal cells in intact rat nucleus pulposus. Spine. 2005; 30(11): 1247-51.

[121] Cappello R, Bird JL, Pfeiffer D, Bayliss MT, Dudhia J. Notochordal cell produce and assemble extracellular matrix in a distinct manner, which may be responsible for the maintenance of healthy nucleus pulposus. Spine. 2006; 31(8): 873-82.

[122] Ishii T, Tsuji H, Sano A, Katoh Y, Matsui H, Terahata N. Histochemical and ultrastructural observations on brown degeneration of human intervertebral disc. J Orthop Res. 1991; 9(1): 78-90.

[123] Hastreiter D, Ozuna RM, Spector M. Regional variations in certain cellular characteristics in human lumbar intervertebral discs, including the presence of a-smooth muscle actin. J Orthop Res. 2001; 19(4): 597-604.

[124] Le Maitre CL, Freemont AJ, Hoyland JA. The role of interleukin-1 in the pathogenesis of human intervertebral disc degeneration. Arthritis Res Ther. 2005; 7(4): R732-45.

[125] Weiler C, Nerlich AG, Bachmeier BE, Boos N. Expression and distribution of tumor necrosis factor alpha in human lumbar intervertebral discs: a study in surgical specimen and autopsy controls. Spine. 2005; 30(1): 44-54.

[126] Roberts S, Caterson B, Menage J, Evans EH, Jaffray DC, Eisenstein SM. Matrix metalloproteinases and agrecanase: their rôle in disorders of the human intervertebral disc. Spine. 2000; 25(23): 3005-13.

[127] Cs-Szabo G, Ragasa-San Juan D, Turumella V, Masuda K, Thonar EJ, An HS. Changes in mRNA and protein levels of proteoglycans of the anulus fibrosus and nucleus pulposus during intervertebral disc degeneration. Spine. 2002; 27(20): 2212-9.

[128] Rannou F, Corvol M, Revel M, Poiraudeau S. Dégénérescence discale et hernie discale: rôle des métalloprotéases et cytokines. Rev Rhum. 2001; 68(10-11): 913-20.

[129] Roberts S, Johnson E. Innervation du disque intervertébral et lombalgie discale. Rev Rhum. 2000b; 67(Suppl 4): 225-32.

[130] Weiler C, Nerlich AG, Zipperer J, Bachmeier BE, Boos N. Expression of major matrix metallo proteinases is associated with disc degradation and resorption. Eur Spine J. 2002; 11(4): 308-20.

[131] Bernick S, Cailliet R. Vertebral end-plate changes with aging of human vertebrae. Spine. 1982; 7(2): 97-102.

[132] Ariga K, Yonenobu K, Nakase T, Hosono N, Okuda S, Meng W, et al. Mechanical stress-induced apoptosis of endplate chondrocytes in organ-cultured mouse intervertebral discs: an ex vivo study. Spine. 2003; 28(14): 1528-33.

[133] Court C, Colliou OK, Chin JR, Liebenberg E, Bradford DS, Lotz JC. The effect of static in vivo bending on the murine intervertebral disc. Spine J. 2001; 1(4): 239-45.

[134] Lotz JC, Chin JR. Intervertebral disc cell death is dependent on the magnitude and duration of spinal loading. Spine. 2000; 25(12): 1477-83.

[135] Johnson WE, Eisenstein SM, Roberts S. Cell cluster formation in degenerate lumbar intervertebral discs is associated with increased disc cell proliferation. Connect Tissue Res. 2001; 42(3): 197-207.

[136] Galbusera F, Schmidt H, Neidlinger-Wilke C, Wilke HJ. The effect of degenerative morphological changes of the intervertebral disc on the lumbar spine biomechanics: a poroelastic finite element investigation. Comput Methods Biomech Biomed Engin. 2011; 14(8): 729-39.

[137] Butler D, Trafimow JH, Andersson GB, McNeill TW, Huckman MS. Discs degenerate before facets. Spine. 1990; 15(2): 111-3.

[138] Prescher A. Anatomy and pathology of the aging spine. Eur J Radiol. 1998; 27(3): 181-95.

[139] Kettler A, Werner K, Wilke HJ. Morphological changes of cervical facet joints in elderly individuals. Eur Spine J. 2007; 16(7): 987-92.

[140] Wilke HJ, Zanker D, Wolfram U. Internal morphology of human facet joints: comparing cervical and lumbar spine with regard to age, gender and the vertebral core. J Anat. 2012; 220(3): 233-41.

[141] Oegema TR, Bradford DS. The inter-relationship of facet joint osteoarthritis and degenerative disc disease. Br J Rheumatol. 1991; 30(Suppl 1): 16-20.

[142] Farfan HF. The pathological anatomy of degenerative spondylolisthesis. A cadaver study. Spine. 1980; 5(5): 412-418.

[143] McDougall JJ. Arthritis and pain. Neurogenic origin of joint pain. Arthritis Res Ther. 2006; 8(6): 220. Review.

[144] Schaible HG, Ebersberger A, Von Banchet GS. Mechanisms of pain in arthritis. Ann N Y Acad Sci. 2002; 966: 343-54.

[145] Yamashita T, Cavanaugh JM, el Bohy AA, Getchell TV, King AI. Mechanosensitive afferent units in the lumbar facet joint. J Bone Joint Surg Am. 1990; 72(6): 865-70.

[146] Yamashita T, Cavanaugh JM, Ozaktay AC, Avramov AI, Getchell TV, King AI. Effect of substance P on mechanosensitive units of tissues around and in the lumbar facet joint. J Orthop Res. 1993; 11(2): 205-14.

[147] Ozaktay AC, Cavanaugh JM, Blagoev DC, Getchell TV, King AI. Effects of a carrageenan-induced inflammation in rabbit lumbar facet joint capsule and adjacent tissues. Neurosci Res. 1994; 20(4): 355-64.

[148] Beaman DN, Graziano GP, Glover RA, Wojtys EM, Chang V. Substance P innervations of lumbar spine facet joints. Spine. 1993; 18(8): 1044-9.

[149] Manchikanti L, Boswell MV, Singh V, Pampati V, Damron KS, Beyer CD. Prevalence of facet joint pain in chronic spinal pain of cervical, thoracic, and lumbar regions. BMC Musculoskelet Disord. 2004 May 28; 5: 15.

[150] Kallakuri S, Singh A, Chen C, Cavanaugh JM. Demonstration of substance P, calcitonin gene-related peptide, and protein gene product 9.5 containing nerve fibers in human cervical facet joint capsules. Spine. 2004; 29: 1182-6.

[151] Krafft M, Kullgren A, Tingvall C, Bostrom O, Fredriksson R. How crash severity in rear impacts influences short- and long-term consequences to the neck. Accid Anal Prev. 2000; 32(2): 187-95.

[152] Chen C, Lu Y, Cavanaugh JM, Kallakuri S, Patwardhan A. Recording of neural activity from goat cervical facet joint capsule using custom-designed miniature electrodes. Spine. 2005; 30(12): 1367-72.

[153] Lu Y, Chen C, Kallakuri S, Patwardhan A, Cavanaugh JM. Development of an in vivo method to investigate biomechanical and neurophysiological properties of spine facet joint capsules. Eur Spine J. 2005; 14(6): 565-72.

[154] Lu Y, Chen C, Kallakuri S, Patwardhan A, Cavanaugh JM. Neurophysiological and biomechanical characterization of goat cervical facet joint capsules. J Orthop Res. 2005a; 23(4): 779-87.

[155] Lu Y, Chen C, Kallakuri S, Patwardhan A, Cavanaugh JM. Neural response of cervical facet joint capsule to stretch: a study of whiplash pain mechanism. Stapp Car Crash Journal. 2005b; 49: 49-56.

[156] Curatolo M, Petersen-Felix S, Arendt-Nielsen L, Giani C, Zbinden AM, Radanov BP. Central hypersensitivity in chronic pain after whiplash injury. Clin J Pain. 2001; 17(4): 306-15.

[157] Kasch H, Stengaard-Pedersen K, Arendt-Nielsen L, Staehelin Jensen T. Pain thresholds and tenderness in neck and head following acute whiplash injury: a prospective study. Cephalalgia. 2001; 21(3): 189-97.

[158] Kirkaldy-Willis WH, Farfan HF. Instability of the lumbar spine. Clin Orthop Relat Res. 1982; (165): 110-23.

[159] Hicks GE, Morone N, Weiner DK. Degenerative lumbar disc and facet disease in older adults: prevalence and clinical correlates. Spine. 2009; 34(12): 1301-6.

[160] Lotz JC, Ulrich JA. Innervation, inflammation, and hypermobility may characterize pathologic disc degeneration: review of animal model data. J Bone Joint Surg Am. 2006; 88(Suppl 2): 76-82. Review.

[161] Fagan A, Moore R, Vernon Roberts B, Blumbergs P, Fraser R. ISSLS prize winner: The innervation of the intervertebral disc: a quantitative analysis. Spine. 2003; 28(23): 2570-6.

[162] McCarthy PW, Carruthers B, Martin D, Petts P. Immunohistochemical demonstration of sensory nerve fibers and endings in lumbar intervertebral discs of the rat. Spine. 1991; 16(6): 653-5.

[163] Willenegger S, Friess AE, Lang J, Stoffel MH. Immunohistochemical demonstration of lumbar intervertebral disc innervation in the dog. Anat Histol Embryol. 2005; 34(2): 123-8.

[164] Ozawa T, Aoki Y, Ohtori S, Takahashi K, Chiba T, Ino H, et al. The dorsal portion of the lumbar intervertebral disc is innervated primarily by small peptide containing dorsal root ganglion neurons in rats. Neurosci Lett. 2003; 344(1): 65-7.

[165] Aoki Y, Ohtori S, Takahashi K, Ino H, Takahashi Y, Chiba T, et al. Innervation of the lumbar intervertebral disc by nerve growth factor-dependent neurons related to inflammatory pain. Spine. 2004; 29(10): 1077-81.

[166] Nakamura SI, Takahashi K, Takahashi Y, Yamagata M, Moriya H. The afferent pathways of discogenic low-back pain. Evaluation of L2 spinal nerve infiltration. J Bone Joint Surg Br. 1996; 78(4): 606-12.

[167] Boswell MV, Shah RV, Everett CR, Sehgal N, Mckenzie-Brown AM, Abdi S, et al. Interventional techniques in the management of chronic spinal pain: Evidence-based practice guidelines. Pain Physician. 2007; 10(1): 7-111.

[168] Grenier N, Kressel HY, Schiebler ML, Grossman RI, Dalinka MK. Normal and degenerative posterior spinal structures: MR imaging. Radiology. 1987; 165(2): 517-25.

[169] Modic MT, Pavlicek W, Weinstein MA, Boumphrey F, Ngo F, Hardy R, et al. Magnetic resonance imaging of intervertebral disk disease. Clinical and pulse sequence considerations. Radiology. 1984; 152(1): 103-11.

[170] Pathria M, Sartoris DJ, Resnick D. Osteoarthritis of the lumbar facet joints: accuracy of oblique radiographic assessment. Radiology. 1987; 164(1): 227-30.

[171] Carrera GF, Haughton VM, Syvertsen A, Williams AL. Computed tomography of the facet joints. Radiology 1980; 134(1): 145-8.

[172] Weishaupt D, Zanetti M, Hodler J, Boos N. Accuracy of routine MR imaging of the lumbar spine in assessment of osteoarthritis of the lumbar facets. Presented at 25th Annual Meeting of the International Society for the Study of the Lumbar Spine, Brussels. 1998. June 9–13.

[173] Kettler A, Wilke HJ. Review of existing grading systems for cervical or lumbar disc and facet joint degeneration. Eur Spine J. 2006; 15(6): 705-18.

[174] Lane NE, Nevitt MC, Genant HK, Hochberg MC. Reliability of new indices of radiographic osteoarthritis of the hand and hip and lumbar disc degeneration. J Rheumatol. 1993; 20(11): 1911-8.

[175] Pfirrmann CW, Metzdorf A, Zanetti M, Hodler J, Boos N. Magnetic resonance classification of lumbar intervertebral disc degeneration. Spine. 2001; 26(17): 1873-8.

[176] Thompson JP, Pearce RH, Schechter MT, Adams ME, Tsang IK, Bishop PB. Preliminary evaluation of a scheme for grading the gross morphology of the human intervertebral disc. Spine. 1990; 15(5): 411-5.

[177] Kellgren JH, Jeffrey MR, Ball J. The epidemiology of chronic rheumatism. vol II: Atlas of standard radiographs of arthritis. Oxford, Blackwell Scientific Publications. 1963.

[178] Weishaupt D, Zanetti M, Boos N, Hodler J. MR imaging and CT in osteoarthritis of the lumbar facet joints. Skeletal Radiol. 1999; 28(4): 215-9.

[179] Delbeke D, Schöder H, Martin WH, Wahl RL. Hybrid imaging (SPECT/CT and PET/CT): improving therapeutic decisions. Semin Nucl Med. 2009; 39(5): 308-40.

[180] Dutton JA, Hughes SP, Peters AM. SPECT in the management of patients with back pain and spondylolysis. Clin Nucl Med. 2000; 25(2): 93-6.

[181] Matar HE, Navalkissoor S, Berovic M, Shetty R, Garlick N, Casey AT, et al. Is hybrid imaging (SPECT/CT) a useful adjunct in the management of suspected facet joints arthropathy? Int Orthop. 2013; 37(5): 865-70.

[182] Willburger RE. Prostaglandin release from lumbar disc and facet joint tissue. Spine 1994; 19(18): 2068-70.

[183] Fernandes JC, Martel-Pelletier J, Pelletier JP. The role of cytokines in osteoarthritis pathophysiology. Biorheology 2002; 39(1-2): 237-46.

[184] Martel-Pelletier J, Alaaeddine N, Pelletier JP. Cytokines and their role in the pathophysiology of osteoarthritis. Front Biosci. 1999; 4: D694-703. Review.

[185] Wittenberg RH. In vitro release of prostaglandins and leukotrienes from synovial tissues, cartilage, and bone in degenerative joint diseases. Arthritis Rheum 1993; 36(10): 1444-50.

[186] Igarashi A, Kikuchi S, Konno S, Olmarker K. Inflammatory cytokines released from the facet joint tissue in degenerative lumbar spinal disorders. Spine. 2004; 29(19): 2091-5.

[187] Igarashi A, Kikuchi S, Konno S. Correlation between inflammatory cytokines released from the lumbar facet joint tissue and symptoms in degenerative lumbar spinal disorders. J Orthop Sci. 2007; 12(2): 154-60.

[188] Xu D, Sun Y, Bao G, Liu W, Zhu X, Cui S, et al. MMP-1 overexpression induced by IL-1β: possible mechanism for inflammation in degenerative lumbar facet joint. J Orthop Sci. 2013; 18(6): 1012-9.

[189] Haro H. The role of matrix metalloproteinases and vascular endothelial growth factor in the resorption process of herniated disc. Spine J 2002; 2(5 Suppl): 106.

[190] Kato T, Haro H, Komori H, Shinomiya K. Sequential dynamics of inflammatory cytokine, angiogenesis inducing factor and matrix degrading enzymes during spontaneous resorption of the herniated disc. J Orthop Res 2004; 22(4): 895-900.

[191] Tolonen J, Grönblad M, Virri J, Seitsalo S, Rytömaa T, Karaharju E. Transforming growth factor beta receptor induction in herniated intervertebral disc tissue: an immunohistochemical study. Eur Spine J 2001; 10(2): 172-6.

[192] Matsui Y, Maeda M, Nakagami W, Iwata H. The involvement of matrix metalloproteinases and inflammation in lumbar disc herniation. Spine. 1998; 23(8): 863-9.

[193] Benneker LM, Heini PF, Anderson SE, Alini M, Ito K. Correlation of radiographic and MRI parameters to morphological and biochemical assessment of intervertebral disc degeneration. Eur Spine J. 2005; 14(1): 27-35.

[194] Kumar A. Thoracic disc prolapse in calcified discs. Orthopedics 1991; 14(1): 98-9.

[195] Gruber HE, Norton HJ, Sun Y, Hanley EN Jr. Crystal deposits in the human intervertebral disc: implications for disc degeneration. Spine J 2007; 7(4): 444-50.

[196] Lagier R, Wildi E. Incidence of chondrocalcinosis in a series of 1,000 surgically excised intervertebral disks. Rev Rheum Mal Osteoartic 1979; 46(5): 303-7.

[197] Chou C. Pathological studies on calcification of the intervertebral discs. Nihon Seikeigeka Gakkai Zasshi. 1982; 56(4): 331-45.

[198] Karamouzian S, Eskandary H, Faramarzee M, Saba M, Safizade H, Ghadipasha M, et al. Frequency of lumbar intervertebral disc calcification and angiogenesis, and their correlation with clinical, surgical, and magnetic resonance imaging findings. Spine. 2010; 35(8): 881-6.

[199] Ariga K, Miyamoto S, Nakase T, Okuda S, Meng W, Yonenobu K, et al. The relationship between apoptosis of endplate chondrocytes and aging and degeneration of the intervertebral disc. Spine. 2001; 26(22): 2414-20.

[200] Gruber HE, Hanley EN Jr. Analysis of aging and degeneration of the human inter-vertebral disc. Comparison of surgical specimens with normal controls. Spine. 1998; 23(7): 751-7.

[201] Kohyama K, Saura R, Doita M, Mizuno K. Intervertebral disc cell apoptosis by nitric oxide: biological understanding of intervertebral disc degeneration. Kobe J Med Sci. 2000; 46(6): 283-95.

[202] Park JB, Lee JK, Park SJ, Kim KW, Riew KD. Mitochondrial involvement in fas-medi-ated apoptosis of human lumbar disc cells. J Bone Joint Surg Am. 2005; 87(6): 1338-42.

[203] Zhao CQ, Jiang LS, Dai LY. Programmed cell death in intervertebral disc degenera-tion. Apoptosis. 2006; 11(12): 2079-88. Review.

[204] Park JB, Chang H, Kim KW. Expression of Fas ligand and apoptosis of disc cells in herniated lumbar disc tissue. Spine. 2001; 26(6): 618-21.

[205] Zhao CQ, Zhang YH, Jiang SD, Jiang LS, Dai LY. Both endoplasmic reticulum and mitochondria are involved in disc cell apoptosis and intervertebral disc degeneration in rats. Age (Dordr). 2010; 32(2): 161-77. Review.

[206] Wang H, Liu H, Zheng ZM, Zhang KB, Wang TP, Sribastav SS, et al. Role of death receptor, mitochondrial and endoplasmic reticulum pathways in different stages of degenerative human lumbar disc. Apoptosis. 2011; 16(10): 990-1003.

[207] Kroeber M, Unglaub F, Guehring T, Nerlich A, Hadi T, Lotz J, et al. Effects of control-led dynamic disc distraction on degenerated intervertebral discs: an in vivo study on the rabbit lumbar spine model. Spine. 2005; 30(2): 181-7.

[208] Ohshima H, Tsuji H, Hirano N, Ishihara H, Katoh Y, Yamada H. Water diffusion pathway, swelling pressure, and biomechanical properties of the intervertebral disc during compression load. Spine. 1989; 14(11): 1234-44.

[209] Bibby SR, Fairbank JC, Urban MR, Urban JP. Cell viability in scoliotic discs in rela-tion to disc deformity and nutrient levels. Spine. 2002; 27(20): 2220-8.

[210] Park JB, Park IC, Park SJ, Jin HO, Lee JK, Riew KD. Antiapoptotic effects of caspase inhibitors on rat intervertebral disc cells. J Bone Joint Surg Am. 2006; 88(4): 771-9.

[211] Ha KY, Koh IJ, Kirpalani PA, Kim YY, Cho YK, Khang GS, et al. The expression of hypoxia inducible factor-1alpha and apoptosis in herniated discs. Spine. 2006; 31(12): 1309-13.

[212] Risbud MV, Fertala J, Vresilovic EJ, Albert TJ, Shapiro IM. Nucleus pulposus cells upregulate PI3K/Akt and MEK/ERK signaling pathways under hypoxic conditions and resist apoptosis induced by serum withdrawal. Spine. 2005; 30(8): 882-9.

[213] Jones P, Gardner L, Menage J, Williams GT, Roberts S. Intervertebral disc cells as competent phagocytes in vitro: implications for cell death in disc degeneration. Ar-thritis Res Ther. 2008; 10(4): R86.

Permissions

All chapters in this book were first published in OSTEOARTHRITIS, by InTech Open; hereby published with permission under the Creative Commons Attribution License or equivalent. Every chapter published in this book has been scrutinized by our experts. Their significance has been extensively debated. The topics covered herein carry significant findings which will fuel the growth of the discipline. They may even be implemented as practical applications or may be referred to as a beginning point for another development.

The contributors of this book come from diverse backgrounds, making this book a truly international effort. This book will bring forth new frontiers with its revolutionizing research information and detailed analysis of the nascent developments around the world.

We would like to thank all the contributing authors for lending their expertise to make the book truly unique. They have played a crucial role in the development of this book. Without their invaluable contributions this book wouldn't have been possible. They have made vital efforts to compile up to date information on the varied aspects of this subject to make this book a valuable addition to the collection of many professionals and students.

This book was conceptualized with the vision of imparting up-to-date information and advanced data in this field. To ensure the same, a matchless editorial board was set up. Every individual on the board went through rigorous rounds of assessment to prove their worth. After which they invested a large part of their time researching and compiling the most relevant data for our readers.

The editorial board has been involved in producing this book since its inception. They have spent rigorous hours researching and exploring the diverse topics which have resulted in the successful publishing of this book. They have passed on their knowledge of decades through this book. To expedite this challenging task, the publisher supported the team at every step. A small team of assistant editors was also appointed to further simplify the editing procedure and attain best results for the readers.

Apart from the editorial board, the designing team has also invested a significant amount of their time in understanding the subject and creating the most relevant covers. They scrutinized every image to scout for the most suitable representation of the subject and create an appropriate cover for the book.

The publishing team has been an ardent support to the editorial, designing and production team. Their endless efforts to recruit the best for this project, has resulted in the accomplishment of this book. They are a veteran in the field of academics and their pool of knowledge is as vast as their experience in printing. Their expertise and guidance has proved useful at every step. Their uncompromising quality standards have made this book an exceptional effort. Their encouragement from time to time has been an inspiration for everyone.

The publisher and the editorial board hope that this book will prove to be a valuable piece of knowledge for researchers, students, practitioners and scholars across the globe.

List of Contributors

Sarah Karrar and Charles Mackworth-Young
Department of Rheumatology, Charing Cross Hospital, Fulham Palace Road, London, UK

Rie Kurose
Department of Orthopaedic Surgery, Hirosaki University Graduate School of Medicine, Hirosaki, Japan

Takashi Sawai
Department of Histopathology, Tohoku University Graduate School of Medicine, Sendai, Japan

Sture Forsgren
Department of Integrative Medical Biology Anatomy Section Umeå University Umeå, Sweden

Veronika Kralj-Iglič
Laboratory of Clinical Biophysics, Faculty of Health Sciences, University of Ljubljana, Ljubljana, Slovenia

Michele Abate and Vincenzo Salini
Department of Medicine and Science of Aging, University G. d'Annunzio, Chieti, Italy

Isabel Andia
BioCruces/Cruces University Hospital, Barakaldo, Spain

Xiaoming Zhang
Department of Anatomy and Cell Biology, University of Kansas School of Medicine, Kansas City, USA

Brian Egan and Jinxi Wang
Department of Orthopedic Surgery, University of Kansas School of Medicine, Kansas City, USA

Xiao-Yu Yuan and Yuqing Wu
State Key Laboratory of Supramolecular Structure and Materials, Jilin University, Changchun, China

Liping Zhang
Grain and Oil Food Processing Key Laboratory of Jilin Province, Jilin Business and Technology College, Changchun, China

Xiaoming Zhang
Department of Anatomy and Cell Biology, University of Kansas School of Medicine, Kansas City, USA

Darryl Blalock and Jinxi Wang
Department of Orthopedic Surgery, University of Kansas School of Medicine, Kansas City, USA

Herng-Sheng Lee
Department of Pathology and Laboratory Medicine, Kaohsiung Veterans General Hospital, Zuoying Dist., Kaohsiung City, Taiwan

Donald M. Salter
Center for Genomics and Experimental Medicine, MRC IGMM, University of Edinburgh, Western General Hospital, Edinburgh EH4 2XU, United Kingdom

Nidhi Sofat and Sharenja Jeyabaladevan
Institute for Infection and Immunity, St George's, University of London, Cranmer Terrace, London, UK

Çalışkan Nurcan and Mevlüde Karadağ
Gazi University, Faculty of Health Sciences, Nursing Department, Ankara, Turkey

Elizabeth Pérez-Hernández
División de Educación e Investigación en Salud, UMAE "Dr. Victorio de la Fuente Narváez", Hospital de Ortopedia, Instituto Mexicano del Seguro Social, Distrito Federal, México

Nury Pérez-Hernández
Escuela Nacional de Medicina y Homeopatía, Instituto Politécnico Nacional, Distrito Federal, México

Ariel Fuerte-Hernández
Escuela Superior de Ingeniería Mecánica y Eléctrica, Instituto Politécnico Nacional, Distrito Federal, México

Index

www.ingramcontent.com/pod-product-compliance
Lightning Source LLC
Chambersburg PA
CBHW080527200326
41458CB00012B/4362